10 — 1|0

# MEDICINE
## AND THE
# GERMAN JEWS

# MEDICINE
AND THE
GERMAN
JEWS
A HISTORY

JOHN M. EFRON

YALE UNIVERSITY PRESS/NEW HAVEN & LONDON

Copyright © 2001 by Yale University. All rights reserved.

This book may not be reproduced, in whole or in part, including illustrations, in any form (beyond that copying permitted by Sections 107 and 108 of the U.S. Copyright Law and except by reviewers for the public press), without written permission from the publishers.

Designed by Mary Valencia

Set in Galliard Old Style type by Integrated Publishing Solutions, LLC.

Printed in the United States of America by Vail-Ballou Press, Binghamton, New York.

Library of Congress Cataloging-in-Publication Data
Efron, John M.
Medicine and the German Jews: a history / John M. Efron.
p.   cm.
Includes bibliographical references and index.
ISBN 0-300-08377-7 (cloth : alk. paper)
1. Jewish physicians—Germany—History 2. Jews—Medicine—Germany—History.
3. Medicine—Germany—History. I. Title
R694 .E376 2001
610'.89'924043—dc21
00-011315

A catalogue record for this book is available from the British Library.

The paper in this book meets the guidelines for permanence and durability of the Committee on Production Guidelines for Book Longevity of the Council on Library Resources.

10 9 8 7 6 5 4 3 2 1

# CONTENTS

| ACKNOWLEDGMENTS | vii |
|---|---|
| INTRODUCTION | 1 |
| 1. THE EMERGENCE OF THE MEDIEVAL JEWISH PHYSICIAN | 13 |
| 2. JEWISH PHYSICIANS: IN AND OUT OF THE GERMAN GHETTO | 34 |
| 3. *HASKALAH* AND HEALING: JEWISH MEDICINE IN THE AGE OF ENLIGHTENMENT | 64 |
| 4. THE JEWISH BODY DEGENERATE? | 105 |
| 5. THE PSYCHOPATHOLOGY OF EVERYDAY JEWISH LIFE | 151 |
| 6. IN PRAISE OF JEWISH RITUAL: MODERN MEDICINE AND THE DEFENSE OF ANCIENT TRADITIONS | 186 |
| 7. BEFORE THE STORM: JEWISH DOCTORS IN THE KAISERREICH AND WEIMAR REPUBLIC | 234 |
| CONCLUSION | 265 |
| NOTES | 271 |
| INDEX | 339 |

# ACKNOWLEDGMENTS

It is a pleasure to recognize the assistance and sustenance I received from institutions, colleagues, friends, and family during the writing of this book. Generous financial support came in the form of a fellowship from the American Council of Learned Societies, and a summer stipend from the National Endowment for the Humanities. At Indiana University, further funds were made available by the Research and University Graduate School, the Robert A. and Sandra S. Borns Jewish Studies Program, and the Department of History.

The historical sources for such a study are scattered far and wide. The librarians and staff at the Edelstein Collection at the Jewish National and University Library, Jerusalem, were ever-obliging. Chava Nowersztern, Francisco Carvahlo-Moreno, and Naomi Alshech made my research there a pleasure. Similarly, the staffs at the Wellcome Institute for the History of Medicine Library in London, the Leo Baeck Institute, and the Jewish Theological Seminary, both in New York, facilitated my work with customary skill and grace.

While the act of writing is a solitary experience, the production of a text is a collaborative enterprise. A host of people read and commented on parts or all of the manuscript. Others heard some of the arguments presented in oral form at conferences, or at invited lectures, and their comments and questions were food for further reflection, and, I hope, improvement. Derek Penslar was a constant source of incisive criticism, encouragement, and good humor. Likewise, Dror Wahrman read and critiqued the manuscript shortly after his move to Bloomington, and I am grateful for his efforts and our late-night discussions. George Alter, Michael Berkowitz, Michael Brenner, Elisheva Carlebach, Ann Carmichael, Elisabeth Domansky, Dyan Elliott, Arthur Field, Ted Fram, Susannah Heschel, Ronnie Po-chia Hsia, Robert Jütte, Herbert H. Kaplan, Werner Kümmel, Olga Litvak, Michael

## ACKNOWLEDGMENTS

A. Meyer, Gina Morantz-Sanchez, David Myers, Hindy Najman, David Ransel, David Ruderman, Thomas Schlich, Haym Soloveitchik, David Sorkin, Jeffrey Veidlinger, Nina Warnke, Steve Weitzman, and Eberhard Wolff all gave of their expertise and helped shape my thinking on a host of issues and historical periods. *A shaynem dank* is due Mikhl Herzog, who many years ago introduced me to Moishe Marcuze, a physician whose work is the subject of analysis in Chapter 3.

A considerable portion of this book was written while I was a visiting scholar at the University of Chicago in 1998. As is his wont, Sander L. Gilman was a gracious host and stimulating conversation partner, helping push this book in directions not originally intended. I am grateful for his encouragement and generosity. Unfortunately, George L. Mosse, of blessed memory, did not live to see the publication of this book. However, we discussed the project at various points, and his intellectual stamp has left its impress on these pages.

To my friends, Jeff Isaac and Bob Orsi, I express my gratitude for the caring and the conversation. They make breakfast the most important and fun meal of the day. My colleague, Carl Ipsen, tracked down a difficult-to-find source in a Roman library, while Libby Katz, Kevin Hughes, and Tim Pursell also offered me important assistance.

Writing this book required a number of research trips to London and New York. In London, John Gerszt and Sue Mandelbaum always provide me with a home away from home. I am deeply grateful to them for their hospitality, generosity, and many years of friendship. If I don't exactly get the key to the city when I stay in New York, my friend Ami Krane nevertheless always gives me the keys to her apartment. She, too, is a gracious host, and I am fortunate to count her among my dearest friends.

My sincere thanks go to Charles Grench, former executive editor of Yale University Press, and editor Otto Bohlmann for their support of this project, and my manuscript editor, Nancy Moore Brochin, for her encouragement and keen sense of literary style.

My children, Hannah and Noah, were toddlers when this book was in its infancy. They grew along with it and remain my pride and joy. I thank them for the hilarity and the *naches* they provide. At every stage, the loving support of Deborah made this book possible. It is my pleasure to dedicate it to her.

# INTRODUCTION

We live in a medicalized world. In the West, health, beauty, fitness, weight, diets, miracle drugs, alternative medicine, and breakthrough surgical procedures all animate a considerable portion of late twentieth-century conversation. And if this is the liturgy of contemporary discourse, then health clubs and gymnasiums are our culture's secularized sites of worship.

Medicine is also big business. Health care costs continue to skyrocket, pharmaceutical giants rake in enormous profits, and people spend vast sums of money on "doctor-recommended" items that range from painkillers to athletic footwear, all in the quest to make the body function or just look better. The medical profession sets the terms of our popular health discourse and behavior, and as such plays an especially commanding role in our lives.

Because of all this, medicine enjoys power. But it is not an authority born merely of its own scientific advances and real therapeutic achievements. Rather, it is also due to the receptivity of popular culture to medicine. Indeed a hallmark of our culture is the public's seemingly insatiable and uncritical appetite for all things medical. We are not merely and unwittingly manipulated by the world of medicine. Rather, we bestow authority upon it by hanging on its every pronouncement. In a genuinely symbiotic way, we are complicit in assisting it to enjoy the significance it does.

While medicine and popular culture enjoyed a new kind of relationship at the end of the twentieth century, one that was enhanced by both the commercial dimension to medicine and a public that craved, and still craves, medical information, the two have always operated in tandem. It seems especially worthwhile, therefore, to illuminate times in the past when culture, both high and low, have intersected with medicine. To this end, scholars who are not, strictly speaking, historians of medicine have turned increasingly to medical history with a view to enlightening social and cultural history.

On the other hand, whereas historians of medicine once sought to catalogue the great discoveries, advances, and personalities of medical science, they are no longer content to do so. Such an interpretation of medicine's past is not only unsatisfying, it is distorting, for it wrenches medicine from the realms of culture and society, leaving it suspended in an imaginary realm of value-free objectivity. It is an environment where only "good" as a moral and material category is accentuated.

To be sure, the history of medicine is indeed about such things as the blessed eradication of smallpox and polio, the emergence of transplant surgery, and the discovery of highly effective psychotropic medications. But it extends well beyond those bounds. In the last few decades scholarship has focused on telling the social and cultural history of medicine as well as the history of culture and society through medicine. To these ends, new topics of investigation have emerged.[1] These include recounting patient narratives from different times and places, the story of women physicians, histories of epidemics and disease; detailing the politicized nature of medical research and treatment; telling the story of empire through an examination of colonial medicine; and, of course, recalling the horrible reality of medical criminality.

The involvement of minority groups in medicine is also beginning to come under historical scrutiny. One such group whose ubiquitous involvement in medicine has for some time been the object of historical inquiry is the Jews. But to date, Jewish medical history has tended to concentrate on biblical and talmudic medicine as well as medical practice among the Jews of medieval and early modern Southern Europe. In contrast to this, the historical association between the Jews of Central and Eastern Europe and medicine has not been documented to anywhere near the same extent.[2] In addition, too few attempts have been made to view Jewish history through the lens of medicine.

This book is about the relationship between the Jews of Germany and medicine as it unfolded from the early modern period through the rise of Hitler. It is not a history of "great contributions" to medicine made by Jews. Such lists—whether in the domains of medicine, sport, or entertainment—tell us little about the Jewish dimension to these achievements. And how can they? The process of scientific discovery, record-shattering achievement, or artistic creativity is universal and is most often (though not always) divorced from the ethnic, racial, or religious identity of the successful individuals. Certainly some meaning—it is rarely made clear and logically plausible exactly what—can be attached to such things, but the compilation of catalogues of boosterism is not the job of the historian. In what follows, I have sought to tell the history of the German Jews' relationship to medicine at those moments in that long history when the Jewishness of physicians and patients actually counted for something meaningful, and was constitutive of a particular historical development or of the formation of a set of ideas about Jews as subjects of medical investigation.

INTRODUCTION

The history of Jews in German medicine stands to teach us much about the culture and values of German Jewry, the relationship of Jews to German culture, and the special ways Jews contributed as major producers and consumers within the German medical community. Such a history may also allow us to see more clearly the extent to which we play a role in shaping contemporary medicine, as much as it seeks to shape us.

Few occupations are as immediately linked to a group as medicine is to the Jews. In the popular realm it has become the stuff of legend and stereotype, both positive and negative, and a source of pride, amusement, entertainment, and folklore. As a people, the Jews have enjoyed an intimate and deeply symbiotic relationship with medicine. As a religion, Judaism has long countenanced it as a respectable and indeed necessary calling, and socially the Jews have long viewed medicine as a path to professional fulfillment and honor within the community.

Germany offers a particularly rich context within which to explore this history, for it is there that one can detect the complex interstices of Jewish identity and medicine. Beginning in the Middle Ages, Germany had a large and well-developed Jewish health care system, with hospitals, hospices, a rabbinic literature on health, methods of medical training, and family dynasties of Jewish physicians. Thus the sociology of Jewish medicine in Germany was similar, though by no means identical, to that found in other parts of Europe. Nevertheless, it resided in the shadows of the medicine practiced by Jews in the Mediterranean world.

By the modern period, however, the situation was quite different, for Germany was then the world's medical leader and home to more Jewish doctors than anywhere else. This had an internal and an external impact. On one hand, the numerical preponderance of Jewish physicians and scientists became a way for German Jewry to define and distinguish itself from other Jewish communities. Science helped German Jewry create a sense of self-worth, and was used as a vehicle for Jewish self-expression and representation. On the other hand, the sheer number of Jewish physicians made them central to the medical culture of modern Germany. In this capacity they were both greatly valued but also rendered highly vulnerable to attack because of their ubiquitous presence.

In this study, I seek principally to shed light on two historical-cultural developments. The first is the place of medicine in German Jewish culture — its centrality and its social and intellectual significance. This involves an examination of the rise of the German Jewish physician, his emergence as a new

INTRODUCTION

kind of Jew in the early modern period—the secular, Jewish intellectual—and the further development of that type into the modern era.

Beyond the production of physicians, it is my contention that medicine and its culture have had a significant impact on the creation of modern Jewish identity. This is to say, the Jews are a people not only of the book, but also of the body.[3] In what follows I explore the ways modern German Jews increasingly expressed themselves in terms of their own bodies (this happened later in other countries as well), and how by the eighteenth century being Jewish meant having not just a spiritual identity, but a physical one as well.

Not only did medicine leave its imprint on Jewish culture, but the Jews played a crucial role in the formation of modern medical discourse and practice. Already in the Middle Ages we see for the first time associations of Jews with particular pathological traits. Most common among these were claims that the Jews had a distinct pallor and foul odor, and that they were prone to quinsy, an inflammation of the tonsils and surrounding tissue, in addition to a multitude of skin diseases, the glandular disorder scrofula, and hemorrhoids.[4] With time, ever more diseases were added to the list. Jews were discovered to be especially "prone" to mental disorders, diabetes, and certain forms of cancer. Added to this, their supposed immunity to alcoholism, tuberculosis, and infectious diseases, among them cholera, typhus, and smallpox, only served to make the Jews medical curiosities, patients of an entirely different order. The identification of these ailments served to distinguish them from the Christian majority.[5]

By the nineteenth century, Jews were seen in Germany as a distinct and separate race, for they seemed to display pathological and psychopathological characteristics that identified them as separate from their Gentile neighbors in significant ways.[6] Jews thereby became the principal reference group for medical and anthropological discussions pertaining to nature versus nurture, and environmental versus biological determinism. Central to the debates, and indeed complicating them, were Jewish doctors. Because there were so many of them, they delicately straddled the line that demarcated scientific observer from observed patient. As Jews and doctors, they were indeed both simultaneously. Yet Jewish doctors were powerless to do anything to change the fact that the epistemological breakthrough of the Middle Ages that labeled the Jews as fundamentally diseased proved an especially tenacious line of thought into the twentieth century.

So deeply entrenched and highly valued in Jewish culture is medicine that in order to write the history of the relationship in Germany, I have chosen

## INTRODUCTION

to adopt a longue durée approach. It is my contention that the history of medical practice among German Jews can best be viewed and explored as a chronological whole. Doing so not only affords us the means to identify innovations and change, but will also permit us to detect continuities and reemerging themes and patterns. Therefore, my starting point traces the rise of medieval and early modern Jewish physicians in order to outline their professional undertakings and position within medieval medicine. More specifically, this perspective permits the delineation of the differences in their modes of practice and relation to their respective communities in Spain, Italy, Poland, and Germany.

As in other European centers of medieval Jewish medical practice, German Jewish physicians enjoyed a certain mystique. Even while they were members of marginalized or even banished communities, Jewish doctors were sought out to treat lay and clerical elites. Among Christians, they developed reputations that were in part based on the overall taboos that attended Jews in medieval society. In a world governed by magical and superstitious beliefs, intimate though potentially "risky" contact with the outcast who was believed to possess enormous power made the Jewish doctor highly desirable.

However, as discussed in Chapter 2, there was one notable difference between the situation as it obtained in Germany and that which was to be found elsewhere. In Germany, the medical establishment confronted the Jewish doctor with an antisemitic campaign of remarkable vehemence. It was defined by the production of a catalogue of accusations and charges that were to last into modern times. Though similar charges had been made in other places, notably Spain, nowhere else in Europe was such a large corpus of medical antisemitica produced and circulated. To a great extent, it is the virulent hostility of German doctors that explains why university-trained Jewish physicians did not appear in Germany until the eighteenth century, that is, some two hundred years after they had been admitted to various Italian medical schools.

Chapter 3 focuses on Jewish medical practitioners who outlined their vision for a healthy Jewish future during the Berlin *Haskalah,* or Jewish Enlightenment of the eighteenth century. This was a time of incipient modernization and secularization, and such historic processes led to a revaluation of many ancient Jewish customs and traditions, particularly when they were perceived as damaging to health. *Maskilic* doctors (proponents of the Haskalah) saw themselves as custodians of the health of the Jewish people, and they sought to introduce changes in such areas as the Jewish diet, child care, and burial practices. Their undertaking was part of an overall program of Jewish physical regeneration, designed to prepare the Jewish masses for political emancipation.

By the middle of the nineteenth century, the Jewish physician became a symbol of the promise as well as the perils that accompanied modernization and the receipt of citizenship. In 1845, a series of articles appeared in the major German Jewish weekly newspaper, the *Allgemeine Zeitung des Judentums*. In these articles, which sought to make the case for a reform of Judaism, the author claimed that scrupulous attention to Jewish ritual was incompatible with citizenship. To be observant was to relinquish any possibility of full acceptance and to forgo the economic advantages of emancipation. As an example, the author related the story of an Orthodox father who permitted his three sons to attend the gymnasium (high school). Having distinguished themselves there, one decided to go on and study medicine, the second, mechanical engineering, while the third went into business. Hardly out of their father's sight, the two that went to university stopped observing Jewish ritual. Clearly this would be a source of disappointment to the father. But for the author of the story, the only question was a rhetorical one: "Could the father really ask the son not to write a prescription on the Sabbath or not to go to a remote village when called?"[7]

With this story, the proponent of religious reform indicates that for observant Jews in Germany, seeking a career in medicine could entail hard and sometimes life-changing choices. Above all, it might necessitate the abandonment of ritual observance. This did not apply to other careers, for medicine was unique. The problems arising from its practice were therefore used to illustrate the dilemmas facing modern Jews. Neither the engineer nor the businessman was bound by a professional code of conduct that would have him render his services when he chose not to. He was not professionally mandated to break the Sabbath if need be in order to fulfill his professional responsibilities. Certainly many did, but this was a matter of choice. Such was not the case for the doctor. The social and professional pressures on him were binding, and stark choices lay before him.

Many obstacles stood in the way of the full acceptance of Jews into German society. In addition to traditional religious and social antisemitism was the belief that Jews possessed a unique set of pathologies and psychopathologies that set them apart from Germans. Whether this was indeed the case was a central debate among medical practitioners and researchers at the end of the nineteenth century, and is explored in Chapters 4 and 5. Examining such discussions today, one can detect the emergence, in Germany, of the

## INTRODUCTION

"Jewish body" as a cultural and scientific idea. One feature of such was the manner by which the constructions of the pathological Jewish body became a site of political, national, and cultural contestation. For the Germans used elaborate descriptions of the Jewish body (by definition, it was defective) to describe their own physical state. By defining themselves in terms of that which they deemed abnormal, the Germans could characterize themselves as healthy paragons of pathological normality.

But the story of modern medicine's encounter with the Jews goes beyond the simple arrangement of Jews as patients and non-Jews as observer-physicians. For another factor that prompted the medical establishment to focus its gaze upon the Jews was the high level of participation of Jews in medicine. Especially in Central Europe, their heavy presence in a profession that focused on the Jews as cultural and medical curiosities only served to increase medicine's preoccupation with them.

In Germany, medicine provided many young Jews with a means of professional and thus social advancement, and it was the prism through which many of the discussions of the Jews' status in Wilhelmine society was filtered. Jewish doctors therefore used the discourse and methodology of contemporary medicine to ponder the place of Jews and the nature of Jewishness in the modern, secular world. Because of their professional training, Jewish physicians became some of the most astute observers of and commentators upon the Jewish condition and body. But as Jews themselves, these physicians blurred the distinction between patient and doctor. By studying the pathology of the Jews, they became both observed and observer. Consequently, any critique of the Jewish body by a Jewish physician, although often issued in imperious and detached tones, was also a passionate critique of the Jewish self.

Even though among Jewish doctors there was a widely accepted premise that the health of the Jews needed to be significantly improved, the very heterogeneity of Jewish society and its physicians often produced highly divergent prescriptions for cures. Secular Jewish critics of the Jewish body tended to ascribe the cause of Jewish illness to the normative structure and practices of rabbinic, or traditional, Judaism, claiming they bred ill health. Thus, a primary theme of such discourse was the suggestion that Jews could attain good health by combining a commitment to personal well-being with Jewish cultural and political modernization and reform.

On the other hand, physicians who subscribed to religious Orthodoxy tended to see the prevalence of physical and mental disease among Jews as the result of the abandonment of rituals held to be salutary, such as the dietary laws, and those pertaining to ritual purity. Zionist medical polemics suggested yet another cure for the ills that beset individual Jews and their communities — the creation of a healthy environment in the Land of Israel. Here, both diaspora disease and mentality would undergo radical change for the better. The personal experience of the influential Zionist thinker A. D. Gordon (1856–1922) is illustrative of the promise. Rejected for Russian army service on the grounds that he was medically unfit, Gordon eventually made his way to Palestine, where, at the age of forty-eight and never having performed any physical labor, he threw himself into agricultural work. A revered figure, Gordon formulated a philosophy that came to be known as "the religion of labor," insisting that the redemption of humanity in general, and the Jews in particular, would come about only through the creation of a direct relationship with nature through physical labor. For Gordon, Jewish "zealots of labor" could emerge only in Palestine, where the transformation, or "redemption," he envisaged would make Jewish culture "healthy" and "vital."[8]

The belief that Jews had to strive to become healthy and vital was central to the project of Jewish modernization and identity formation, and Jewish medical practitioners and social scientists played a crucial role in that undertaking. In particular, the language of medical regeneration and the metaphors of health and disease were most assiduously employed by Zionist physicians to characterize contemporary Jewish society. Zionists recognized that their task involved the regeneration of the Jews and the revivification of a Jewish society they regarded as having undergone stultification during the long course of their dispersion. By representing the exilic state of the Jews as one that promoted ill health, Zionist polemicists established antipodal diagnostic categories of "normal" and "abnormal" to describe the individual and collective ills afflicting Jews and Jewish society. Consequently, the languages of medicine and the natural sciences, perhaps as much as any other borrowed discourses, came to shape and define the political language of Zionism, providing it with a rich array of metaphors and long-lived images about Jews.[9]

The linguistic and visual semiotics of the Zionist enterprise were informed by fin-de-siècle notions of health, disease, strength, weakness, masculinity, and femininity — categories rooted in modern medicine. That this should be so was no accident, given the high percentage of Zionist polemicists who were also medical practitioners. In both Germany and Eastern Europe, Zionist physicians were highly influential in their writings and contributed to the formation of Zionist culture and ideology, invoking medical references and metaphors to describe both the Jews and their political and social condition.[10]

## INTRODUCTION

One of the most remarkable features of the nineteenth-century discourse about the Jews' body was that although it showed Jews as healthier, living longer, and enjoying a lower mortality rate than non-Jews, at the very same time, the stereotype of the weak and sickly Jew came into being. Christians and Jews from all walks of life made political and ideological hay from this stereotype. What permitted its rise in the face of scientific evidence to the contrary was the notion that Jews, as an overwhelmingly urban, commercial, and intellectual group, led lifestyles that went against the grain of accepted European norms of health and vigor, themselves based first and foremost upon a Christian, masculine ideal. And Jews simply did not conform. Thus they could be classified as ill because even sickness, whether imagined or real, can be invested with gendered and culturally proscribed meanings. For example, in contemporary society, breast cancer is largely perceived as befalling only women. Yet men, too, suffer from it and in increasing numbers. But broadening public perception of the disease would entail the difficult task of breaking down deeply engrained assumptions. The modern Jews' body (always male unless otherwise specified) was gendered as effeminate, that is, frail and vulnerable. Despite descriptions of them as "tenacious," "persistent," and "resistant," modern Jews, because of their social and cultural proclivities, have often been labeled "fragile," "sickly," and "diseased." This, like popular assumptions about breast cancer, is a deeply engrained pattern of thought.

Such thinking became a staple of the mythology about Jews, a core belief brought into especially sharp relief by the Zionist experience. According to early ideologues, only Eretz Yisrael could (and did) create healthy Jews imbued with a martial spirit. This line of thought is connected to another foundational myth of the modern Jewish experience, namely that it was only in Palestine and, later, Israel that Jewish politics first emerged, the claim being that the two-thousand-year-long Diaspora had witnessed Jewish political powerlessness, a sure sign of national "sickness." Now, as with claims about Jewish ill health, this one was made contrary to the historical evidence testifying to an ancient and sophisticated Jewish political history. With the rise of the nation-state in the nineteenth century, politics became a measure of a "healthy" nationhood and, by extension, the perceived absence of such in the case of the Jews entailed a denial of their national normalcy and well-being.[11]

In the wake of the Enlightenment of the eighteenth century, Jews were under considerable pressure to assimilate to German life. In fact their political emancipation was conditional upon the extent to which Jews rid themselves of the most particularistic elements of their culture. The response of German Jewry was to modify and then later abandon many religious practices, for much in the repertoire of Jewish customs and rituals contributed to a sense that the Jews were in some essential way different from the Germans, and intended to remain apart from them.

Many Jews, therefore, criticized the most separatist religious acts as being out of step with modern sensibilities and an impediment to Jewish integration. Worse still, many from among the educated German elite, particularly Protestant professors of early Christianity, as well as rabble-rousing antisemites, saw in these rituals "proof" of the atavistic nature of Judaism, decrying the rituals as antiquated, separatist, and even barbaric.

Yet in contrast, as shown in Chapter 6, important Jewish voices mounted a vigorous defense of religious customs. It was natural that German Jewry, with its high proportion of physicians, would defend the most corporeal (and attacked) of Jewish rituals—*kashrut* (dietary laws), *shehitah* (ritual animal slaughter), and *brit milah* (circumcision)—on the basis of science. They sought to give scientific evidence before the bar of history as to why such customs did not run counter to prevailing German notions of morality, ethics, and rationality.

Very often, the texts such doctors produced to defend ancient Jewish ritual appear to be presentations of dry, scientific data. Similarly, the detailed description of experiments bears little relation to Jewish apologetic literature of the past. This is the case because the point of reference for such texts is modern science, not the traditional, Jewish canon. Nevertheless, modern German Jewish physicians were in the midst of creating a new kind of Jewish literature—a secular and scientific Jewish apologia.

The creation of such was made necessary and possible only by the emerging constellation of factors concerning Jews, medicine, and the growth of antisemitism at the end of the nineteenth century. This is the subject of Chapter 7. From the 1870s until the rise of the Third Reich, German and Austrian Jews flocked to the field of medicine in unprecedented numbers. Their unmistakable presence, especially in the cities, significantly changed the face of German medicine and Jewish society. What both precipitated and facilitated the entrance of German Jews into science was the development among them of what Thorstein Veblen called "a skeptical frame of mind." With their moorings to tradition cut loose, Jews were free to enter the intellectual world of science and medicine to an extent never before seen in Jewish history.[12] As a consequence, the sheer number of Jews with scientific or medical training helped recast German Jewry from a tradition-bound

INTRODUCTION

community to one that expressed modern—indeed, scientifically avant-garde—ideas.

Because they had arisen in the context of medical specialization, a preferential mode of practice for Jewish doctors, some of these "ideas" led to accusations by their opponents that the Jews were destroying "traditional" German medicine. In addition, overcrowding in the medical profession, and changes in insurance laws that made for intense economic competition, set the stage for a hostile backlash against Jewish physicians. As a result, the fin-de-siècle saw the resurrection of malicious, medieval charges against Jewish doctors. Modified and secularized, Jewish doctors were again portrayed as prime agents in a conspiracy to kill Christian patients. As in the distant past, they were again accused of using their expertise to conquer Germany by spreading plague, performing medical experimentation on Christians, and causing the ruination of German doctors through unfair business practices.

The intimate relationship of German Jewry to medical practice came to an end with the rise of Hitler. On one hand, the propaganda and ideology behind the Nazi persecution of Jewish doctors drew on negative, medieval German stereotypes of Jewish physicians. On the other, it was novel in that by seeking to build the "therapeutic racial-state," Nazi Germany signaled its intention to purify the world. To create their utopian paradise of the fit and healthy, the Nazis eliminated those they deemed unworthy of life. Central to the experiment was the elimination of the Jews, whom they declared biologically inferior. Jewish doctors were an important subgroup among the persecuted. According to Gerhard Wagner, head of the Nazi Physicians' League, "The Führer considered the cleansing of the German medical profession more important than for example that of the civil service, as the task of a physician was in his opinion one of leadership or should be such."[13]

Founded upon perverted biological and medical notions, the Third Reich bestowed upon "Aryan" doctors enormous responsibilities as guardians of the nation's racial health. In that spirit, the campaign against Jewish physicians was accorded particular importance, for not only were Jewish doctors identified as usurpers of German scientific culture, they represented for the Nazis better than any other group a potential source of "race defilement," given their intimate access to the German people. Further motivation for Hitler came from the fact that one of the earliest and leading sources of resistance to the Nazi menace came from the Association of Socialist Physicians, originally founded in 1913 by Ignaz Zadek, the brother-in-law of the Jewish socialist theoretician and politician, Eduard Bernstein. The association, with its majority Jewish membership, supported a wide range of social causes and advised Socialist parties in the Reichstag on health care policy.[14]

Concerned with identifying the underlying social causes of disease, not just with treating illness itself, Socialist physicians eschewed race-based diagnoses of ill health, opting instead for environmental explanations. Politically and medically they were a thorn in the side of the conservative German medical establishment long before Hitler's rise. Such doctors were ubiquitous, and astute social commentators such as the great Yiddish novelist Israel Joshua Singer brilliantly captured the sentiments of left-wing German Jewish physicians in the father and daughter characters Fritz and Elsa Landau in his epic novel, *The Family Carnovsky*. They lived and tended to the sick in a working-class neighborhood in Berlin where everyone "knew the odd couple." Many of the residents "addressed him not as Herr Doctor but as Comrade Doctor," and her patients, too, called Elsa "Comrade Doctor." When Fritz Landau returned the greeting, "The men smiled proudly because the doctor called them Comrade. They were proud that he belonged to their party and attended meetings at Petersile's beer hall." Later, when she was elected to the Reichstag as a Socialist deputy, Elsa was constantly tormented and humiliated by Nazis, eventually fleeing to New York with her aging father.[15]

The Association of Socialist Physicians, which included many Jews, constituted a bright ray of hope in a medical community that had by and large come to regard Nazism as a source of its own salvation and reward. For Hitler, who had long since identified the "Judeo-Bolshevik" enemy as Germany's greatest foe, Jewish physicians, a majority of whom were Social Democrats, came to embody in his mind the principal enemy within the enemy. It is for all these reasons that Hitler considered the elimination of the German Jewish doctor "exceptionally necessary and urgent."[16]

# CHAPTER 1

# THE EMERGENCE OF THE MEDIEVAL JEWISH PHYSICIAN

The social link between the Jews and medicine dates to the Middle Ages, for it was then that medicine began to be practiced by significant numbers of Jews. One reason for the profession's popularity among Jews was that from the medieval period until the eighteenth century, physician-rabbis were highly visible figures on the Jewish social landscape. This had a decided effect on the culture and value system of the Jews, bolstering the prestige of medicine, securing its image as a noble undertaking, validating medicine's compatibility with traditional Judaism, and helping its more illustrious practitioners become beloved within their communities. In other words, from early on, doctors became role models for Jews. Moreover, for both Jews and Gentiles, the cognitive and cultural association of Jews with medicine, which persists down to our own time, was also formed during the Middle Ages.

In Western Europe, the transition of Jewish culture from one that was theologically amenable to medicine to one that actually boasted a disproportionate number of physicians was relatively abrupt.[1] From about 1250, medicine came to occupy a central place in the array of professions engaged in by medieval Jewry. At this time, Jews constituted about 1 percent of European society, with slightly higher percentages in larger towns and cities. At various times, however, Jews accounted for as much as 50 percent of the physicians in a given locale.[2]

This is somewhat ironic because although Judaism wholeheartedly sanctions and encourages medicine, there has never been a field designated "Jewish medicine." While the Bible and Talmud certainly address such subjects as human anatomy, hygiene, and the nature of disease and its causes, medical discussions by the rabbis were generally entered into for the purposes of making a halakhic, or legalistic, interpretation.[3] Ancient Jewish disquisitions about the body were not part of a self-contained therapeutic discourse.

This is because an independent, secular, Jewish medical tradition akin to that possessed by the Greeks, the Arabs, the Chinese, or the Indians simply has never existed.[4] There were no Jewish medical schools in the talmudic age, nor were there any medical textbooks and treatises written in Hebrew, save the *Sefer Asaf,* a medical compendium assumed to have been written in Palestine between the third and fifth centuries, but possibly compiled in Byzantium as late as the tenth.[5] Indeed, the dearth of ancient medical literature in Hebrew was even recognized and bemoaned by medieval Jewish translators.[6]

And while the Talmud is full of remedies, treatments, and discussions of physicians, later generations of rabbis specifically warned against using rabbinic literature as medical texts.[7] Just as Moses Maimonides (1135–1204) had warned that the astronomical knowledge of the rabbis was no match for that of the experts, somewhat later no less a figure than Jacob ben Moses Möllin (1365–1427), the most distinguished talmudist of his generation and head of the Jewish communities of Germany, Austria, and Bohemia, argued that: "One should not try any of the medicines, prescriptions or exorcisms recommended in the Talmud because no one today knows how they should be applied. If they should be tried nevertheless and found ineffective, the words of our sages would be exposed to ridicule."[8]

It is all the more remarkable, then, that medicine became so closely associated with Jews, given that no system of medicine derived from Judaism. The history of "Jewish medicine" is mostly the history of its doctors and that of Jews as objects of medical observation. It is a story that spans the medieval and modern periods. The roots of the relationship of Jews to medicine struck deepest in Mediterranean lands, for there perhaps thousands of Jewish doctors ministered to the sick, both Jewish and Gentile, throughout the course of the Middle Ages and early modern periods. While their story, which has been rendered in large brushstrokes, may lack some detail, it nevertheless fills a rather large canvas. It is not the aim of this book to repeat that story. Rather, some general aspects of it serve as necessary, comparative background before moving on to examine the history of medicine among the Jews of Germany.[9]

Generally speaking, the most important developments in medical training and practice between the seventh and eleventh centuries took place in the Muslim world and Southern Europe. Islamic intellectual culture absorbed Greek philosophy, science, and medicine, building on them to create a majestic flowering of knowledge and high culture. Arab physicians elaborated on Greek medicine, composed medical encyclopedias, and led the world in the description and treatment of various diseases.[10]

It is not surprising, then, that prior to 1250 and the rise of the Jewish physician in the West, the greatest concentration of Jewish doctors was to be found in the Islamic world of the eleventh and twelfth centuries.[11] Historian Shlomo Dov Goitein has further observed that under Islam, "an almost unbroken succession of medical men constituted both the actual and official leadership of one of the two minority groups in Egypt and the adjacent countries during the whole of the High Middle Ages and far beyond."[12] Moses Maimonides, the rabbinic authority, philosopher, and court physician, is the most famous such character of this type.[13] As in so many areas of human endeavor, there was a symbiotic quality to the relationship between Arabs and Jews when it came to medicine. Arab medicine played an influential role in Jewish life and culture under Islam, providing it with professional and intellectual inspiration; in turn, Judaism's positive attitudes toward medicine were clearly incorporated into Islam itself, contributing to the prominence of Arab medicine.

While they eventually became important as practitioners, Jewish physicians at the beginning of the twelfth century exerted their greatest influence on the development of later medieval medicine in their role as translators and transmitters of Greek and Arabic medical texts into Hebrew (Jews had already translated an enormous number of Arabic philosophical texts into Hebrew).[14]

Carried by Jewish immigrants to Southern and Western Europe, the Hebrew translations were picked up by Jewish medical practitioners, who in turn developed a keen reputation for their medical knowledge.[15] By 1400, Jews had translated all the most important Arabic medical texts, and the most recent ones in Latin. The consequence of the enterprise of translation was threefold. First, the Jewish physician came to be held in high esteem because he was privy to the wisdom of both Greek and Islamic medicine. Second, the building of what has been called the "Hebrew medical library" meant that the High Middle Ages marks the beginning of a culture of professional medicine among the Jews.[16] This is not a uniquely Jewish story. The creation of a professional medical corps was a European phenomenon — one that saw the imposition of very strict licensing procedures for physicians, and the development of what has been termed the overall "medicalization of society."[17] Nevertheless, it is a further indication that medieval Jewish society was open to Christian innovation and custom. And third, medicine as a course of study exposed the Jewish doctor to other related disciplines such as astronomy, biology, botany, mathematics, and physics. Thus in addition to doctors, a quiet epistemological revolution had its first stirrings in Jewish society with the production of a new type of intellectual: the Jew who could boast philosophical and/or scientific literacy.

To be sure, "Jewish medicine" was a somewhat circumscribed phenomenon. By concentrating on translation, the production of original works of medical scholarship in Hebrew was minimal. In fact, after 1400 Jewish physicians became dependent on Christian medical knowledge and the scholastic model of instruction.[18] By an act of omission, wherein no Jewish authors are mentioned, we are given insight into the limited, intellectual contribution of "Jewish medicine" in the Middle Ages by recalling the description of the ideal physician in the prologue to the *Canterbury Tales*. Chaucer had him well-versed in Escalapius, Hippocrates, Rufus, Dioscorides, Galen, Rhazes, Hali, Serapion, Averroes, Avicenna, Constantine, Scotch Bernard, John of Gaddesden, and Gilbertine. Not a Jewish author among them. And as if to underscore the point, Chaucer declared of the physician, "He did not read the Bible much."[19] Nevertheless, before 1400, the Jewish translation project was of decisive importance, for Christian students would have come to many of these texts by way of the Latin translations by Jews.

Moreover, those medical treatises were the primary sources used in the education of Jewish physicians during the Middle Ages. In Southern Europe, Jews were largely excluded from universities before the middle of the fourteenth century. Therefore, aspiring Jewish medical students had to seek private instruction, and despite some contact with faculty at universities such as Salerno and Montpellier, the majority of Jewish physicians practicing around the Mediterranean throughout the Middle Ages learned their art from Jewish doctors in a one-to-one apprenticeship, and by studying the Hebrew translations. And rabbinic dicta about the dependency of the community on the physician notwithstanding — the Talmud admonishes that "it is forbidden to live in a city without a physician" — the cost of medical studies was borne solely by the family.[20] It was not a communal responsibility. Very often, the existence of medical dynasties among Jews meant that sons would study medicine under their fathers, or sometimes, the promise of a bride's father to teach medicine to his prospective son-in-law was even written into the marriage contract.[21]

Throughout the Middle Ages and the early modern period, the popular reputation Jews built for themselves as doctors derived principally from their role as practitioners.[22] Two features of medieval Jewish medical practice help explain how this was achieved. The first stems from the relatively large number of Jewish physicians, all engaged in patient observation and treatment. Their exposure to so many sick people provided them with invaluable experience and knowledge. A related point involves the peripatetic nature of medieval Jewish doctors. In their travels to many communities and correspondence with a wide array of medical and rabbinical personalities from all over Europe, Jewish doctors shared a vast quantity of information with one another, thereby bringing wider attention and expertise to a variety of medical conditions. The same, of course, holds true for treatment protocol.[23] The result of the vast circulation of medical knowledge among Jews was, at the very least, a widely held impression that Jews were in possession of a sophisticated body of medical knowledge that enabled them to provide a superior level of medical care compared to Gentile physicians. The fact that the medieval Jewish (and Gentile) doctor was powerless to cure most illnesses is immaterial, for his contemporaries, Christian and Jewish, believed otherwise. It was their faith in his talents that led them to form the enduring stereotype of the Jewish doctor capable of effecting cures.

As a consequence, Jewish doctors enjoyed public recognition both within the narrow confines of Jewish society and far beyond its limits. As is well known, Jewish physicians all over Europe were called upon to be court physicians in the service of kings, princes, and members of the aristocracy. Christian clergy also made use of Jewish doctors, to the extent that the majority of late medieval and Renaissance Popes had Jewish physicians in the medical retinues at their service.[24]

Although temporal and church officials employed Jewish physicians to care for them, they expressly forbade the Christian populace at large from being treated by Jewish doctors. The church council at Béziers (1246) threatened to excommunicate Christians who sought medical treatment from Jews, and similar councils at Alby (1254) and Vienna (1267) excluded Jews from the free practice of medicine. Synods at Avignon (1326 and 1337), Freising (1440), and Bamberg (1491) all reinforced the ban on Christians using the services of Jewish physicians.[25] (Mutual suspicion reigned, as the rabbi likewise passed injunctions against Jews using the services of Christian doctors.) What is paradoxical here is that the felt need of the Church to reimpose the bans time and again indicates that Christian common folk had few qualms about securing the services of Jewish doctors. Nor, would it seem, did they hesitate to defy Church policy when it was in their personal interest to do so.

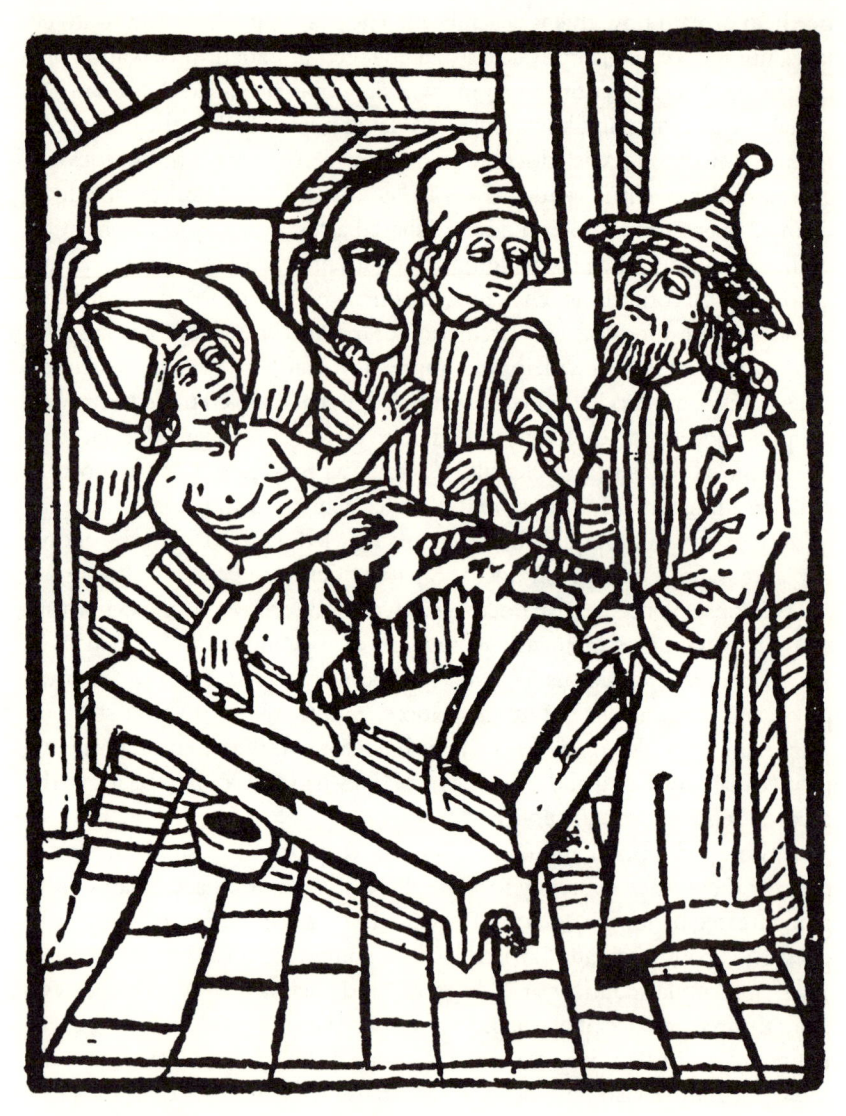

FIGURE 1. Throughout the Middle Ages, despite Church decrees and royal ordinances forbidding Jewish physicians from treating Christian patients, it was common for lay and clerical elites to seek treatment from Jews. In this illustration from Hans Schobser's *Plenarium* (Augsburg, 1487), St. Basil is being attended to by his Jewish physician, Ephraim. Although Basil lived in fourth-century Caesarea, Ephraim is depicted as a German Jew in medieval attire. Source: Harry Friedenwald, *The Jews and Medicine* (Baltimore, 1944).

Their intimate proximity to seats of power served to expand the role played by Jewish doctors. They were not only called upon to heal, but soon became royal confidants, advisors, and even shapers of policy. In addition, when necessary, they were able to use their positions to intercede on behalf of the Jewish community. To a great extent, their role as communal advocates mitigated the resentment fellow Jews expressed toward physicians as a result of the royal privileges they enjoyed, such as exemption from communal taxes, or special dispensation from wearing the distinctive and humiliating clothing and markings other Jews were required to display.

The way both clerical and secular powers used Jewish physicians was also a result of the creation of university medical faculties during the thirteenth century, and the introduction of medical licensing that occurred between the twelfth and sixteenth centuries. The effect of licensing was to reduce the number of individuals who could offer health care. Further reductions were the result of guild protectionism, which also succeeded in preventing or severely controlling the medical practice of non-university-trained personnel.[26] Especially affected were the activities of women, who, it can be assumed, were primary health care providers.

While comparatively little is known of women doctors in the Middle Ages, recent historical research makes it clear that they did not confine themselves to treating other women but offered their services to men as well, and could generally be found across the spectrum of medical specialization. However, the newly imposed conditions of practice that effectively excluded women from universities also took a decided toll on the number of women medical practitioners. Available figures reveal extremely small numbers. In France between the twelfth and fifteenth centuries, women constituted only about 1.5 percent of physicians. In England from the eighth to the sixteenth century, only eight female physicians have been identified. Although no comprehensive study of Italy exists as yet, the results of local investigations seem consistent with the findings for France and England. Medieval German women physicians also probably existed in similarly small numbers.[27]

It is certain that many more women practiced medicine than the meager historical record reflects. They may simply never have had their names recorded, or they may have, as a result of the professions' tightened regulations, congregated in specialties that lacked prestige and thus interest for the chronicler. Whatever the case, the fact is that while there were certainly more women doctors than we know about, women were not numerically well represented in the medical profession, a condition that may actually have worsened over time. Perhaps an unintended beneficiary of this development was the Jewish physician. In a society characterized by staggering rates of infant mortality, short life expectancy, violence, disease, filth, and overcrowding, it is wholly to be expected that municipal officials would rely on the services of Jewish doctors, both male and female, when there were simply too few Christian male practitioners to serve the people.

Ironically, in the Middle Ages and early modern period, a number of Jewish women achieved considerable reputations as excellent physicians and teachers.[28] This may have been because like Christian women and Jewish men, they had also been excluded from university study and thus may have continued to provide medical services that university-trained physicians considered peripheral to the profession. In addition, we must consider whether medieval Jewish society was more accepting of women physicians than was Christian society because of Jews' fear of being treated by Gentiles. Did medieval Jews prefer that Jewish bodies be tended to by Jewish women rather than by Christian men?

The written record that does exist concerning Jewish women doctors reflects their favorable status in relation to Gentile society, a most significant achievement for that day and age. A contract signed in Marseilles and dated 1326 indicates an arrangement between the Jewish Sara de Saint Gilles and the Christian Salvet de Bourgneuf, wherein she agreed to teach him "*artem medicine et phisice*" for a period of seven months. She was also duty-bound to provide him with board and clothing. In return, Salvet was obliged to turn over to Sara all fees he earned from treating patients for the duration of his apprenticeship.[29]

Perhaps because of the backwardness of formal medical education in Central Europe, and the paucity of physicians there, the largest number of Jewish women doctors was to be found in Germany. In one study focusing on Frankfurt am Main for the years between 1387 and 1497, it was found that of the fifteen women medical practitioners operating in the city, a majority were Jewish.[30]

Sara, in the bishopric of Würzburg, Zerlin, an eye doctor in Frankfurt am Main around 1430, and Frau Morada in Günzburg are three of the better-known individuals whose activities were recorded. The first, Sara, who was granted a license by municipal authorities to practice medicine in 1419, for which she paid an annual tax of 10 florins, was so successful that she was able to accumulate a considerable fortune — enough to buy a manor house. In Frankfurt, Zerlin's skills were so prized that she was permitted to reside among Christians outside the *Judengasse*, while in 1542, a book on

Jewish customs was dedicated to Frau Morada, the inscription reading, "modest Frau Morada, doctor of the art of medicine, resident of Günspurg."[31] Like their male counterparts, and Christian women, Jewish women learned their craft as apprentices, the standard method of instruction until the sixteenth century, after which time Jewish men from Germany began to obtain formal instruction at Italian and Dutch medical schools.

But even before this trend began, there is no doubt that during the Middle Ages a mystique developed about the Jewish doctor. The roots of this sense that the Jewish doctor was somehow special — he was both highly regarded and deeply feared — can be traced to the Janus-faced representation of the Jewish physician in Gentile imagination. The mystique derives from the fact that on the one hand, the Jewish doctor was clearly a respected individual. His ennobled and clerical employers are testament to that. Moreover, he was held in esteem because his knowledge of Hebrew was believed to have provided him with access to privileged and quite possibly esoteric information.[32]

Ironically, that which Christians feared most about Jews, their otherness and exoticness, provided a source of comfort and hope to Gentile patients. Thus, much like today's Westerners in need of medical treatment who, having unsuccessfully exhausted mainstream medical therapies in search of a cure, seek out faith healers or non-Western medical practitioners, Christians of the Middle Ages and early modern period turned optimistically to Jews for treatment.

The core religious difference between the two groups also attracted non-Jews to the Jewish physician, for this difference could have practical consequences. The Fourth Lateran Council of 1215 explicitly declared that the Christian doctor attending a sick bed had first to take care of the patient's soul, by calling upon a priest to attend the house-call. The idea that bodily cures depended on the health of the soul was taken seriously by Christian physicians until the scientization of medicine during the Enlightenment. As German physician Jakob Martini wrote in a diatribe against Jewish doctors in 1636, "A doctor may, with full right and all fairness occasionally abandon the sick, if the patient is a godless and malicious person, unaware that his sickness is a punishment from God for his godless character. . . . Such a person is not worth the merest good deed, let alone being attended to in his illness by a doctor who should care for his health."[33] It is precisely because of their different religious faith that Jewish physicians were completely unconcerned with matters spiritual on the Christian sickbed. Consequently, to the Christian patient, all the healing powers of Jewish doctors could be concentrated on ensuring physical recovery, with theological issues not interfering in or even preventing the commission of the treatment.

For many, Jewish doctors possessed other qualities that could be perceived as positive. Some Christians held that they had supernatural powers, a notion that was part of a well-established set of beliefs concerning the magical and kabbalistic proficiency of Jews.[34] Writing in the nineteenth century, Sir Walter Scott, in describing his Jewish heroine, the physician Rebecca, expounded on popular medieval beliefs about Jewish doctors in his classic, *Ivanhoe*:

> But the Jews, both male and female, possessed and practised the medical science in all its branches, and the monarchs and powerful barons of the time frequently committed themselves to the charge of some experienced sage among the despised people, when wounded or in sickness. The aid of the Jewish physicians was not less eagerly sought after, though a general belief prevailed among the Christians, that the Jewish Rabbis were deeply acquainted with the occult sciences, and particularly with the cabalistical art which had its name and origin in the studies of the sages of Israel. . . . It is besides probable, considering the wonderful cures they are said to have performed, that the Jews possessed some secrets of the healing art peculiar to themselves, and which, with the exclusive spirit arising out of their condition, they took great care to conceal from the Christians amongst whom they dwelt.[35]

Accounts of the occult healing practices of the Jews existed in medieval Christian folklore. For example, it was said of Zedekiah, court physician to Emperor Charles the Bald at the end of the ninth century, that he could fly. His legend grew with time. In 1378, Johannes, Abbot of Trittenheim, declared that Zedekiah once "threw a man into the air, tore him there into pieces, piled his organs into a heap, and then joined them together again." All this was said to have occurred without the slightest harm having come to the man.[36] This claim, and others like it, was related to the widespread medieval belief that the Jews were proficient demonologists and in league with the Devil. Although the charge was a general one, and applied equally to all Jews, very often Jewish doctors, especially those in medieval and Reformation Germany, were the specific targets of such accusations (see Chapter 2).

While the charge of demonology can be denied, it is nevertheless true that Jews, like their Christian neighbors, did believe in demons and their ability to affect human behavior and health. They considered illness to be evidence of demonic forces at work.[37] In order to counteract the evil doings of malign spirits, medieval Jewish medical practice, like its Christian counterpart, resorted to magic and superstition.[38] Indeed, despite biblical injunctions against the use of incantations, Judaism, often with rabbinic sanction, permitted the use of magic and sorcery to combat illness believed to have been caused by evil spirits. The hesitant sanctioning of this occurred because of Judaism's imperative that everything short of idolatry, incest, or murder be done to save a patient. Thus was Judaism's elaborate magical and superstitious tradition, plus that borrowed from the surrounding cultures, employed to heal the sick.

Among Jewish doctors, the use of magical healing oscillated between the use of generic magic and specific Jewish forms. Very often, the principle behind the use of certain treatments was that if they were disgusting to humans, then surely they would have the same effect on demons.[39] Among Jews, some of these were referred to as *segullot*, or remedies that defy rational explanation. Thus among Jewish and Christian healers we see employed, among other things, the milk and urine of humans and donkeys, hot animal bile, snake soup, and fresh animal blood obtained immediately after slaughter.[40]

Among the *segullot* with a particular Jewish dimension, there were occasions when talmudic incantations were employed. It is said that the Maharil Jacob ben Moses Möllin, who warned against using talmudic cures, made one exception, invoking the dictum of like cures: "When a bone sticks in one's throat he should place a similar bone on his head and say, One, one, gone down, swallowed, swallowed, gone down, one, one. This cure is tested and proven, and is therefore the only one that may be used."[41] Given the firmly held conviction that disease was sent as punishment for sin, Jews believed that illness could be warded off by charity, prayer, change of conduct, and a fourth, ingenious way. In order to cheat satanic, disease-bearing forces, Jews changed their names, the aim being to fool the demons. This practice was especially observed among German Jews. New names were generally chosen from the Bible, according to some authorities, preferably without any letters that were contained in the person's original name. Because Jews are known by their parents' names (son of, or daughter of), they were also symbolically changed in order to prevent detection by evil forces. In a solemn ceremony, the name of the patient was changed in the synagogue in the presence of a quorum of ten males over the age of thirteen. The metamorphosis was effected according to a specific formula, while the officiant held a Torah scroll. In more modern times in Germany, names were chosen that indicated a long life, in the hope that the Angel of Death would be dissuaded from exacting punishment on one who had already lived so long. These names included Haim (life), Alter (old man), and Zayde (grandfather). All such names had their female equivalents.[42]

There was also a host of specifically Jewish treatments to cure certain illnesses. To combat weak eyes, a common therapy involved bathing them in wine that had been used at the *havdalah* service, the candle-lighting ceremony marking the close of the Sabbath. Similarly, staring long and hard at the flames of Sabbath candles was said to ward off ocular disease. Another homeopathic treatment common among medieval German Jews to prevent excessive bleeding after a circumcision entailed using a cotton poultice that had been smeared with egg-yolk, the mother's pubic hairs, the ashes of a burned feather, and a piece of cloth that had been soaked in blood from the wound. Less bizarre was the common Jewish practice of placing a Torah scroll on a suffering patient, or bringing one into the room where he or she rested, and then reading from it. Related to this is the venerable tradition among Jews of using amulets to prevent illness or to effect the recovery process, a practice that is still very much alive today, especially among Jews of Middle Eastern origin.[43]

The opposite view of Jewish physicians as expert healers was that of Jewish physicians as causing disease and deliberately seeking to harm Gentiles. The first piece of circumstantial evidence brought to bear against them was they were members of a despised and accursed race who had killed Jesus Christ. If the Jews had been bold enough to have committed deicide, it was naturally assumed that their aim was to kill common Christians. Who better to accomplish this goal than Jewish doctors? The standard medieval charge against them was that they knowingly used their position and knowledge to kill their non-Jewish patients.[44] In Chapter 2, this is discussed in much more detail as it pertains to the focal point of such charges, Germany.

Those Jewish physicians most obviously at risk in this accusatory climate were those whose Christian patients had died. In Bohemia in 1161, as a warning to doctors, eighty-six Jews who apparently knew that Jewish physicians had poisoned their patients were collectively punished by being burned at the stake. Farther west, in France, Philip the Fair, at the end of the thirteenth century, ordered the bailiff of Rouen to confiscate the property of Jewish physicians whose patients had died after consuming a prescribed medication.[45] The most notorious accusation of this type was that made during the Black Death of 1348–1350, when Jews were charged with having poisoned the drinking wells of Europe.[46]

# EMERGENCE OF THE MEDIEVAL JEWISH PHYSICIAN

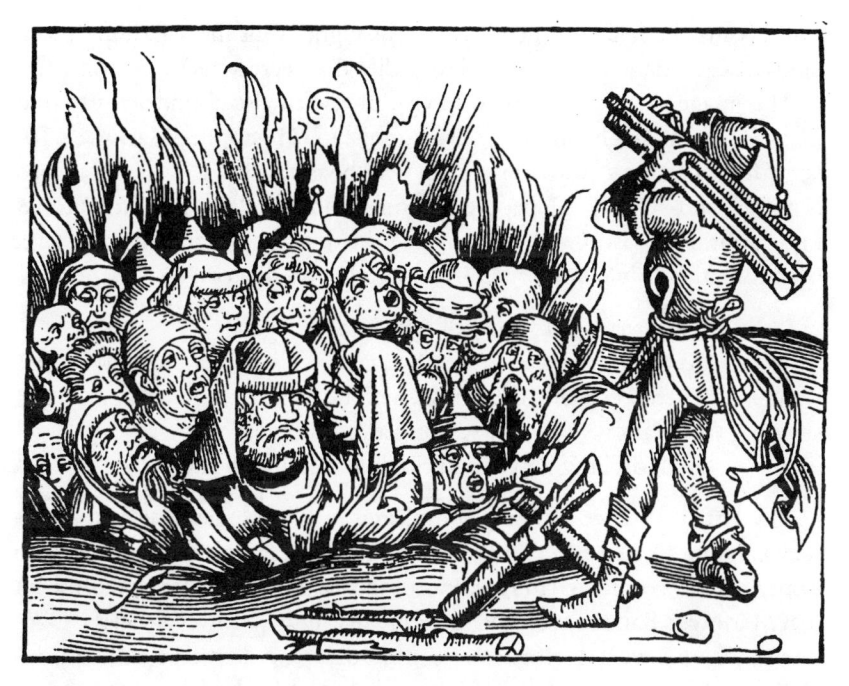

FIGURE 2. This fifteenth-century woodcut depicts Jews being burned alive for having allegedly caused the plague in 1348. The text accompanying the picture stated, "All the Jews in German lands were burned in the year of Christ MCCCXLVIII, accused of having poisoned wells, to which crime many of them confessed." From Hartmann Schedel's *Liber Chronicarum* (Nuremberg, 1493). Source: Georg Hermann Theodor Liebe, *Das Judentum in der deutschen Vergangenheit* (Leipzig, 1903).

Jewish doctors were said not only to have intentionally poisoned their Christian patients, but also to have celebrated it. According to the Reformation leader Martin Luther, "If they [the Jews] could kill us all, they would gladly do so, aye, and often do it, especially those who profess to be physicians. They know all that is known about medicine in Germany; they can give poison to a man of which he will die in an hour, or in ten or twenty years; they thoroughly understand this art."[47] Luther's Catholic antagonist, Johannes Eck, claimed that when Jewish doctors "come together at their festivals, each boasts of the number of Christians he has killed with his medicine; and the one who has killed the most is honored."[48] From Italy came the comment of Saint Bernadino of Siena, founder of the sect of the Holy Name of Jesus. He claimed to be actually relating the deathbed confession of a Jewish doctor from Avignon who "at his last hour declared he died a happy man because he had had the pleasure, throughout his life, of killing thousands of Christians with so-called remedies that were actually poisons."[49]

The image of the murderous Jewish physician also found its way into Elizabethan drama. Barabas, the protagonist in Christopher Marlowe's *The Jew of Malta*, was an avaricious villain who boasted that he walked "abroad o' nights, and kill[ed] sick people groaning under walls," while "sometimes I go about and poison wells." Gloatingly, he described to the Turkish slave, Ithamore, the early phase of his career as a Jewish doctor:

> Being young, I studied Physicke and began
> To practice first upon the Italian;
> There I enrich'd the Priests with burials,
> And always kept the sexton's arms in ure
> With digging graves and ringing dead men's knells.[50]

The virtual absence of Jewish physicians in Elizabethan England—notwithstanding Queen Elizabeth's Portuguese Marrano physician, Roderigo Lopez, who was executed in 1594 on trumped up charges of treason—meant that Marlowe's Barabas is in fact only a literary figure. However, on the Continent, where Jewish doctors were commonplace, polemicists and authorities consistently propounded the idea that Jewish physicians were to be feared because of their supposedly murderous inclinations.

Nowhere were fears about Jewish doctors expressed more often than in Germany. For example, in 1602, two Jewish doctors in Frankfurt, Aaron Rosen and Samuel Lamm, applied for physician's licenses to the authorities. Their requests were granted, and they were sworn in with a special Jewish oath. However, for the purposes of protecting Christian patients from possibly being poisoned by Jewish pharmacists, and to curb competition, Aaron and Samuel also had to agree that they would never prepare any medicines at home. If they wished to do so, the prescriptions had to be made with ingredients purchased at a Christian apothecary.[51]

Such fears were given expression in the Austrian capital as well. In 1610, the medical faculty of the University of Vienna bluntly stated that the secret code of Jewish physicians obligated them to "kill every tenth Christian patient by poisoning."[52] The prevailing Central European view of many was best summed up by the local clergy in Swabia in 1657, who upon hearing of the application of a Jewish physician named Hirsch to practice in the city of Hall, declared that "it is better to die with Christ than to be healed by a Jew-doctor [in league] with the devil."[53]

So, contemporaneous with the spectacular rise to medical prominence of Jewish physicians, charges of malpractice and murder were leveled against them. The Middle Ages and early modern period saw the Jewish doctor become, at one and the same time, a savior and a threat, a dangerous, malevolent individual, and an exotic healer. It is these dichotomous representations that gave Jewish physicians their mystique, making them so sought after on the one hand, and so feared on the other.

Just as the Middle Ages saw the creation of the stereotype wherein Jews were associated with usury specifically and commerce more generally, it was also at this time that Jews became intimately linked with the practice of medicine. The stereotype was formed on a kernel of truth. Business and medicine were exempted from the wide array of occupational restrictions imposed upon Jews during the Middle Ages. When the Jews' proficiency and talent in both endeavors was taken into account, along with the social reality of overrepresentation, the ingredients for the formation of deep-seated associations were set in place. These even include proto-racial ones that spoke of a particular "aptitude" of the Jews for such occupations. According to Converso physician Juan Huarte de San Juan, in his *Inquiry into the Nature and Kinds of Intelligence* (1575), a combination of geography, climate, diet, and historical experience created among ancient Israelites a specific kind of temperament and imagination that made them superior physicians.[54]

Such views were long-lived. In the nineteenth century, a historian of Jewish medicine, Eliakim Carmoly, made a similar claim for his own day by recalling that "the superiority of Jewish physicians over other physicians was so generally recognised, that Huarte, one of the best minds that the Spanish nation has produced, has endeavoured to prove, that by the [G]alenical theories, [the Jews'] temperament is that which was most adapted to medicine."[55] Also writing during the nineteenth century, the era of scientific racism, another author, reflecting on the Jewish experience in medieval Spain, quoted an officer of Montpellier University who had declared that "the reputation of Jewish physicians was such, that at one time it was believed essential to skill in medicine to be of Jewish descent."[56]

A measure of the extent to which medicine became associated with the Jews in the public mind is the fact that in Spain, the word *physician* actually became a derogatory code word for *Jew*. One of the reasons for this was that long after the expulsion of the Jews at the end of the fifteenth century, an inordinate number of physicians were to be found among the little-trusted New Christians. One of the bases for the association of the two words—

*Jew* and *doctor*—in the minds of Spanish authorities may have been the fact that into the seventeenth century, the Inquisition prosecuted physicians in large numbers for Judaizing.[57]

The noticeable presence of Jewish doctors may also have indirectly added to medicine's contribution to the terror apparatus of Inquisitorial Spain. According to one scholar, medicine played an active role in the persecution process, for it was "allied with the inquisitorial authorities in the task of corporally and morally disciplining sixteenth-century Spanish society."[58] In other words, as would happen later in Nazi Germany when medicine played such a prominent role in the destruction process of the Jews, doctors in early modern Spain not only collaborated with the state but also may have played a specifically retributive and punitive role, inspired by the disproportionate number of physicians of Jewish origin in Spain.[59]

That Spanish Jews held medicine in particularly high regard is evidenced by the fact that for centuries after the expulsion, successive generations of doctors among Iberian Jewish families carried on the profession in their new domiciles.[60] The Iberian Peninsula's medical loss was Turkey's, Italy's, Holland's, Germany's, Poland's, and North Africa's gain.[61]

The immediate and most important locus of post-expulsion Jewish medical practice in Europe was Italy.[62] From the sixteenth until the eighteenth century, the premier European institution for the training of Jewish medical students was the University of Padua, which attracted Jewish students from all over Europe and Turkey, despite their having to pay higher tuition fees than non-Jews.[63] Only at the end of this period did Northern Europe—initially Holland, and then Germany—assume the lion's share of Jewish students seeking medical degrees.

Padua provided the Jewish student with a host of options, possibilities, and even temptations that were unimaginable for most Jews of that era. Intellectually, their horizons were broadened by exposure to a vast liberal arts curriculum and the latest medical and scientific texts. Additionally, they obtained rich clinical and surgical experience. Socially, their stay at Padua was just as significant. Not only did they mingle with former Conversos from the Iberian Peninsula, but their fellow Jewish medical students also came from Germany, Poland, and Russia. Nor were Jewish students separated from Gentile ones. Padua divided up its student body into "nations," and while the Jews possessed no official "national" designation, and most lived among and were supported by the local Jewish community, the Jewish medical students certainly studied and freely mingled with their non-Jewish classmates.[64] This intense experience was reinforced by the fact that after returning home to practice medicine in their respective countries, the Jewish students continued to maintain contact with one another. A principal factor guaranteeing that such ties were maintained after matriculation was that many of the graduates hailed from the same family. Such lines often extended from the sixteenth to the eighteenth century.[65]

The "Padua experience" was lived by approximately 320 Jews between 1617 and 1816.[66] But the cultural and social significance of this story goes beyond the mere training of Jewish physicians. David Ruderman is correct when he writes that Padua's medical school "represented a major vehicle for the diffusion of secular culture, especially scientific culture, within the pre-emancipatory Jewish communities of Europe."[67] Having acquired an intimate knowledge of secular fields of inquiry, cultivating non-Jewish modes of behavior and deportment, and reconsidering Jewish values in light of their immersion in the culture of the Christian university, these young men returned to their homes as changed Jews.

However, their encounter with the secular and scientific world, as well as their social engagement with non-Jewish medical students, was not without cost. The deliberate choice to dedicate one's life to the pursuit of medicine or science instead of Torah was interpreted by traditionalists as a rejectionist stance. In response, the physicians answered their critics by demonstrating that science was deeply embedded in Judaism and was not contrary to it. According to David Nieto (1654–1728), philosopher, first rabbi of London's Bevis Marks Synagogue, hakham of the Spanish and Portuguese congregation, and Padua medical school graduate, science in fact originated with the Jews. "The source of the sciences went out from us and our holy Torah includes them all."[68]

A second argument employed by the young Jewish doctors involved the creation of a theology of nature. They suggested that just as studying God's words (Torah) was a religious obligation, so too was arriving at a fuller appreciation and deeper understanding of His creation, the natural world. To do so would make manifest God's greatness and incomparability. As David Ruderman states, all of this served "as a satisfying rationalization for Jewish doctor-scientists to view their medical pursuits within the safe confines of Jewish tradition itself."[69]

Nonetheless, despite the claims for the easy compatibility of science and Judaism by these Italian Jewish doctors, their encounter with science in a university setting occasioned a crisis of confidence in the Jewish tradition. The cultural world from whence they came now appeared minuscule. The sea of the Talmud was reduced to an intellectual trickle, and the giants of science and secular philosophy seemed to dwarf the rabbis. Not only did scientists such as David Gans, Joseph Shlomo Delmedigo, and Tobias Cohen express feelings of Jewish cultural inferiority, but even the rabbinical luminaries Moses Isserles in Poland and the Maharal of Prague, both of whom encouraged young Jews to acquire scientific knowledge, struggled to explain away the fact that what the rabbis knew about science seemed to be so paltry, a sign of their cultural insularity.[70]

A wide gulf separates the experience of the early modern from the modern Jewish doctor. In addition to those who studied astronomy, primarily in order to calculate with accuracy the Jewish lunar calendar, Italian rabbis such as Simone Luzzatto, Judah Assael del bene, and Azariah Figo took the first steps toward an appreciation of the secular sciences.[71] Others, such as the peripatetic and one-time yeshiva student Tobias Cohen, pursued medicine. While such men cleared the path for generations of Jews to follow, the crucial difference between these early-moderns and their successors is the fact that the modern Jewish physician, as he appeared in Germany, did not come to the laboratory by way of the yeshiva.

On the threshold of the modern period, one that has seen the production of more Jewish doctors in real and percentage terms than ever before, it is early modern Italy that holds the key to understanding the mind-set of the modern Jewish physician. More than this, it is to Italy, where from the end of the fifteenth century foreign Jews had studied medicine at the universities of Naples, Bologna, Pisa, Pavia, and Perugia, that one can trace the roots of the crucial preference taken by intellectually gifted young Jews for medical over rabbinical studies. But as these roots spread, they struck deepest in Germany, the country to which many of the Jewish graduates returned. It is there that we see the true legacy and development of the "Padua experience."

Still, the culture that made room for secular knowledge in the intellectual arsenal of the Italian Jew took considerable time to burst forth in Central Europe. The following example serves to illustrate how different was the attitude toward physicians in Germany compared to Italy. Moreover, it makes clear the sharp distinction in Germany between religious and scientific authority. The above-mentioned valorizing of Christian scientific wisdom that many early modern European Jewish intellectuals engaged in did not find an echo in Germany. In fact, there, communal elders were positively fearful of the potentially corrosive effect on the Jewish masses of secular ideas borne by university-trained Jewish physicians. Concerned that the doctors' learning and prestige could be used to undermine its authority and power, the Jewish leadership in seventeenth-century Frankfurt, for example, openly declared that Jewish doctors would not be permitted to exercise the same influence over their co-religionists as Gentile physicians did in Christian society.

To achieve their ends, the leadership forbade Jewish physicians to invite other Jews to settle in Frankfurt, Germany's largest Jewish city, without the consent of the community. Furthermore, in the economic realm, the community enforced a class-based fee structure for patients in order to prevent physicians from overcharging. The poor were to be treated for free, the well-to-do had to pay a certain fixed sum, and only the rich had to pay whatever the doctor asked. Finally, contact between Jews and doctors was limited. Physicians were forbidden to visit community members more than necessary, nor were they permitted to attend to a patient without first having been summoned.[72]

The physician-rabbi, found so commonly in the Near East and in the southern part of the European continent, was neither as ubiquitous nor as prominent in Central and Eastern Europe. By the eighteenth century, the physician-rabbi had largely disappeared from the social world of European Jewry, and if he can be said to have ever existed as a genuine social type in Germany, his demise probably precedes this date by at least one hundred years, if not more.

Secularization, though slow, proved inexorable, and by the 1750s the desire for political acceptance, social equality, and cultural enrichment had become powerful forces among Germany's Jewish elites. There, the attainment of social status no longer came through mastery of rabbinic texts, but through commercial and professional success. The struggle of early modern Jewish doctors to reconcile talmudic and scientific learning, or even to justify the former, turned into a nonissue in Central Europe. Perched high on the ladder of social accomplishment and authority, the German Jewish physician was a scientist from a minority culture — and only that. He was not a hybrid doctor and rabbinic scholar.

However, this is not to say that medicine in Germany, even into the twentieth century, ever became a wholly secular affair. As this book demonstrates, religious and ethnic concerns informed the medical practice of many Jewish physicians. What happened is that Jewish doctors in Germany employed Judaism and Jewishness in new ways in order to discuss and treat the various afflictions, real or imagined, suffered by the Jewish collectivity.

The ancient teachings on medicine and its widespread practice beginning in the Middle Ages had firmly established medical practice among Jews as one of the most socially and culturally viable occupational choices for them. The religious and social roots of medicine among the Jews led to its designation as a "Jewish occupation," by Jew and Gentile alike. When German Jews first went abroad to study medicine in the seventeenth century, or began to do so in significant numbers at home in the eighteenth century, they did so laden with the cultural baggage of the ancient association of Jews and medicine. When that journey was over, they had succeeded in fashioning a new type of Jewish doctor.

In the two hundred years immediately prior to the Holocaust, Germany became for Jewish physicians what Egypt had been for them in the eleventh century, the Mediterranean in the thirteenth and fourteenth centuries, and Italy from the sixteenth to the eighteenth century. It was in German-speaking Europe that they practiced in very large numbers, were disproportionately found in certain specialties, and produced a very large Jewish medical library. And unlike the Jewish physicians who had written and translated general medical treatises before them, many Jewish doctors in Germany actually wrote on Jews and their physical and psychological maladies. This corpus of writings on the Jews comprised scores of learned monographs, hundreds of scientific articles, a long-running journal on medical issues concerning the Jewish people, and even fictional and dramatic accounts of Jewish doctors and diseases. Many German Jewish physicians worked in Jewish hospitals, tended primarily to Jewish patients, and incorporated into their research on the Jewish body contemporary Jewish political and ideological agendas. And so, if Italy was the birthplace of the modern Jewish physician, Central Europe was where he grew to adulthood.

To be sure, by the late nineteenth century very few Jewish doctors in Germany would have been attuned to the place of medicine within the Jewish religious tradition. They may have been aware that there had been many Jewish doctors in the past, but their knowledge of Judaism's theology of healing was probably not very keen. They were, after all, not well versed in Jewish religious culture. However, new Jewish concerns such as racial antisemitism, Zionism, assimilation, and the impact of economic competition among doctors touched the lives of German Jewish physicians and affected them in myriad personal and professional ways—ways that are illuminated in memoir literature and in contemporary scientific and popular writings. What becomes clear is that the ancient engagement of Jews and medicine, while continuing in modern Germany—even increasing exponentially—underwent a categorical change, wherein the old struggle over the reconciliation of science and religion metamorphosed into one that saw medicine now linked not to faith per se, but to ethnicity.

This process developed first and foremost in Germany during the Haskalah, or Jewish Enlightenment of the eighteenth century. From that time on, through to the twentieth century, a host of social, political, and cultural forces coalesced to produce Jewish physicians who sought, by employing their professional skills, to modernize and regenerate the Jewish body and by extension, the Jewish body politic.

This process was slow in developing, for the emergence in the eighteenth and nineteenth centuries of the modern Jewish doctor in Germany was a protracted affair. If we are to properly understand the social role and intellectual impact that resulted from his evolution, we must first appreciate the rich legacy and unique burdens he bore.

CHAPTER 2

# JEWISH PHYSICIANS
## IN AND OUT OF THE GERMAN GHETTO

For 1,140 years, from the first mention of an anonymous Jewish doctor in the service of Archbishop Arno of Salzburg in 798 CE to the decertification of Jewish doctors under the Nazis in September 1938, the presence of Jewish medical practitioners in German-speaking Europe had been constant.[1] While their story is less well documented than that of their co-religionists in Southern Europe, Jewish doctors were also prevalent throughout German lands during the course of the Middle Ages. Like their medieval Spanish and Italian contemporaries, with whom they were in contact, Jewish doctors in Germany were trained in an apprenticeship system, studied Hebrew translations of classical medical texts, and built familial dynasties of physicians.[2]

Unfortunately, there is very little documentary evidence that attests to the personages or activities of medieval German Jewish physicians. However, certain fragments pieced together from disparate sources may provide a window onto the life of the medieval German Jewish doctor. Perhaps because of the paucity of documentation, as well as the glittering contemporary Jewish culture of Southern Europe, there is a perception that medieval Jewish medicine in Central Europe was in some ways backward. But from the scant evidence that we do possess, a more nuanced and revised picture can be drawn.

We begin with medical literature. The Bodleian manuscript of the *Sefer Asaf,* also known as the *Book of Remedies,* an important Hebrew medical compendium dating from the early Middle Ages, indicates paleographic and linguistic evidence that the codex was written in Germany around 1150. First, the script itself closely resembles that of contemporary German Jewish works. Second, specific mention of the town names of Worms (where an important Jewish community resided) and the more difficult-to-identify Neuhausen strongly suggest the German origin of this manuscript. Most revealing of all, the text contains dozens of German words for herbs and minerals, transliterated into Hebrew. Moreover, those German words are punctuated so as to permit the Jewish user to correctly pronounce the names of those medicaments and medical supplies that Jews must have been buying from non-Jews.[3] Scholars have determined that the book, which was most likely used by at least the five Jewish doctors mentioned in it, offered medical care based on the "anatomy, physiology, and uroscopy developed and refined by authorities like Galen, Hippocrates, and Dioscorides."[4] This would mean that, intellectually speaking, these German Jews were providing medical care based on a sophisticated body of knowledge that was identical to that employed by their Mediterranean brethren.

Another sketch of the Jewish doctor in Germany appears in the *Sefer Hasidim* (Book of the pious). In that compendium of some two thousand moral and ethical stories written in the Rhineland around the year 1200, approximately twelve of the stories have to do with doctors and their patients.[5] Precisely because it is not a medical text but a guidebook to the religious culture of medieval Jewish pietism in Germany, the several references to physicians tend to reflect social attitudes toward (and of) doctors and the services they offered, and thus serves as an important guide to the era's attitudes toward the human body and healers.

From the references to medicine in *Sefer Hasidim*, it appears that medieval Ashkenazic medical practice was syncretistic. It was characterized by a combination of two differing approaches to healing. On the one hand, magic and medical folkways were employed, while on the other, there are indications that Rhineland Jewry around the year 1200 was aware of and subscribed to the newly emerging ethos of medical professionalization.

Although some magical approaches to Jewish healing have been identified in Chapter 1, here we must note that the *Sefer Hasidim* provided specific instruction on how to perform magic in order to effect cure. "Women would take herbs to boil for their children when they became sick and would perform (magic, saying): 'If he is to live, then let him be cured within nine days, and if to die, then let him die within nine days.'" However, it is clear that only Jewish magic would suffice to cure the Jewish patient. The story is told of a Jewish woman whose son was ill. She refused the offer of a Christian woman who told her: "Give your son to drink upon this stone and he will be cured." When the Jewish women inquired about the nature of the stone, the Christian replied that "it was brought from the pit [the Holy Sepulchre] and it is part of the stone in which [Jesus] was buried." The Jewish woman refused the offer for this very reason, although she had been assured that sick Christians had been cured by these means.[6] In fact, it should be noted that the rabbis took very seriously the issue of whether it was permissible for sick Jews to use the incantations of Gentiles. Many responded in the affirmative, concocting a post-modern justification for such usage, namely, that only the sound of certain words has therapeutic value, and that the words themselves are without inherent quality. Consequently, it was even permitted to invoke the name of Jesus or various saints.[7]

Two other components, when combined with the belief in magic, clearly indicate the dualistic nature of medical practice in medieval Germany. These are the techniques employed to diagnose and heal, and the references to fees and payments for services rendered. Mention is made in *Sefer Hasidim* of doctors (*rofim*) examining the urine of the patient, a standard medieval diagnostic technique, performing surgery, and resorting to medical textbooks for reference. One also finds discussion of physician responsibility, obligation to the sick poor, and payment methods. Taken together, magic, contemporary science, and medical economics exist in a complementary way to suggest that the treatment methods, financial expectations, and moral worldview of the medieval German Jewish physician were not that different from his Southern European counterparts.[8]

Like the Sephardim, Ashkenazic doctors also served nobility and clergy at the same time that church councils forbade Christians from being treated by Jewish doctors and taking the medicines they prescribed.[9] Yet the conciliar bans against Jewish doctors treating Christian patients—while important for understanding the ideology that inscribed dominant notions about the Christian body and by extension, the relation of Jews to it—were honored mostly in the breach.[10] Jewish physicians, it appears, were sought out by Germany's lower orders. In a society where the Jew was generally reviled, the widespread use of Jewish doctors is an intriguing irony. Their popularity stemmed from several quarters. Free of guild restrictions, they offered a wide array of medical treatments, ranging from diagnosis to minor surgery. Moreover, they tended to render their services at cheaper rates than did Christian physicians, thus providing a viable option in the medical marketplace. In addition, contrary to the law, Jewish doctors most likely filled prescriptions, and again, for less than Christian apothecaries charged.

The cruelly coercive nature of pre-modern society meant that the punishment meted out for malpractice by a Jewish physician could fall on the entire community. Alert to this overwhelming sense of responsibility placed on the shoulders of the Jewish doctor, Christian patients expressed a certain confidence in Jewish healers that they were extra careful in their treatment procedures. Another attractive feature for the German commoner revolved around the type of diagnostic treatment offered by Jewish physicians, one that at a certain point distinguished them from their Christian counterparts. By the late sixteenth century, university-trained Gentile physicians gradually stopped employing uroscopy as a diagnostic tool, claiming that it was unreliable and unscientific.[11] Many Jews, on the other hand, continued to use the technique. And for the public, the observable "performance" of the examination appealed to patients, providing them with a sense that their doctor was actually "doing something" to relieve their suffering. As we shall see later in this chapter, divergent sources of medical knowledge—university study versus practical apprenticeship—and subsequent forms of medical practice between Jewish and Christian physicians were crucial markers of Jewish medical inferiority in the eyes of German doctors.

It was not only individual Christian elites and commoners who elected to use Jewish doctors. Beginning in the Middle Ages, secular German authorities appointed Jews to the post of city physician, resulting from a shortage of qualified personnel.[12] Many Jews enjoyed such positions, and the 25 pounds annual salary paid to Yosel of Basle around 1373, the 18 pounds paid to his successor, Gutleben, or the permission granting Jacob of Strasbourg, who worked in Frankfurt, the right to reside outside the *Judengasse* were not unusual remunerations.[13] The skills of Jewish physicians were required, and no matter what official Church policy was, social necessity took precedence over theology.[14]

In addition to individual healers, from the Middle Ages on, German Jews (as was the pattern all over Europe) could also boast of an expansive network of social service institutions that included hospices, hospitals, and sick care societies. These were established and run by the Jewish community council, called the *kahal*. This governing body also ensured that communities had physicians, surgeons, apothecaries, and bathhouses.[15] Moreover, the *kahal* officially supervised the activities of wet-nurses and ritual circumcisers, or *mohelim*.

Sick care facilities were not only geared up to treat patients in times of ordinary need. In terms of health, the medieval period saw extraordinary demands made with frequent regularity. For example, the community councils in Germany devised elaborate quarantine and treatment procedures to be implemented in times of plague and epidemic, even making special religious and social provisions for individuals who had taken ill. Generally taking the form of release from certain obligations, dispensations included not having to attend synagogue or pay taxes. Respected community members who were poor and had become sick were provided with small subventions, after the council had examined each individual applicant and voted. Sick transients were also regarded as the community's responsibility and were provided with a night's lodging in the hospice. When they were well enough, they were moved on to the next town or village, thus dispersing the health care costs among several communities rather than placing the onus on just one. This procedure was not free of problems. Very often, when one of these patients died after being sent on to a new community, lawsuits were filed to recover expenses incurred for medical care and subsequent burial.[16]

The costs involved in providing such a wide range of health care facilities were very high. To meet their financial obligations, Jewish communal authorities in Germany made special Sabbath and High Holiday appeals to congregants in synagogues. Another source of revenue came from men called to the Torah during a synagogue service; in return for the honor they made donations to a specific sick care society or to a general fund for ailing members of the community. A common method of tapping community resources occurred after Sabbath, when wealthy individuals were expected to fill out blank subscription forms that had been left for them with the amount they wished to donate.[17]

Care for the sick, in all its dimensions, was the responsibility of the entire community, irrespective of income levels or social status. Yet the division between wealthy and poor and their relative abilities to assist in caring for the community's sick was sometimes a source of grievance and class conflict. In 1760 in Holland, just such an example was also exacerbated by ethnic antagonism. In that year, Naftali Hirsch Goslar wrote from Amsterdam to his son in Halberstadt: "The Portuguese Jews are the richest here and very philanthropic, but they prefer to support the sick, the lame, and the blind than poor Jewish scholars, since, as the Polish Jews say, they are conscious of the fact that they will sooner become sick, lame, or blind before they themselves become Jewish scholars!"[18]

The Jewish community's obligations to the ill went beyond providing them with funds and health services. The *kehillah*, or community, was also responsible for the appointment and licensing of Jewish physicians, although the state played a significant role in this as well. For example, from 1579, any Jewish physician seeking to practice in Frankfurt, even if he possessed a university degree, had to present himself for examination before a commission composed of three city councilors and two doctors. This was the result of malpractice charges brought against a Jewish doctor who in 1574 had been elevated to the post of town physician.[19]

While some major Jewish communities permitted independent practitioners to ply their skills, most Jewish physicians were formally retained by either the communities or the *hevrei kadisha* (burial societies).[20] In the hiring of a communal physician, the *kehill*'s practices mirrored those of society at large, for German towns also employed physicians to care for the poor. For example, the contracts of Jewish physicians in Germany generally stipulated that they were to treat the poor and needy free of charge, or at greatly reduced fees. Similarly, allowing for the peculiarities of Jewish social arrangement and custom, salaries for Jewish physicians were governed by the *Medizinalordnungen* (medical ordinances) of German towns during the seventeenth and eighteenth centuries, and thus tended to be akin to those of non-Jews.[21]

Certain specificities, however, did appear in the contracts of Jewish physicians. From 1619, records of fees and salaries began to be kept in Prague, and we are given a good sense of the earning capacity of Jewish physicians in Central Europe into the eighteenth century. Generally speaking, earning levels were considerable, with Jewish communal physicians earning the bulk of their livelihood not from their official retainer but from the extra fees they charged the well-to-do. Salaries differed widely from community to community. Some features affecting pay scales included the size and wealth of the community in which they practiced, the custom of doctors themselves having to pay for patient medication (as practiced in Breslau), or the need to factor in transportation expenses (as was the case in Vienna).[22] The particular mode of remuneration was also structured differently from place to place. In Posen, doctors were granted tax exemptions, while other towns provided Jewish physicians with free living accommodations.[23]

The topics covered in contracts between the Jewish physician and the community included the physicians' residence obligations — most stipulated that he could not leave the city without permission, a measure designed to prevent his flight during epidemics — fee scale, his specific treatment duties toward community members, and the nature of his relations with the *kahal* board. The wording of contracts was often exact and specific. For example, in the contract of the distinguished Joseph Shlomo Delmedigo, drawn up on Friday March 14, 1631, in Frankfurt, the following stipulations appeared. Delmedigo was expressly forbidden to refuse to treat the sick (a striking difference from the views of his contemporary, Jakob Martini, expressed in Chapter 1), was obliged to offer identical treatment to rich and poor, and was not allowed to leave the city without permission. Moreover, the contract noted that while he was currently exempt from taxation, this privilege would be rescinded should he ever become rich. Two years later, in 1633, an addendum to the original contract stipulated that Delmedigo was to receive one half florin for a first visit to a patient, but that he was to make an additional daily house call free of charge. For home visits he made between the hours of 10 AM and 5 PM he was to receive extra money.[24]

From the three-year contract signed between the *hevra kadisha* (burial society) of Breslau and Dr. Abraham Kisch in 1767, we learn that "he is to visit the poor sick in the local Jewish hospital twice daily . . . [that] all payments for medicaments required for the cure of the poor are to be taken care of by the doctor out of his own pocket and [are] to be given for nothing." For his services, Dr. Kisch was paid an annual cash sum of 300 Reichstaler in two installments. After agreeing to all the terms, Kisch agreed not to amend any of the conditions to which he had hitherto agreed, or otherwise pay a fine to the government of 200 specie ducats.[25]

The specificity of these contracts, despite their formulaic niceties, seem to indicate a certain unease on the part of community officials toward Jewish physicians. It would appear that these officials were deeply concerned with asserting control over the doctors. This becomes clear in the case of Frankfurt, when in 1656, the community issued a *Hanhagat ha-Rofim,* a "Conduct of Physicians" document, spelling out doctor's fees, duties, and obligations. Most interestingly, a postscript was appended to this document, which declared that a physician was to be denied community membership until he agreed never to become a leading functionary (*parnas*) of the Jewish community council. However, if the man was over sixty years of age and had retired from medical practice, he was permitted to seek the position.[26]

This deliberate barring of physicians from holding political office suggests a deep-seated fear on the part of the traditional authorities that too much power would be concentrated in the hands of doctors, were communal appointments made open to them. Doctors had long been politically and socially influential individuals in Jewish society. We have already noted their acquisition of power by virtue of their skills and service to Gentile elites during the Middle Ages. In both early modern Italy and Eastern Europe, the physician-rabbi wielded immense authority. What was different about Germany? Why when doctors were so revered in other Jewish communities and were possessed of political authority were community notables in Germany so determined to block Jewish physicians' access to power?

The first reason has to do with the typology of the early modern Jewish doctor.[27] As noted at the conclusion of Chapter 1, in the seventeenth century those physicians who had attended Padua and a host of other universities in Italy and elsewhere had become imbued with secular learning. Their mere potential to disseminate, and perhaps their actual desire to promote the spread of such knowledge among their co-religionists at home, posed a threat to the deeply conservative, traditional pattern of religious existence in Germany. When coupled with the reality of the physicians' relatively open access to the Jewish masses—access the Jewish authorities tried to strictly regulate—the traditional leadership regarded the doctors as poised to indoctrinate the masses with "new" and "insidious" ideas. Already blessed with social and intellectual authority derived from their status as physicians, these men constituted a potent challenge to the security and personal authority of the traditional leadership, as well as a larger threat to the integral culture of the ghetto.

But surely, one would imagine that Jewish leaders in Italy and Eastern Europe also had the same fears as their German counterparts. However, conditions in all three places were so different that physicians with identical credentials and similar worldviews were perceived very differently in their respective communities. On the Continent, Italian Jewry was in general the community most hospitable to secular culture. There, the ghetto was never hermetically sealed, and whether it was in the realm of popular culture, music, or science, Italian Jewish lay and religious leaders generally recognized and condoned the potentially symbiotic relationship between Jewish and general culture.[28] Thus it was possible for the Jewish physician in Italy to also hold political office, for very often in that country the doctor's authority was derived not merely from his credentials as a man of science but also from his standing as a rabbinic scholar.

By contrast, in early modern Poland, it was not intellectual affinity with Gentile culture but pure pragmatism that led to the emergence of the physician who also maintained a position of leadership within the community. Although scientific pursuits, especially astronomy, were permitted and sometimes encouraged—principally in order to assist with the scrupulous calculation of the new moon—science was always seen as a "subspecialty" of talmudic study and was never formally incorporated into the curriculum of the Polish yeshiva.[29]

The social and economic devastation exacted on Polish Jewry during the Chmielnicki massacres (1648–1650) and subsequent wars of the mid-seventeenth century saw a decline in rabbinic scholarship in that country. The intellectual fields in which Jews incurred losses included science—in particular, astronomy. By the eighteenth century, Polish talmudists no longer studied the subject. Thus, given that the epistemological basis for the study of science had been halakhic observance to begin with, and that this particular intellectual *engagement* was only really coterminous with the century-long, Golden Age of Polish Jewry — circa 1550–1648 — the scientist was a marginal, barely existent figure on the social landscape.

On the other hand, physicians came to occupy what David Fishman has labeled "the only group in Old Polish Jewry resembling a non-rabbinic intellectual elite," constituting "a highly prestigious and powerful class in Jewish society."[30] Barred from studying at the universities of Cracow and Vilna, young Polish Jewish doctors returned from their studies abroad and served Polish rulers — very often the same ones who had initially sponsored their expensive Italian studies. Thus, in the seventeenth century, their activities came to resemble those of medieval Jewish doctors in the Mediterranean region. In addition to their medical duties, they became courtiers, financial advisors, moneylenders, and court emissaries. They were permitted free travel, residence, and farming rights.[31] As a result, Jewish communities often appointed physicians to represent them at court. Thus they took on the role of *shtadlan*, or communal intercessor, and, in contrast to the contemporary situation in Germany, some doctors even served as *parnasim*, or representatives to the Council of Four Lands, the central governing institution of Polish-Lithuanian Jewry from the sixteenth century until its dissolution in 1764.[32] Other physicians served as presiding officers in large communities such as Posen, Cracow, and Vilna.[33]

What allowed for this situation to develop in Poland is the fact that precisely because secular knowledge was so undervalued, Jewish physicians had only minimal intellectual impact on Polish Jewry. Supreme intellectual authority in early modern Poland resided with the talmudic scholar. He who knew *halakha*, not Hippocrates, was assured pride of place in Jewish society. Thus, as David Fishman notes, physicians never became "role models or ideal types" among Poland's Jews.[34] In actuality, the fact that they could become doctors to begin with placed them outside the sociological norms of the larger group. Their ability to finance expensive studies abroad, their mastery of foreign languages and sciences, and the very fact that they chose to exercise their intellectual muscle in the name of science and not Torah branded them as radically different from the vast majority of Polish Jews.

Polish Jewish society accorded these men honor and respect and even rewarded them with community positions, but not because they were seen as part of an intellectual vanguard. Their medical knowledge was inconsequential in terms of the dominant scale of intellectual values. Now the *kehillah*, it is true, bestowed upon physicians considerable respect and certain dignities, flattering them with special titles, such as "our teacher," upon their being called to the Torah — a practice, the distinguished historian Jacob Katz tells us in his memoirs, continued into the twentieth century in his native Hungary.[35] But all of this occurred principally because of the utilitarian function early modern physicians served as *shtadlanim*. Charged with the all-important task of representing the community before the Gentile authorities, the intercessors were talented, articulate, and urbane men, able to negotiate their way in Christian society.[36] Thus, *kehillah* leaders permitted physicians to occupy official positions of community service because their skills made them indispensable. In fact, even after the disasters of 1648, the rabbinic culture of Poland was so strong and the hierarchies of social prestige so fixed that the Jewish physician, with his secular wisdom acquired abroad, was not perceived of as a cultural menace to Jewish society or a political threat to its traditional leadership.

Now we are in a position to appreciate more fully how different the situation was in seventeenth- and early eighteenth-century Germany. In that country, the stipulation that physicians could not occupy the office of *parnas* was enacted because, unlike Italy, there was no cultural space in Germany for the Jewish physician and his secular ideas. Religious and social conservatism ran deep, and a threatened leadership actively sought to curb secular influences.[37] This trend deepened after 1648 and the regeneration of German Jewish communities following the Thirty Years' War (1618–1648), when Germany emerged as a center of rabbinic learning. The simultaneous decline of the Polish communities witnessed the opening up of major *yeshivot* in places such as Hamburg, Fürth, Halberstadt, Nikolsburg, Eisenstadt, and Mannheim.[38] Yet the new situation was tenuous. Time and circumstance prevented the development of a Polish-style certainty and confidence about the impregnability of early modern Jewish culture. Thus, rather than talmudic culture being an ancient fortress, as was the case in Poland, in Germany it must be viewed as having been a garrison of recent vintage. One other feature that militated against German Jewish authorities bestowing upon communal physicians sensitive political tasks was the fact that many of the Jewish physicians there, especially in the north of the country, were Iberian Conversos. This experience, together with their ethnicity, served to make them the objects of mistrust.

And in contrast to Poland, there was no practical need for the Jewish physician-cum-political-functionary in Germany. While the office of shtadlan was found principally in Poland, Lithuania, and Moravia, in Germany the activities of the shtadlan were generally performed by the parnas.[39] But by

1650, again as a result of the Thirty Years' War, there had arisen in Germany a new Jewish clique — military provisioners and financiers, known as Court Jews (*Hofjuden*). These men served simultaneously as agents of the states and as Jewish community leaders.[40] Their intimacy with the court allowed for their standing in the community, and consequently they filled the same political post very often occupied by Jewish physicians in Italy and Poland.

Despite the inferior status of those who practiced medicine in Germany, the country still offered promising career opportunities and the possibility of a handsome livelihood to young Jews. Nevertheless, it took a considerable amount of time for German Jews to become professionally attracted to the field of medicine. There are four principal reasons for this: restrictions on Jews graduating from Protestant universities; entrance restrictions against Jews at Catholic institutions; medical antisemitism; and the slow development of professional medicine in Germany.

As to the first reason, until the second decade of the eighteenth century, Jews were not permitted to graduate from Protestant medical schools. The first Jew to do so was Moses Salomon Gomperz, who took his medical degree at Frankfurt an der Oder in 1721.[41] Jews had, however, been attending such medical schools for some forty years before this date. In 1678, the first Jews admitted to study at a German medical school were Tobias Cohen and Gabriel Felix, both from Poland. They had been specifically admitted by order of Elector Frederick William the Great of Brandenburg. The Elector's tolerance should not be overstated, and his desire to admit Jews was not merely part of the consolidation of German states after the Thirty Years' War, and the concomitant growth of the universities as training grounds for state bureaucrats. For the Elector made it quite clear that his long-term objective was to effect the conversion of Jewish medical students to Christianity. This would come about "when they interact with Christians, form a better opinion of the Christian faith, and perhaps, through the grace of God, convert."[42] Although this hoped-for scenario never came to fruition, Cohen, Felix, and others like them who first gained admission to Protestant universities such as Halle (1695), Gießen (1697), Duisberg (1708), and Marburg (1710) took courses at these institutions but actually completed their degrees principally at either Padua or Leiden.[43] As a consequence of German admissions barriers, only seventeen Jews from Germany took medical degrees at foreign universities between 1678 and 1721, the period for which we have fairly accurate figures.[44]

The second feature inhibiting the entrance of Jews into the German medical profession was the fact that Catholic institutions of higher learning denied Jews admission until the last third of the eighteenth century. Jewish medical students were only first accepted at Mainz in 1770, Würzburg in 1786, and Bonn in 1786. In Austria the Toleranzpatent of 1782, issued by Joseph II, undid the edict of 1740, issued by his mother (Maria Theresa), which specifically barred non-Catholics from studying medicine at Habsburg universities.[45] In 1789, Abraham Samuel Ackord became the first Jewish medical school graduate of the University of Vienna. However, Ackord's graduation did not signify the dawning of an unrestricted day. Jewish students were admitted only on an officially "tolerated" basis, and only then, if they had some familial connection with "tolerated" families already residing in the Imperial capital.[46] Because so many Catholic universities had been simply off limits to Jews for so long, medicine as a course of study was open only to those elite strata that could either afford to send their sons abroad or meet the residence requirements open to descendants of Court Jews.

A third reason, and most likely the fundamental cause of the above-mentioned, restricted admissions policies, was antisemitism.[47] Here Germany proved exceptional. Speaking in general terms about early modern German attitudes toward the Jews, Reformation scholar Heiko Oberman has observed that "during the sixteenth century, Europe made a hesitant but significant transition to modern times." And in Northern Europe, he further noted, this meant "a marked step forward in the understanding of human rights and in the advocacy of tolerance." But then he added the qualification that "the ideal of tolerance grew very much at the expense of the Jews in Northern Europe, particularly in Germany—at the expense of their social role, their legal status, and their religious liberties."[48] This situation had a decisive impact on the relatively late emergence of the university-trained Jewish doctor in Germany.

While universities in Italy from the sixteenth century and those in Holland from the seventeenth century displayed tolerance in accepting Jewish medical students, with some discrimination notwithstanding, Germany was home not only to an exclusivist admissions policy but also to a hostile and sustained campaign specifically directed against the Jewish physician.[49] A sizable corpus of viciously antisemitic tracts about Jewish medical practitioners began to appear from about 1530, and reappeared with regularity into the Nazi period. The roots of German medical antisemitism of the nineteenth and twentieth centuries were struck deep in soil that had been tilled by antisemitic medical adversaries of the early modern era. This is not to trace a simplistic, straight line from Luther's antisemitism to Hitler's. To follow the philosopher Karl Japsers' dictum that "Hitler's entire program was to be found in Luther's teachings" is to stretch the limits of historical explanation.[50] Nevertheless, discursive patterns, particularly ancient ones, have, in their cultural transmissibility, significance and power. Referring to a recent declaration of contrition made by the German Lutheran Church vis-à-vis its own history of antisemitism, one theologian has recently noted that "it cannot be concluded that modern anti-Semitism has nothing to do with the anti-Judaism of the sixteenth century."[51] The larger discussion of German antisemitism as a cultural and political force in German history cannot be adequately addressed here. What I am prepared to say is that in at least one specific area of antisemitic discourse — that involving Jewish doctors — Germany developed in the sixteenth century a vocabulary and a canonized set of beliefs about the Jewish physician that remained a permanent fixture of German antisemitism into the modern period, long after other antisemitic tropes had been dispensed with.

Thanks to this early modern polemical literature, an indelible image was created of the Jewish doctor as a murderously evil charlatan, a professional incompetent, an introducer of the devil to Germany, a vice-ridden, depraved, criminal locked in ruthless competition with German physicians. An examination of such texts reveals the discursive climate in Germany as it related to Jewish doctors.

Paracelsus, one of the sixteenth century's most distinguished physicians, decried Jewish doctors in his *Labyrinthus Medicorum* (1538), noting that they had no particular aptitude for medicine. "What is their medicine?" he asked, "What do they have? What do they do? What do they know from their books? From their deeds [it is clear] they know nothing but how to defraud." He mocked them for claiming to be the foremost and most ancient medical practitioners among all peoples, when in fact they were merely "the oldest rogues among all nations." Not to the Jews, he concluded, but "to the Gentiles was medicine given. They are the most ancient doctors."[52] Paracelsus' claims did not go unanswered. Exactly fifty years later, David de Pomis, an Italian Jewish physician, wrote in response: "Did not the art of medicine exist among the Jews nearly 1,500 years before the time of Apollo, Aesculapius and Hippocrates — as is clear to him who studies the Law of Moses? . . . [M]edicine was discovered first among the Jews, only later among the other nations."[53]

One year after Paracelsus' *Labyrinthus Medicorum*, in 1539, the city physician of Worms, Philipp Begardi, published his *Index Sanitatis,* a medical self-help manual. In addition to the advice he provided, Begardi took the opportunity to rail against an array of characters whom he classified as medical impostors and charlatans. Among them, he included monks, Paracelsus, whom he called a "revolutionary," alchemists, apothecaries, witches, and magicians. But it was the Jews, whom he referred to as "captains of the charade," who were the worst of medical impostors.[54] Like others who would come after him, Begardi singled out German Jewish doctors for opprobrium, contrasting them unfavorably with Jewish doctors from Southern Europe. There, according to the author, one could find some learned ones, while in Germany they were all "swindlers and great knaves."[55] For this claim he provides as evidence the fact that a Jewish doctor with whom he was once conversing supposedly told him that "it is no art to help the sick, but it is an art to prize money from people."[56]

And yet despite the charges, Christian patients kept coming.[57] If Jewish doctors were so incompetent and so greedy, why were they able to elicit such loyalty from Christians? Begardi himself suggests two possible reasons. The first was that they promised the patient that his or her health could be restored. Although Begardi saw this as an act of hubris or fraud on the part of the doctor, it could also be interpreted as an expression of the physician's self-confidence. Moreover, it is possible that the trust Christians placed in their Jewish doctors (something Begardi acknowledged) derived from the fact that the optimism Jewish doctors instilled in their patients may have contributed to their recovery, in turn validating the patients' trust and confidence. The second reason that perhaps contributed to the loyalty displayed by Gentile patients was the widely held conviction, deserved or otherwise, that "Jewish physicians are the best doctors."[58] Yet in suggesting why they are not deserving of this reputation, Begardi may have inadvertently provided a clue to the successful reputations enjoyed by Jewish doctors. "And yet consider this," he wrote, "truly they have no real skill other than small experiments and experience." Endorsing the Hippocratic aphorism, Begardi noted that "experimentation is deception," and that it was principally Jewish doctors, and even some Christians wishing to be called physicians, who engaged in such practice. "They deceive you," warned Begardi, "with their subtle craftiness and roguishness and you will find that in the end, they endanger not only your body, but also your soul." He pleaded, "Believe me, you will have neither good fortune nor a cure from them." What was to be done? Begardi insisted that Christians be forbidden to have any contact with Jews. Just as Jews had, in the past, been prohibited social intercourse with heathens and Samaritans, so too were Christians now forbidden to accept medicines from Jews, and those that did were to be punished by being made pariahs.[59] Deeply convinced of the destructive influence of the Jews, Begardi advocated the most far-reaching program of social and professional separation of Jews and Germans.

Also in 1539, the Reformation leader, Martin Luther, laid similar charges against Jewish doctors, claiming that: "The Jews, who pass themselves off as doctors, kill Christians, who need to be healed by them, for they believe they serve God when they severely injure them and secretly kill them. And we, crazy fools, in danger of our lives, take refuge among our enemies and hateful [opponents], and thus tempt God."[60]

Prior to the modern period, magic, piety, religion, demonology, health, and sickness were inextricably bound up with one another. Especially in his later years, Luther displayed a vehement opposition to magic, especially that practiced by Jews.[61] Not only did he hold the firm belief that Jews practiced all sorts of chicanery, he even thought them capable of spreading disease through magic. In 1543, the same year he published his notorious *On the Jews and Their Lies,* as well as the anti-Kabbalistic *On the Ineffable Name, Vom Schem Hamphoras,* Luther told of an incident that had occurred on one of his travels. With a heavy streak of paranoia, Luther recounted how a community of Jews had employed magic to make him sick. About his recent trip to the town of Eisleben, Luther wrote to his wife, Katherina: "I became ill on my way just before reaching Eisleben. It was really my own fault. But if you had been there, you would have said it must have been the fault of the Jews or their God. We had to pass through a village before reaching Eisleben, which was inhabited by many Jews. Perhaps they were blowing hard at me [*hart anblasen*] . . . and it was done. When I passed through the village, a cold draft came into the wagon and almost froze my head, I swear."[62] So here Luther recapitulated the earlier trope of the easily duped Christian who, through either his inherently trusting nature or his complete lack of awareness, would turn himself into easy prey for malevolent Jews. In Luther's mind, just outside of Eisleben the Jews had singled him out for attack and had conspired to make him sick by spreading their germs to him.

While the Reformation engendered intra-Christian disputatiousness and deep, permanent division, bitter enemies on both sides of the religious dispute were nevertheless able to agree on the supposed evil of the Jewish physician. Luther's charges, for example, were repeated by his arch nemesis, Johannes Eck. In his *Ains Jüden büechelins verlegung* (1541), a vicious "*summa* of the anti-Jewish literature of the Middle Ages, leaving out no accusation of genocide, blasphemy or treason," the author lambasted Christians who naively put their trust in poorly trained Jewish physicians, the aim of whom it was to murder them.[63] In particular, he wrote: "I am speaking of disloyal

German Jews, and not those foreign Jews who studied medicine in other countries. How can [an untrained German] Jew know anything more than an old woman herbalist [*ain jedes alts kreüterweyb*]. Alone they study from experimentation and practice.... How can they become good doctors if they are not scholars and do not know the art of the inherent quality of things and their effect."[64]

In 1564, the city physician of Frankfurt, Adam Lonicer, published his monumental *Kreuterbuch* (Book of herbs). In this encyclopedic work of some seven hundred pages on the medicinal use of herbs, the author devoted almost half the introduction to a diatribe against Jewish doctors. Although he mentioned that the "noticeable corruption of the people" had been brought on by the medical quackery of "country folk" and "impertinent old women," it was "especially" the case because of "the Jews." It is a startling comment on the obsessive nature of medical antisemitism in Germany that Lonicer not only singled Jews out among a cast of characters perceived as dubious healers but also went on to rail against them at such length that he threw his own book's introduction out of balance.

Lonicer repeated medieval charges about the allegedly anti-Christian teachings in the Talmud, the murderous inclination of Jewish doctors, and their overcharging for medications.[65] In sum, Lonicer declared, "the Jews sucked the blood of Christians through usury and medicine." He endorsed the Church ban on Jews and Christians eating together and that against Christians using medications prescribed by Jews. And why? "Because they are all untutored, stupid asses who have not studied philosophy, do not know the characteristics of the complexion, the fundamental causes of weakness, or have knowledge of medicine, do not know a word of Latin aside from that which they have falsely noted and remembered from German tractates."[66]

The deceitfulness and trickery of Jewish physicians were the principal themes hammered home by the hateful lawyer and physician Ludwig von Hörnigk. His *Medicaster Apella oder Juden Artzt* (The doctor Apella, or the Jewish doctor) (1631) was a diatribe against medical impostors and charlatans. In this tract, the Jews occupied pride of place in his list of evildoers. "A common expression says: Wherever Christ our Lord builds his church, next door does the devil build his chapel. The same can be said of the noble art of medicine."[67] For alongside responsible medical practitioners, there were, according to von Hörnigk, a host of culprits practicing quackery for gain, or even worse. Among them, he included money-hungry, shady doctors, unscrupulous veterinarians, adulation-seeking priests and extortionate clerics, bankrupt shopkeepers, lazy, drunken artisans, gratitude-soliciting and flattering ladies-in-waiting, swindling dentists, "and above all, godless, accursed, Christian-hating Jews." While von Hörnigk saw all those he accused as one and the same, he noted that "Jewish doctors in Germany" (*Judenärtzten in Deutschland*) were worse than the others and also represented a group that had degenerated from its "excellent" status as God-fearing and God-beloved, during the "time of the Old Testament." They had become in the eyes of God and the whole world "a maledicted and damnable people."[68]

Despite his reputation for possessing remarkable curative talents, the Jewish doctor labored under the negative image that Christian polemicists constructed. With the claim that Jews were proficient demonologists and in league with the Devil, they were said to have used their position as doctors — more often the literature accused them of being impostors — to harm Christian patients. As the Protestant preacher Bernhard Waldschmidt said in his polemic against those who employed magic and incantations to heal, *Pythonissa Endorea . . . Hexen- und Gespenst-Predigten* (Witches and ghost sermons) (1660): "Among us [Christians] there are so many who . . . in their illness seek the help and advice of Jewish doctors . . . in case God, through His means, does not bring quick relief, or does not respond with real help when they ask His advice, or do not use Christian doctors first. [In such cases] they give up on God and turn to the devil and his tools, Jewish doctors."[69] Like Martin Luther, nearly one hundred years earlier, some polemicists continued to make accusations of Jewish medical malpractice based on the association of Jews and Kabbalah. In 1634, and in a second edition, which appeared as late as 1721, Ananius Horer in his *Artzney-Teuffel* (Devil's medicine) told his readers that: "Without conscience, [Jews] slander and defame Christ on a daily basis, as they do all Christians, whom they also kill . . . primarily with medicine . . . which they learn along with philosophy, from their secret laws, which are codified in books, but have transmitted orally to their progeny. For that reason, to this day, they can bring forth none of these [murderous skills] without their Kabbalah and Talmud, which are nothing more than a patchwork, beggar's-coat of lies."[70]

In addition to theological charges, economics was also a motivating factor in the German attacks on Jewish doctors. Beginning in the 1590s and throughout the seventeenth century, the northern port city of Hamburg was home to an important settlement of Portuguese Jewish refugee families.[71] Vital participants in the burgeoning commercial world of Hamburg, the Sephardic community numbered several hundred members by 1650,

## JEWISH PHYSICIANS: IN AND OUT OF THE GHETTO

with many new individuals continuing to migrate to it from Northern Europe's premier Sephardic center—Amsterdam. In addition to their prominent role as merchants, this community had more than its share of doctors. A consequence of this was the development of a bitter rivalry between Sephardic and Christian medical practitioners. It is against this background that one must read *Apella Medicaster Bullatus oder Juden Artzt* (1636, 2d edition, 1733), the work of Hamburg physician Jakob Martini. Locked in competition himself with Hamburg's Sephardic physicians, the author was at pains to demonstrate the peculiar relationship between the Jews and medicine. He noted that the profession provided the perfect opportunity for the Jews to give full expression to their inherently charlatan-like behavior. His allusion to disguise, true identity, and social status was an implicit comment on Hamburg's Iberian Jews: "It is an avaricious, Jewish trick to pass oneself off as a doctor, and not as any other educated man, for the Jew knows that no other discipline will serve him as well in his greed as does medicine." In particular, continued Martini, Jews preferred to serve the upper classes and other prominent people, for it is among them that their greed can be most conveniently satisfied.[72] Preference and practice can of course differ, and in the case of these Jewish physicians it did. The fact that the Jews offered their services to the lower classes (which is most likely one of the principal bases of the dispute) was, in the context of the polemic, of little concern to Martini. His aim was to characterize the Jewish physician by recourse to older, generic, anti-Jewish accusations of greed and chicanery.

From Austria came similar charges and uncompromisingly vile images. In his general diatribe against all forms of medical quackery, *Wehmühtige Klag* (The wistful lament) (1677), physician and author Johann Christoph Bitterkraut related the story of one Jewish physician's malpractice. Bitterkraut regaled the reader with the sorry episode of "one careless, stinking Jew, who through his swindling uroscopy in Delft in Holland" horribly botched his treatment of one sick woman. He examined her urine and prescribed a strong purgative for what appeared to be ailing her. Tragically, he failed to observe that she was also pregnant. The consequence of the treatment was that the twins she was carrying were stillborn and she too died a couple of days later.[73] If we accept the story as true, then the Jewish doctor was clearly negligent. But, most important, Bitterkraut would have us take this one case as representative of the medical services offered by all Jews. In portraying the doctor as a cold, insensitive child-murderer, the story echoes the medieval accusations of Jewish ritual murder of Christian children. Thus while

Bitterkraut's text can be situated within a larger genre of medieval antisemitic literature, its focus on professional abuse and medical malpractice also endows it with a "modern" quality.

Doubtless, one of the most uncompromisingly virulent diatribes against Jewish physicians was *Gewissen-loser Juden-Doctor* (The unscrupulous Jewish doctor) (1698), written under the pseudonym Christian Treumundt. In the extremeness of its language, and in the relentlessly vile images the author conjures up, the text does not really find its echo until the advent of the vulgar, antisemitic book *Judenspiegel* (The Jews' mirror) (1819), by Hartwig von Hundt-Radowsky.[74]

Treumundt raised a number of themes that became future staples of antisemitic discourse, particularly that which was aimed at Jewish doctors. The first is repulsiveness. He painted a disgusting picture of the Jewish medical student, repeatedly referring to him as an "impudent," "stinking," "snotty-nosed Jew-boy" (*Rotz-Näsigte Jüden-Bub*).

In addition, he talked about the attraction of Jews to medicine. According to Treumundt, the first thing that motivated the Jewish medical student was the opportunity to clean out or hold the urine-glass of an older "accursed Jewish doctor," the one under whom the student had passed his apprenticeship.[75] Now, because excreta, in all forms, were thought to be "bad humors," the examination thereof was standard diagnostic practice in the Middle Ages.[76] But it was the examination of urine in particular that was at the core of patient diagnosis. Scores of brief textbooks and color charts indicating disease symptomatology on the basis of urine color and smell were published as ready references for physicians. When hired, city physicians were often contractually obliged to examine the urine of any citizen who wished to have the service performed.[77] In other words, when Jewish physicians engaged in this activity, they were merely following the medical conventions of the day.

Yet Treumundt's claim about the Jews' "desire" was part of a larger and older German, coprophilic iconography and discourse about the Jews. The most notorious example of this was the infamous *Judensau,* vile images of Jews engaged in various acts of bestiality. From the thirteenth to the sixteenth century, architectural sculpture depicted vivid representations of Jews suckling the teats, drinking the urine, and eating the feces of pigs. These were most often carved into church exteriors and on the undersides of wooden pews, and served as ornamentation on bridges and town halls. In addition, such images were distributed in the form of illustrations into the nineteenth century.[78] It was into this vein of representation that Treu-

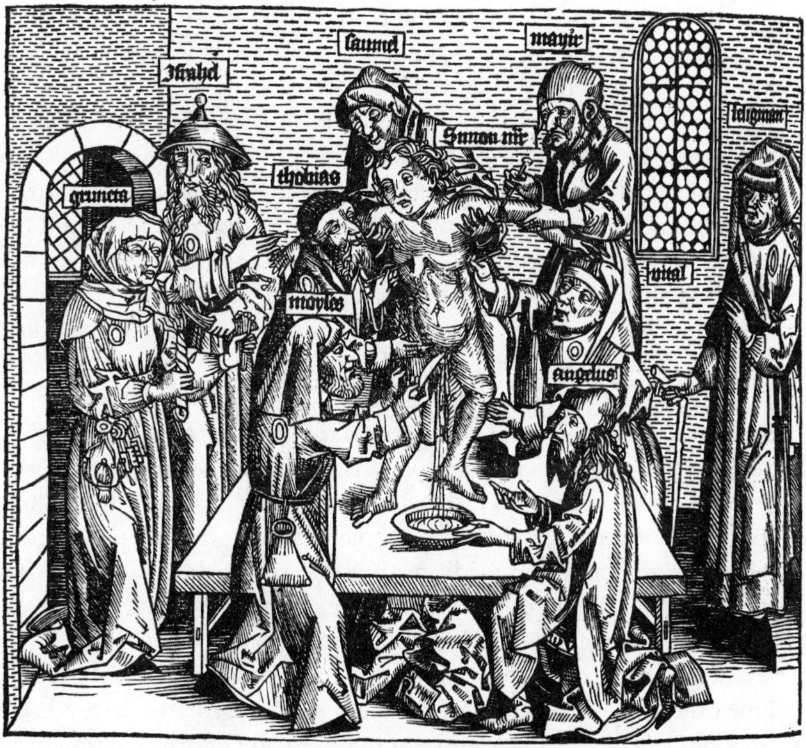

FIGURE 3. Also from Hartmann Schedel's *Liber Chronicarum* (Nuremberg, 1493), this illustration depicts Jews ritually drawing blood from the child Simon of Trent. Note the round Jewish badges on the cloaks of the Jews, and the distinctive Jew's hat worn by the man standing in the doorway. As if to confirm the canard of Jewish doctors committing acts of malfeasance against innocent Christians, the woman walking through the portal bearing needles to stick in Simon is the Jewish physician Brunetta. Source: Georg Hermann Theodor Liebe, *Das Judentum in der deutschen Vergangenheit* (Leipzig, 1903).

mundt tapped when making reference to the alleged urophiliac proclivities of Jewish medical students.

Like others of his ilk, Treumundt accused Jewish doctors of being motivated by excessive greed. He claimed that it is for the mere sake of gain that "Jewish parents encourage their children to enter this money-making profession," graphically adding that "through unacceptable, yet transparent means, they devilishly suck money from Christians."[79] Relying here on positively medieval imagery, the author portrayed the Jewish doctor as vampire and usurer, "bleeding" Gentiles of their money. And finally, there was the supposed ignorance of Jews, manifest by their inability to speak and write Latin. Calling them "donkeys," Treumundt complained that Jews *"mauschel,"* that is, they spoke German with a Yiddish accent.[80]

When the term *mauschel* first appeared in 1622 in a broadside against Christian minters of coin, it referred to the secret language they are said to have spoken when transacting business. Yet the word *mauschel* derives from the Jewish proper name Moshe, and means, in this context, to act and behave like a Jew—that is, deceitfully and stupidly.[81] Treumundt used the word to decry the ignorance of Jewish doctors, drawing special attention to the orthographic and discursive Latin errors they supposedly made, belittling their linguistic and medical skills when he unfavorably compared these with what he deemed to be the superior faculties of the Christian physician.[82]

Treumundt's accusation is reminiscent of that made by the Hamburg pastor, theologian, and school inspector Johann Müller in his *Judaismus oder Jüdenthum* (Judaism or Jewry) (1644). There, Müller conceded that "it may be that a few of them [Jewish doctors] have studied well and thoroughly, and even written books on medicine, but that is extremely rare." In what would become a standard trope of German antisemitism, the author remarked that "the majority are inexperienced asses *who hardly know how to write and read a line of German,* not to mention the simplest word in Latin and the other languages necessary for medicine."[83] Again, we detect that it was not all Jews who were found wanting, just all German Jewish physicians. The specificity with which the polemicists singled out German Jewry is most significant, for it highlights the widespread professional anxiety and cultural ambivalence that was unique to the German setting.

The ideas expressed by these virulent critics of Jewish physicians were not the isolated opinions of a handful. Scores of German texts—many written by nonphysicians, and many not even specifically aimed at Jewish doctors—contained whole passages or even chapters that referred unfavorably to the Jewish physician. Even at the turn of the eighteenth century, the notorious *Entdecktes Judentum* (Judaism revealed) (1700), by Johann Andreas Eisenmenger, devoted significant space to the purported calumnies of the Jewish physician. And just as he had selectively drawn on passages from the Talmud to demonstrate the supposed disdain Judaism expressed toward other religions—which in his day he interpreted as Christianity—so too did Eisenmenger make use of the antisemitic writings about Jewish doctors by Jewish converts.[84]

In fact, in the corpus of medical antisemitica, the Jewish doctor came in for especially harsh condemnation at the hands of Jewish converts, who, as one-time insiders, represented themselves as being able to speak on the topic of Jewish medical malpractice with indisputable "authority."[85] By issuing warning calls and graphically "exposing" the supposedly conspiratorial activities of the Jewish physician, the convert, driven by the desire to prove himself a loyal Christian, created an image for himself as the hero, poised to snatch the unsuspecting Christian patient from certain death at the hands of the Jewish doctor.

The first Jewish convert to rail publicly against Jewish physicians was Antonius Margaritha, grandson of Jacob Margoliot, the famed halakhist and rabbi of Regensburg. In 1530 Margaritha published an ethnographic book ridiculing Jewish religious practices and beliefs, *Der gantz jüdisch Glaub* (The complete Jewish faith).[86] Not long after the book's appearance, the author demanded a public religious disputation with the leader of the German Jewish community, Josel of Rosheim. During the debate, hosted by Emperor Charles V and held at the Diet of Augsburg in 1530, Josel was able to resoundingly defeat the apostate. Margaritha was summarily arrested and banished from Augsburg. One year later, he left the Catholic faith, underwent his second conversion, and became a Protestant.[87]

Among the many charges in *Der gantz jüdisch Glaub,* Margaritha claimed that Jewish prayers preached hostility toward Christianity, that the Jews had sought converts, and that they had committed treason.[88] These accusations were fundamental when he came to discuss the Jewish physician, for they were said to characterize the type of treatment the Gentile patient could expect to receive. Moreover, the Jewish doctor was a type, according to the author, whose poor training guaranteed his inferiority, made him qualitatively different from his Christian counterpart, and designated him as a clear and present danger to German patients. Deriding the poor Latin spoken by Jewish doctors and their substandard education, Margaritha maintained that "there has never been a German, Bohemian, or Hungarian Jewish doctor who even saw a Hebrew translation of Avicenna, Galen, and Hippocrates, let alone read one, and even less likely in Latin. Nor have they read any other medical books. . . . They have a few small [medical] books in German, written in Hebrew characters, and have some knowledge of roots and herbs, which they learned from their fathers and grandfathers."[89] By contrast, he lauded the Hebrew, Greek, and Latin learning of Jewish physicians from Sicily, Spain, and Italy, and he even described in a complimentary fashion a dissection class he personally observed at Pavia, which had been directed by a senior Jewish doctor.[90]

Perhaps most interestingly, Margaritha's most vigorous denunciation of the German Jewish doctor appears abruptly, near the conclusion of a chapter entitled, "On Their Slaughtering." In this section in which he provides his Gentile readership with a straightforward, if simplistic, description of the Jewish method of animal slaughter, Margaritha suddenly breaks off the discussion to encourage his readers to "ask all Jews who pass themselves off as doctors if they are not also a *shochet* and *bodek* [the words appear in Hebrew script and mean *slaughterer* and *inspector*, respectively]; that is, if they cannot grab the cow [saying something] in Hebrew and kill it. They will all answer yes. As soon as he can, he then passes himself off as a doctor due to the fact that he knows what constitutes sickness and health in cattle, and can speak about it. He is of the opinion that he knows enough to fool Christians by speaking about their illnesses. I wish therefore to warn all Christian people against German Jewish doctors who travel about the land, for their medicine has no basis and substance."[91] This association of Jewish modes of ritual slaughter with the supposedly murderous inclinations and practices of Jews lasted into the twentieth century. Perhaps not as specifically as Margaritha, who focused only on Jewish physicians, but certainly following closely in his tradition, modern antisemites have cast a wider net and detected in all Jews a bloodthirstiness toward fellow human beings, born of religious rituals surrounding the killing of animals.[92] This theme is discussed at greater length in Chapter 6. For now, it is sufficient to note that the origins of modern denunciation of kosher animal slaughter are to be found in sixteenth-century diatribes against Jewish physicians.

Viktor von Carben, who claimed to have been a rabbi prior to his conversion at the age of forty-nine, had also engaged in a public disputation, this time before the archbishop of Cologne, and had also served as an expert witness in the Pfeffercorn-Reuchlin controversy over the confiscation of the Talmud (1509–1510). He warned his readers in his *Juden Büchlein* (Little Jewish book) (1519, 1550) that "some [Jewish doctors] had never read a medical book and yet prescribe medicaments for the poor and through these ruin and kill Christians, as well as cheat them. And I say truthfully that no Jew is to be trusted, especially the friendly ones."[93]

We find the Bavarian Samuel Friedrich Brenz, who had converted to Christianity in Feuchtwangen in 1601, informing his readers in his anti-Jewish polemic, *Jüdischer abgestreiffter Schlangen-Balg* (The Jewish snake skin that has been shed) (1614), that "the more Goyim the Jewish doctor kills the higher into Grace he comes — that is, in heaven or paradise. Such a doctor should be compared to a Mohel, that is, one who circumcises Jewish boys. For the Kabbalah says that he who circumcises as many children as correspond to the numerical value of his Hebrew name receives a reward as a *ben olam habbo* [a child of the world to come]. Such is the same for a Jewish doctor. When he kills as many Christian patients as correspond to the numerical value of his Hebrew name, so does he receive the same reward as one who circumcises Jewish children."[94] Finally, Brenz also introduced a concomitant scenario of the Jewish doctor harming the Christian patient — the Jewish patient recovering as a result of the nefarious use of Christian blood. Employing a variant on the medieval blood accusation, Brenz claimed: "When a Jewish woman is in childbirth and cannot be delivered, the rabbi takes three strips of parchment made of doe skin, writes something on them and places one upon the head, the other two in the hands of the suffering woman."[95] He opined that the ink used to write the inscriptions on the parchment was most likely the blood of a Christian.

The few texts mentioned above could easily be expanded into an even longer catalogue of hate. But such documentation would take us far afield. The point has been to give a sense of the deep fear and loathing expressed by German polemicists toward the Jewish physician. The themes of animus were pervasive, the sentiments widely shared. But before moving on, we would be remiss if we did not mention some of the responses of Jewish physicians to the calumnies hurled at them. Their ability to attract a broad Christian clientele did not blind Jewish doctors to the fact that for many European elites, especially in Germany, they constituted a despised class.

From Italy, for example, came one of the earliest Jewish replies to such discrimination, *De Medico Hebraeo Enarratio Apologica* (Venice, 1588), by the above-mentioned Italian Jewish physician David de Pomis. Confidently, the author stated that "No one has ever witnessed any crime by a Jewish physician. . . . It is only because of a common prejudice that we are accused and suffer injury." Further on, he asks wryly: "Why have princes and prelates sought Jewish physicians? Because of their crimes and wrong-doings or because of their ability and their good treatment?"[96]

The Marrano physician and Jewish apologist Isaac Cardoso's impassioned apologia, *Las excelencias y Calunias de los Hebreos* (Amsterdam, 1679), is principally concerned with antisemitism on the Iberian Peninsula, although, one must hasten to add that like de Pomis' apologia, it addresses, even if by default, many of the specific accusations made by the German polemicists. Although there is no direct evidence that Cardoso was familiar with the German material, he was certainly aware of the principal themes, and may even have been alerted to the tenor of the German argument, for as a Sephardic physician in Amsterdam, he would have been aware of the competitive struggle engaged in by his brethren in Hamburg. Moreover,

German polemics bore fundamental similarities to the charges found in the Iberian literature, sharing, in addition to specific charges, certain tonal qualities. Vis-à-vis antisemitic discourse in general, Yosef Yerushalmi has observed that *only* the German literature of the day "approached the Hispano-Portuguese in its virulence."[97]

Of all the Jewish apologists with origins in the Iberian Peninsula, it was Benedict de Castro of Hamburg who responded most forcefully and directly to a German detractor. De Castro's *Flagellum calumniatum* of 1631 was a rebuttal of Joachim Curtius' diatribe against Jewish physicians, *Exhortatio celeberr. et excellentis* (1631). Additionally, Ludwig von Hörnigk's *Medicaster Apella oder Juden Artzt* was also published in 1631. And, to repeat, de Castro's response may well have been prompted in part by the generally tense atmosphere that existed between German and Sephardic physicians in Hamburg—one that prompted the appearance of Jakob Martini's hateful text, *Apella Medicaster Bullatus oder Juden Artzt* (1636).

Without doubt, the Jewish response to Samuel Brenz's accusations of 1614 by Salomon Zevi Hirsch of Uffenhausen struck the most bitter and indignant tone. In 1615, Hirsch published a vigorous response in Judeo-German entitled *Yudisher Teriyak* (The Jewish cure). Referring to Brenz as a "liar" and his work as that "poisonous book by the baptized Jew," Hirsch organized his own book into seven chapters just as Brenz had done, in order to refute him point for point.[98]

*Yudisher Teriyak* is the work of an exceptionally learned man that illustrates the false distinction between the elite, learned Hebrew writer, and the supposedly ill-educated, populist Yiddish man or woman of letters.[99] The author's erudition is on display throughout, as the text is replete with references directing the reader to passages from a vast array of rabbinic literatures that support his systematic refutation of Brenz's charge, that Judaism displays contempt for Christianity. When the subject turns to "*yudn rofim*," or Jewish doctors, Hirsch barely conceals his anger. After laying out Brenz's accusation that Jewish physicians regard it as a "*mitzvah*," a commandment, to "kill" Christian patients, Hirsch tersely, yet forcefully declares, "Thou shalt not kill. That is the law of the Jews."[100]

The charges against Jewish doctors enjoyed tremendous longevity in Germany. Nearly all the medieval and early modern ideas pertaining to Jewish medical wizardry, quackery, avariciousness, murderousness, and incompetence are repeated with striking faithfulness to the original charges well into the twentieth century. Such was the ill feeling toward Jews as physicians, and so elaborate the German stereotype of them, that it is little wonder that while Jews were welcome students at medical schools in other parts of Europe in the early modern period, the doors of German universities remained closed to them until the eighteenth century.

A fourth and final feature needs to be taken into consideration when accounting for the relatively late arrival to prominence of the German Jewish doctor, and this has to do with the slow development of medical science in Germany itself. Throughout the seventeenth century, university-trained doctors were to be found only in Germany's larger cities. Small towns and rural areas had very few doctors, and medical care was mostly in the hands of barber-surgeons, faith healers, and midwives.[101] Given that these informally trained health care providers were held in low esteem, medicine as a profession and a course of study was overlooked to a great extent because of its association with these types of practitioners.

Moreover, the growth of the German states led to a demand for suitably trained civil servants.[102] Consequently, the most popular university faculties were those of law and theology, not medicine. While members of the military and commercial classes occupied the highest positions in the state bureaucracy, lawyers who proved indispensable, particularly in jurisdiction at the local level, occupied subordinate offices. The state also used the Church as a tool to shore up its own authority. It made much of religious morality as a means to enforce a code of temporal conduct. Thus, ministers of the Church were often looked upon as state functionaries, and from their pulpits, served as conduits for information from the government to the masses.[103] Entering the clergy, therefore, was a popular choice among men in search of a career wherein their services and religious inclinations could be put at the state's disposal.

Thus, the nature of the autocratic state in Germany and its demand for bureaucrats meant that enrollments in medical faculties at German universities lagged far behind those of law and theology. The low level of medical instruction meant that as a course of study it was ridiculed. Consequently, it attracted only about 10 percent of all Germany's university students in the eighteenth century.[104] A measure of the unpopularity of medicine is the fact that at the turn of the eighteenth century, few universities had more than two or three members on a medical faculty, and the standard left something to be desired. Teachers taught almost exclusively medical theory, with no anatomical or clinical work—a pedagogic method that remained largely unchanged until the nineteenth century.[105]

Even though things had changed radically by the end of the eighteenth century, with far greater resources employed in the service of medical education, the actual number of students remained very small throughout the century.[106] For example, in Vienna in 1723 there were only 25 medical students, while at Göttingen between 1767 and 1778 somewhere between 50 and 80 students were enrolled per year. In 1768 Jena had only 17 medical students, a number that rose to 42 in 1773. For the period 1623–1794, Altdorf could manage only 386 medical students, a little more than 2 doctors per annum for 171 years. By contrast, Leiden and Edinburgh, two of Europe's premier medical schools, could boast between 300 and 400 medical students per annum for the course of the eighteenth century. In Italy, the university at Pavia had 2,000 students in total, 200 of whom were in its distinguished medical school.[107]

Thus cultural prejudice and structural backwardness were responsible for the belated emergence of the German Jewish doctor. But even after the fundamental policy change, which resulted in the graduation of Jewish medical students from German universities after 1721, significant obstacles remained in place, all of which served to remind the young Jewish doctor that he was tolerated more than he was accepted. What remained at issue was not if, but how the graduating Jewish doctor would be recognized for his achievements. Rather than expressing pride in their Jewish graduates, the German medical schools looked upon them with shame and embarrassment. For example, Heidelberg's first Jewish graduate was Elkan Seligmann Bacharach. In 1728, his graduation ceremony was said to have taken place *"sine solemnitate in des promotoris hauss,"* (without the celebratory feast in the promotion hall) in the presence of the city's mayor and rabbi, the latter administering to Bacharach a special Jewish oath for physicians.[108] At the University of Erlangen, the statute of the medical faculty stated that Jews could not publicly take their Rigorosum, the oral examination for the degree of doctor, as was the norm. Other prohibitions about where and in what manner Jewish medical students could take their final exams were to be found at Halle, and Mainz, where Wilhelm von Humboldt reported that the ceremony for the first Jew to graduate with a medical degree, Joseph Hamburg (1787), "took place not in public, but in the anatomy theater."[109]

Nor were Jews permitted to print the names of their examiners on their dissertations, the faculty fearing guilt by association with a Jew. In addition, to avoid confusion, inaugural dissertations written by Jews often carried the words *"Judaeus"* or *"Hebraeus"* after the name of the author, for biblical names were common among Christians at that time in Germany. As a measure of how unwelcome these freshly minted Jewish doctors were, they were expressly forbidden to take up low-level positions as university teachers (*Pri-*

*vatdozenten*), an option open to Christian graduates in the eighteenth century.[110] Finally, many had to expressly agree never to practice in Germany, and it is for this reason that significant numbers of German Jewish physicians found work in the more tolerant environment of Poland.[111]

Despite these humiliations, the number of Jewish doctors trained in Germany increased significantly. Although exact figures are not available, it is certain that at least half of the approximately 500 Jews who graduated from German universities between 1721 and 1800 studied medicine.[112] The impetus for the policy change that allowed Jews to become doctors in Germany came from the Enlightenment and the more liberal spirit it promoted. Jewish physicians emerged at the same time the German state underwent a transformation, which saw the rise of a centralized, political entity characterized by increasing commercial activity and industrial output.[113]

One of the first new social groups to arise in this changing environment was a "bourgeoisie of education."[114] The guiding ideal of this order was *Bildung*, a multilayered word approximating the English term "self-cultivation." It entailed the formation of reason and aesthetic taste, through the development and realization of one's inherent abilities. The ongoing process of acquiring Bildung was one in which through education, the individual achieved harmony of personality and an elevated and healthy sense of self-worth.

Bildung became the cultural and social currency of Germany's rising middle classes, principally composed of civil servants, clergy, the professoriate, and commercial groups. Its emergence in the eighteenth century as "a new secular form of individual salvation" came to define German high culture, and did so just at that time the Jews were emancipated.[115] Because of its optimistic, Enlightenment presuppositions about the human potential for inner development and improvement, German Jews, according to George Mosse, "wholeheartedly accepted the ideal of Bildung as a new faith suited to their German citizenship."[116]

For many Jews, the study of medicine became a popular means to acquire Bildung. To be sure, medicine's honored status as a free profession, its noble heritage among Jews, and the fact that in the eighteenth century doctors began to enjoy high social standing and earned handsome salaries were also attractive incentives to Jews seeking a university education. But perhaps most important, medicine's inherently inquisitive and rational nature, its curative mission, and its emphasis, particularly in the eighteenth century, on disease prevention and an improvement in public health meant that for Jews, its ideals embodied the practical application of Bildung better than almost any other vocation.[117]

## JEWISH PHYSICIANS: IN AND OUT OF THE GHETTO

Medicine was a profession perfectly suited, both intellectually and aesthetically, to this new Age of Emancipation. For so many German Jews—first men, and later women as well—doctors served as role models for a newly emerging Jewish community. It was an undertaking with deep cultural roots in Judaism, but unlike the traditional path of rabbinical scholarship for the thinking elite, it was one that also offered the possibility for recognition and acceptance outside the framework of the ghetto. And similarly, unlike commerce, it was respectable. Moreover, medicine could and did serve as a propaedeutic and hortatory device. Consequently, Jewish doctors, both implicitly and (as Chapter 3 demonstrates) explicitly helped create modern forms of Jewish identity. It has been little recognized, but the thousands of German Jews who became physicians after the eighteenth century were instrumental in the vast project that called forth a refashioning of Jewish *mentalités*.

What prompted such a metamorphosis was a host of forces that first appeared in Germany in the eighteenth century. These included the Enlightenment, incipient secularization, religious reform, occupational diversification, political emancipation, and nationalism. Prior to this time, the Jews had been treated as a totally separate minority, often referred to as the "Jewish Nation." Their religious and cultural separateness was taken as a fundamental expression of their distinct national status. But this situation was incompatible with the expectations that arose as a result of emancipation, for although the Prussian state had first emancipated the Jews in 1812, it was the German nation that the German Jews confronted thereafter. Jewish separateness could not be tolerated under these changed circumstances, and therefore a prerequisite of membership in the nation was Jewish assimilation. This was true not just for Jews, but for all minority groups. The unifying forces unleashed by the nation meant that ethnic heterogeneity would have to be passed over in favor of national homogeneity.[118]

Europeans cultivated nationhood through the creation of a set of unifying symbols such as flags, anthems, rites of commemoration, and national monuments. In the world that Jews entered into after the removal of their civic disabilities, they too rallied around these symbols, eagerly adopting them as their own. During the Enlightenment, as provincial German mentalités were in the process of being altered to suit the demands of the unified nation, the Jews began to respond similarly. The older trappings of Jewish nationhood and longing for Zion were either tempered or exorcised completely from Jewish modes of self-expression. This was but one aspect of the refashioning of Jewish mentalités.

## JEWISH PHYSICIANS: IN AND OUT OF THE GHETTO

Related to this is the fact that the nation expressed itself primarily in the adoption of a set of cultural values and norms to which all members were expected to subscribe. Such ideals were the fundamental ingredients of the formation of national character. In Germany, especially after the Napoleonic Wars, the stereotypical German was said to express the virtues of simplicity, honesty, bravery, strength, and virility. National identity in Germany had a markedly physical dimension to it. Aesthetic value judgments concerning male beauty, complexion, and physical proportion were central to the creation of the ideal German type. Anyone who did not fit this abstract ideal was said to embody physical characteristics and qualities directly opposed to it.

Perceived as physically unhealthy, Jews were an obvious target of such judgments. As a consequence, Jewish physicians in the eighteenth century began to suggest a host of changes in Jewish culture that would have a positive effect on the physical nature of what it meant to be Jewish. From the eighteenth century, then, under pressure from the dominant value system they so much wanted to celebrate, and influenced by the admonitions of Jewish physicians who saw themselves as responsible for securing the physical changes necessary to make Jews suitable for incorporation into the nation, Jews began to consider the physical nature of Jewishness in ways that they had never done before.

This process entailed a cognitive shift of considerable proportions, for the drive to assimilate dictated that German Jews needed to begin to consider themselves differently from the way they had previously. They were no longer members of a "Jewish Nation," nor were they merely members of a religious group. Rather, the focus on their physical state meant that from the last third of the eighteenth century, Jews came to see their own bodies in relation to what constituted the "normal" and stereotypical bodies as celebrated by German national culture. Aiming to help Jews conform to the new national ideal, Jewish doctors of the Enlightenment were central to this program of corporeal self-assessment, for it was they who sought to help create the new, healthy Jew.

CHAPTER 3

# *HASKALAH* AND HEALING
## JEWISH MEDICINE IN THE AGE OF ENLIGHTENMENT

The modern Jewish doctor, that is, the physician who expressed Jewish concerns in the course of his medical practice, first appeared in Germany in the eighteenth century. These were men who took up the cause of Jewish health, their aim being to alleviate the medical lot of the Jewish people. Emerging in this era of heightened social and political expectations, these Jewish physicians were infused with the intellectual energy of the Enlightenment. They were ideologically optimistic, faithful to science, and dedicated to serving their people as loyally as their predecessors had once treated royalty and clergy.

One of the important features distinguishing these Jewish physicians from their forebears was that their clinical concerns were limited not to the care and cure of the individual but to the Jews as a group. What accounts for the eighteenth-century emergence of the Jewish physician, and what intellectually preoccupied him as a Jew, as a physician, and as a Jewish physician are the themes explored in this chapter.

The greatest impulse for the creation of the modern Jewish doctor was the quest for political emancipation and the cultural process Jews instituted to help bring this about — the Jewish Enlightenment, or *Haskalah*. Dating from the last third of the eighteenth century, the Haskalah in Germany sought to effect changes in the relationship of Jews to their surroundings by achieving nothing less than a transformation of Jewish life itself. According to Naphtali Herz Wessely (one of the founders of the Haskalah), and many others, these changes were to be introduced by way of educational reforms.[1]

Wessely's *Divrei Shalom ve-Emet* (Words of peace and truth) (1782), considered to be the clearest exposition of the ideology of the early Haskalah, posited two distinct varieties of knowledge: *Torat ha-adam*, secular knowledge, and *Torat adonai*, the teaching of God. It was believed that familiarity with the former realm would enhance the capacity of the Jew to appreciate better the Divine teachings. Secular knowledge was held to be ennobling because of its therapeutic qualities. According to Wessely, secular knowledge is "comprised of etiquette, the ways of morality and good character, courtesy, proper syntax, and purity of expression."[2] Wessely and other proponents of the Haskalah, known as *maskilim,* sought to have Jews conform to a universally accepted code of conduct whereby their Judaism, now redefined through a reinvigorated educational curriculum, would assist them in the attainment of emancipation and, eventually, citizenship.[3]

As a consequence of the Haskalah's explicit goals of educational and religious reform, historians have tended to focus on the ideology's social, intellectual, educational, and even political aspects.[4] David Sorkin has faulted the traditional approach, noting that "whatever the differences in their methods, evaluations or dating, scholars have continued to place the *Haskalah* in a limited, one might say parochial context, treating the broader society and general culture only as a set of influences upon it, or the immediate setting in which it took shape."[5] In other words, Haskalah scholarship needs to make room for greater contextualization, and to expand the terms of the debates over the Haskalah so as to allow for fresher conceptual approaches.

Largely, the history of the Haskalah, in both Western and later Eastern Europe, has been presented as a battle to win over the minds of Jews. However, there was also another component, less obviously enunciated but nevertheless germane to the reformist impulse of the Jewish Enlightenment: its concern with the Jewish body. As an ideology, the Haskalah not only sought to remake Jews by exposing them to secular culture but also aimed at restoring to the Jews control over their bodies. As a close reading of the work of eighteenth-century maskilic physicians indicates, there existed a certain strain in Haskalah thinking that held that Jews had ceded control of their bodies to nothing less than Judaism itself.[6]

In keeping with the Enlightenment's stress on the need for individuals to free themselves from the tyranny of institutions, particularly religious ones, Jewish doctors such as Elcan Isaac Wolf, Moishe Marcuze, and Marcus Herz maintained that Judaism, and the way it was practiced in eighteenth century Germany and Poland, was the fundamental cause of myriad health problems afflicting the Jews. To reform Judaism — that is, to emancipate Jewish individuals from the shackles of traditional Jewish life — would guarantee the physical and mental well-being of the Jews. It is true that few physicians were involved in the movement for religious reform.[7] This then makes the work of the Jewish doctors examined here all the more significant. They constituted a vanguard among their fellow Jewish physicians by advocating some modification, not radical reform. Their importance lay in the fact that polemics and calls for change from such elevated members of Jewish society had an intellectual impact beyond the numbers involved.

Before proceeding, an explanation of that category of individual I call the "maskilic physician" is necessary. To be sure, not all Jewish reformers in the eighteenth century can be called maskilim, nor are the approximately three hundred Jewish doctors who obtained their degrees in the eighteenth century automatically entitled to the appellation.[8] However, for a number of reasons, the physicians studied here are deserving of that title. First, they advocated the reform of the Jews and attacked certain aspects of Judaism that they felt to be in sore need of modernization. Second, they aspired to lead, in place of rabbis. In their view, their possession of scientific knowledge entitled them to positions of authority and leadership. Third, they used Enlightenment categories of social construction and analysis to make their claims about Jewish society. And fourth, they employed medical theory in the service of the Haskalah, a feature that distinguishes them from earlier Jewish physicians who were far less concerned with Jewish health problems. In the hands of these maskilic physicians, the Haskalah's critique of traditional Jewish society also included a damning evaluation of the physical condition of the Jewish people. The message the maskilim were attempting to convey was that there was a direct link between sickness and lifestyle, and that the former could be avoided by transforming the latter.

Another connection between the Haskalah and medicine that needs to be stressed in this context is the important role the Jewish physician was accorded in Jewish popular culture. For Haskalah authors, the doctor as maskilic hero became a familiar character in both Yiddish and Hebrew fiction.[9] He posed as a representative of the newly emerging Jewish *Gelehrtenstand*, cultured in the European fashion, linguistically proficient in the vernacular, and religiously moderate. In Isaac Euchel's *Reb Henekh oder vus tut men damit* (Reb Henekh or what is to be done about it) (c. 1793), the earliest known Yiddish comedy of the Haskalah, the author's complex use of language—wherein the various characters speak Yiddish, German, French, and English—casts the Jewish doctor in the role of secular modernizer. Speaking a fluent but not flawless German, Euchel's parvenu Jewish doctor represents the bright, forward-looking maskilic scientist, standing in sharp contrast to the Yiddish-speaking, tradition-bound moneylender of the play's title, Reb Henekh.[10]

## HASKALAH AND HEALING

From the Eastern European Haskalah, a somewhat more skeptical and less flattering view of the Jewish doctor appears in the satire "*Gilgul Nefesh*" (Transmigration of the soul), by the Galician Hebrew writer and physician Yitshak Erter (1792–1851). In this piece, the opinions about wealthy doctors voiced by the one physician who does not have a commercially successful practice provides a fascinating window onto the hallowed position of the doctor in Jewish society. In addition to delineating the complex fact of intraprofessional animus, Erter highlights the impressionable gullibility of the Jewish masses: "A physician am I, and it is my duty to heal the wounds, and to procure a remedy for every disease of the body. It is true that my colleagues, who can boast of possessing high-sounding titles, look down upon me with a certain contempt. . . . But I am, nevertheless, as well qualified a medical practitioner as they are, and my patients do not fare worse than theirs. The only difference between them and me is that I go about on foot and they rattle around in carriages with a driver. The more horses the more medical knowledge. For according to the people of Israel, if one acquires such wisdom with just one horse, how much more does a physician possess if he owns seven horses."[11]

Here issues of class conflict and professional jealousy clash to produce a doctor-hero that differs markedly from his Berlin counterpart in *Reb Henekh*. Erter's doctor actually tends to resemble Reb Henekh more than he does Euchel's maskilic physician. He is bound to the masses and dedicated to treating them with a sense of loyalty that is reminiscent of Reb Henekh's faithfulness to the culture of the people. While the more cynical approach of Erter reflects the self-parodic and more intimate nature of the Galician Haskalah, both texts portray their respective physicians as cool rationalists, as agents of moral authority, modernity, and Jewish societal transformation. This is precisely the way the physicians addressed here represented themselves to their Jewish patients.

The first Jewish physician to employ his credentials in the name of Jewish physical improvement was Elcan Isaac Wolf, who did so in his discussion of the medical condition of the Jews, *Von den Krankheiten der Juden* (On the illnesses of the Jews) (1777). Wolf took his medical degree at Gießen in 1763, moved to Alsace, where he practiced medicine in Metz, and eventually settled in the German town of Mannheim. Metz was the most important Jewish city in pre-Revolution eastern France.[12] And because Wolf identified poverty as one of the chief culprits responsible for the ruination of Jewish health, his experience in the French context is decisive. When Wolf published his study of Jewish illnesses, the Jewish population of Metz was approximately two thousand. By 1780, despite the existence of some very wealthy individuals, the community was exceptionally poor, and becoming even more so.[13] The situation was so dire that the Royal Academy in Metz ran an essay competition in 1785 based on the question, "Are there means of making the Jews happy and more useful in France?" a direct reference to the desperate social conditions under which the Jews of the city lived. Two years later, the committee of judges announced the names of the three joint-winners: a liberal cleric, Abbé Henri Grégoire; a Protestant, Adolphe Thiéry; and a Polish Jew, Zalkind-Hourwitz. Essentially, all three answered the question in the affirmative, advancing the thesis that persecution was the cause of whatever was wrong with the Jews, and that the eradication of maltreatment would result in Jews who were indeed "happy and useful."[14]

What is most important in the context of the present discussion is the title of Grégoire's submission, *An Essay on the Physical, Moral and Political Regeneration of the Jews* (1789). For as outspoken a supporter of Jewish emancipation as he was, Grégoire was firmly convinced that the Jews were physically and psychologically debased, exhibiting such tendencies as chronic onanism, nymphomania, effeminacy, and melancholia.[15] The essay contest was only a formal episode in a protracted public discourse in ancien régime France and Germany about the Jewish body and the connection between it and the desirability or even possibility of Jewish emancipation.[16] Elcan Isaac Wolf's discussion of Jewish illnesses must therefore be seen against the backdrop of the poverty he witnessed among the Jews in both France and Germany, its effect on their health, and the open debate about their physical and moral qualities.

Wolf displayed the optimism typical of a reformer. In spite of the bleak picture he drew of Jewish life in Germany, he was extremely hopeful about the prospects for the Jewish future. Unable to conceal his joy, he wrote: "How fortunate are we Jews to live in this century. We are ruled by gracious humanitarians, and live quietly, for the most part, among civilized Christians. Prejudices against our religion have been displaced by humane sentiments."[17]

This passage is full of implications for the arguments that Wolf went on to make. Writing in this vein was not merely an eighteenth-century literary convention. The author was making the heartfelt claim that Christian society had reformed itself, as manifested in the newfound respect he seemed to think it accorded Judaism. For Wolf, one measure of this would have been the graduation of Jews such as himself from German medical schools. As he suggested throughout the text, it was now up to the Jews to rehabilitate themselves. They had to show good will to the beneficent Christians among whom they lived. For Wolf, this meant creating healthy and productive Jews, Jews who would be a credit both to themselves, and to what he called the "Palestine of the Palatine" (93–94). This was to be the obligation of the Jewish party in the emancipation contract.

*On the Illnesses of the Jews* is divided into three main sections. The first deals with the illnesses of Jewish newborns, young children, those of marriageable age, and the elderly. The second part of the book focuses on the means by which poverty, the major cause of disease, can be eliminated, and the third section is entitled "Political Means." In it, Wolf suggested those transformations in the political and social realm that should be brought about in order to ameliorate the Jewish condition.

The maskilim and the reformers who followed them centered their attention on prayer, ritual, and education and the need to modernize them. So too did maskilic physicians. For example, Wolf was opposed to the "Jewish mode of prayer," maintaining that it was responsible for Jewish insanity.[18] Nevertheless he was not averse to all Jewish ritual.

Rather, much of Wolf's concern has to do with the detrimental effects of the Jewish diet. His aim was not to do away with dietary laws. On the contrary, he even recommended the introduction of a new *halakhic* (Jewish legal) prohibition against sweets, one that would be as stringently applied and followed as that against pork (48). In fact, believing Judaism to be a rational religion, he wondered whether "our holy Laws had not eternally banned [the consumption] of pork just for [health] reasons" (18).

Wolf was of the particular opinion that pregnant Jewish women, to their own detriment and that of their unborn children, ate too many sweets and consumed too much fatty and spicy food. But how could this be prevented? It was, after all, the late eighteenth century, and coercive communal means to effect behavioral compliance no longer existed. Somewhat ironically, the maskil, Wolf, suggested over and over again a traditional Jewish response to excess—the passage of sumptuary laws. But the ancient social and legal mechanism for enforcing such a regimen, Jewish self-government, was a thing of the past. And the traditional reason for the sumptuary laws—to curb ostentatiousness and its consequence, antisemitism—was not a primary concern of Wolf, who, as he stated at the beginning of his book, lived among civilized and tolerant Christians. Rather, Wolf was a physician, and it was to science and reason that he would appeal. And thus when he requested that his Jewish brethren stop eating this or practicing that, the aim was to bring his recently acquired secular knowledge to bear on the unenlightened Jews. He sought neither to undermine Jewish law nor even to significantly reform Judaism: for him, science and faith were perfectly compatible, and because of the reasonableness inherent in Judaism, science was poised to complement it. Instead, it was the Jews who had become irrational, and it was his desire to radically transform them. It was their behavior that needed modifying and correcting, for their health and well-being depended on it.

Wolf devotes a considerable portion of his book to the question of nutrition. In complaining about the Jewish diet, Wolf anticipated similar charges by other physicians. Around 1781, a French doctor named Le Jau in the town of Phalsbourg in Lorraine, wrote a tract entitled "Remarks on the Diseases of the Jews," in which he decried the types of foods eaten by the Jews of northern France and western Germany. He charged that their tea and coffee consumption was too high, such beverages being "injurious to certain kinds of temperaments." Interestingly, he specifically notes that "among the foods they very much like are those made with flour; they often eat unleavened bread, and have a passion for cakes, pastries and other delicacies [*ils aiment beaucoup les farineux, mangent souvent du pain azime et sont passionnés pour les gâteaux, les pâtisseries et autres friandises*]. . . . They permit their children and young people to take part in these domestic excesses, making them susceptible to diseases caused by crudity of the upper bowels, and by the viscosity and putridity of their humors."[19]

What is striking about Wolf's complaint and that of Le Jau is their willingness to isolate Jews and their culinary habits from those of the host society. Jews were portrayed as the only consumers of such foods, when in fact these authors must have been aware that this was not the case. Very little serious historical work has considered the development and nature of Jewish diets, apart from their ritual aspects. Nearly one hundred years ago, Israel Abrahams discussed the particular character of foods eaten by Jews on the Sabbath and at festivals during the Middle Ages. Religious particularisms aside, the variety of ingredients used to make these preparations were by and large identical to those used by Gentiles. And Robert Bonfil has noted with regard to Jews in the Italian Renaissance that they "cooked and ate for the most part like their Christian neighbors."[20] Doubtless, the same could be said for Central and Northern European Jewry of the eighteenth century.

Although research in the area of European food history maintains that a rise in population accompanied by a decline in purchasing power caused the majority of Europeans to eat a nutritionally worse and less varied diet in the eighteenth and nineteenth centuries than they had in previous times, it is also true that the refinement of courtly culture and the slow but steady rise of a commercial, industrial, and administrative bourgeoisie in both France and Germany between 1680 and 1770 resulted in an increased demand for luxury beverages and foodstuffs, such as tea, coffee, sugar, and chocolate.[21] According to food historian Hans Teuteberg, the period from 1770 to 1850 eventually saw the overwhelming acceptance by the rural population of the urban food innovations of the previous period.[22] Also, discussion about the impact of these foodstuffs on European health was taken up in important centers of science. Between 1672 and 1733, the medical faculty of Paris sponsored some nineteen public disputations about the medical effects and therapeutic uses of a variety of food and beverage items as well as tobacco. In most cases the discussants favored the products discussed.[23] In addition, the eighteenth century saw a proliferation of books by doctors wherein specific foods were associated with disease prevention or cure.[24]

The emergence of such items onto the European market was accompanied by the development of new social and commercial settings such as coffeehouses and restaurants — public places where the new delicacies could be enjoyed.[25] The availability of these goods and the slow emergence of a bourgeois lifestyle also led to aesthetic developments in the area of pastry cooking and dessert creation. It became the custom in the eighteenth century to consume hot drinks such as tea and coffee with sugar, accompanied by pastries.[26]

In France and Germany — two nations enjoying unrivaled reputations (then and now) in the art of *pâtisserie* — it is to be expected that the increasingly bourgeois Jews of the eighteenth century also celebrated this aspect of the dominant culinary culture. While they may not have frequented the bakeries and pastry shops of non-Jews, there is nothing inherent in the ingredients of the widely available delicacies that would have prevented Jews from preparing their own versions, which they doubtless did. And if Jews were consuming more sweets than some doctors thought good for them, they most likely did so at a rate no different from that of their neighbors. The Enlightenment poet Friedrich Nicolai described the Habsburg capital thus: "The feasting and luxurious living in Vienna is known to all the world. . . . One would imagine that the tables of distinguished and rich people are full of many and special meals, but one has no idea how far feasting and gluttony have spread among the lower classes unless one has seen it."[27] Nicolai was obviously speaking of the population as a whole, but such a picture is not even hinted at in the polemical medical literature on Jewish diets. Jews stood alone, their collective sweet tooth a function of their peculiar "religion, morals, nourishment, and occupations."[28]

The object of Wolf's criticism was not *kashrut* (Jewish dietary laws) but the larger, and what he deems unique, culinary culture of Central European Jewry. Despite Wolf's claims, records show that the Jews at that time consumed a rather varied and interesting diet.[29] The long list of foods included savory items such as "legumes, onions, garlic, and sharp cheese. . . . Sweets bought at either the bakery or prepared at home were made of sugar, and flavored with cinnamon, almonds or lemon and orange rind" (45–47). The damage caused by such items as "cakes and pretzels" made from "butter, milk, and flour" were a new phenomenon, according to Wolf. His proof was that "in the description of the journeys of the Israelites in the desert we do not read about such illnesses because mannah and clean spring water were their only food" (49). As a result of recent culinary innovations, Wolf wanted to impose greater restrictions on the Jewish diet for health reasons, just as "Moses, that godly man, in his great wisdom, would have banned confectioners had they lived in his day" (49). The implication, of course, is that while ancient Jews had displayed a prophylactic dietary instinct, modern Jewry, given what it chose to consume, had lost it.

Wolf expended as much polemical energy as he did on the subject of the Jewish diet for two principal reasons: the first to do with science, the second involving culture. Intellectually, he was deeply concerned with the process of digestion, an interest he had displayed early on, having written his inaugural dissertation on *De vermibus intestinorum* (On intestinal worms) (1763). When Wolf attended medical school in the eighteenth century, the curriculum had been fundamentally influenced by the findings on metabolism and nutrition of the great clinical teacher at the University of Leiden, Hermann Boerhaave (1688–1738), and his Swiss pupil, Albrecht von Haller (1708–1777). Both scientists regarded nutrition as a physiological process, maintaining that food constituents replaced body parts that were continuously "wasted" and destroyed "by several actions of life." Under the impact of mechanistic models of the universe as expounded by Galileo and Newton, Boerhaave and Haller sought to explain the function of the human body in similar terms. The continuous change the body experiences (metabolism) and its need for replenishment (nutrition) were regarded as purely mechanical phenomena.[30] Thanks to these discoveries and the later work on oxidation and respiration by the Frenchmen Antoine Laurent Lavoisier and Pierre-Simon Laplace, which provided a chemical as opposed to mechanical explanation for transformations occurring in living organisms, areas such as nutrition and diet became crucial topics in medical studies from the eighteenth century.[31] Wolf's discussion of the Jewish diet therefore needs to be seen against this larger backdrop of scientific innovation in the fields of physiology and chemistry. The exciting new discoveries were soon incorporated into the medical school curriculum. In an eager young doctor such as Wolf, the latest nutritional ideas found an enthusiastic promoter, one who sought to encourage changes in the diet of the Jews based upon the discoveries to which he had been exposed at Gießen.

The cultural imperative for Wolf to have discussed diet to the extent he did derived from contemporary developments in bourgeois culture as they pertained to food. In the eighteenth century, diet was included as part of a larger *Lebensphilosophie* literature. Around since antiquity and enjoying enormous popularity today, authors such as Berlin physician Christoph Wilhelm Hufeland, who wrote *Macrobiotics or the Art of Extending Human Life* (1796), sought to achieve their goal by promoting a harmonious balance between body and soul.[32] One source for the dissemination of such ideas was the cookbook, which became increasingly popular, particularly after the invention of printing.[33] Often, such texts openly stressed the link between health and diet. "It is better," declared an early cookbook, "to get one's medicine out of the kitchen than from the apothecary." Günter Wiegelmann, a leading sociologist who studies people's relation to food, is surely correct in his observation that "cuisine and curing [were] only two sides of the same coin."[34]

Diet and nourishment were also part of a much larger literature on housekeeping and home economics, and this also influenced Wolf's view of the Jewish diet. In pre-industrial Germany, a veritable library of practical guides had been produced, covering topics as varied as praying, cooking, bee-keeping, agricultural work, and health. Appearing from the end of the sixteenth century until the middle of the nineteenth, this literature was meant to assist a man and his wife maintain an orderly, simple, Christian household.

By the eighteenth century, the literature was steeped in the rationalist philosophy of the German Enlightenment, or *Aufklärung*, serving as a guide to the creation of an efficient, systematically run house.[35] The Christian component of these developments notwithstanding, Wolf sought to promote the values of this *Hausväterliteratur* (householder's literature) among Jews. As distinct from the courtly manners and consumption patterns celebrated in medieval cookbooks and the like, the eighteenth-century versions extolled the values of simplicity and bourgeois moderation. It was precisely such qualities that Wolf hoped would eventually dominate Jewish culture. For example, Wolf charged that a major factor contributing to the poor digestive health of Jews stemmed from their preoccupation with business, which forced them to either eat on the run or skip meals altogether (39). This behavior was in marked contrast to the new table manners that had come into vogue in Europe. Beginning in the late Middle Ages and taking their final form in the eighteenth century, the ritualization of European eating habits and the development of table etiquette, including the institutionalization of set mealtimes, the use of cutlery, tablecloths, and napkins all became central to the bourgeois project.[36] It is no accident that with Jews on the verge of emancipation, Wolf, as both a physician and representative of the Jewish *Bildungsbürgertum* (bourgeoisie of education), would ask his fellow Jews to adopt the mores and refined table manners of their Christian neighbors. It was both a matter of their health and social well-being.

Elsewhere, Wolf was happy to recognize and celebrate aspects of traditional Jewish law that were characterized by therapeutic qualities and legislated exhortations to moderation. He noted that circumcision, "although a painful operation," was nothing that he had ever observed to cause illness. "On the contrary," he wrote, "it is ultimately useful for propagation" (20–21). Among the other therapeutic benefits to Jewish law were its prohibitions against drunkenness and licentious and excessive sexual intercourse, its rules for fasting, and its laws concerning female ritual purity. For Wolf, all these had a beneficial effect on the "morals, health, and propagation of the Jews" (44). Within Wolf's worldview, ancient traditions, provided they could be given a rational interpretation and were compatible with new cultural standards, were legitimized.

The same cannot be said regarding Wolf's views of the traditional Jewish education system. However, unlike many of his Haskalah contemporaries, he never expressed any discontent with what Jewish children were being taught at school. He did not seek a curriculum change. As he stated categorically, "No, my brothers! I do not want to assert . . . that we should educate our children like unreasonable animals, according to the rules of the dangerous Rousseau. I know and understand very well the holy purpose of this tradition of ours [that is, early education]" (30).

Wolf was a physician, not an educator, and therefore his primary concern lay with the physical side effects of attendance at the *heder*, or elementary school. Wolf was convinced that adults who had excessively devoted themselves to study were subject to weight loss and irregular digestion. Moreover, those who were learned were "bound to the chains of hypochondria," their health often having faded while they were still young. "Childhood," declared Wolf, "must be full of games, the youth full of laughter, and one should only become serious as one approaches adulthood" (29–30).

Nevertheless, Wolf was not an iconoclast. He appreciated the centrality of education in traditional Jewish society and was cognizant of the beneficial effects of the system, such as its role in the transmission of time-honored knowledge and values to posterity.[37] However, the consequences (as he observed them) led him to question whether future generations of young Jews who had been schooled in the traditional way would be vigorous and healthy enough to take their rightful place in a society that had just begun to make room for them.

According to Wolf, the Jewish emphasis on scholarship continued into adolescence and at that age, those who had not experienced fading health because of their studies would instead succumb to the pressures of business. In linking occupation and ill health, Wolf displayed the considerable extent to which Jewish social critics repeated Gentile misgivings about the over-representation of Jews in trade. For example, Wolf echoes a complaint earlier made by the Italian physician Bernadino Ramazzini in his *Discourse on the Diseases of Workers* (1700). There, the Paduan doctor noted that the Jews "are a lazy race, but active in business." He complained that "[the Jews] do not plough, harrow, or sow," wryly adding, "but they always reap."[38] This farming metaphor was not one chosen arbitrarily; it was part of a larger discourse throughout Europe about Jews and their place in modern society. It also must be recalled that in the eighteenth century, three-quarters of the population in Germany led rural lives, and the countryside was, in W. H. Bruford's felicitous phrase, "the principal material foundation of German civilization in that age."[39]

That the Jews did not farm and thus enjoy the benefits of the elements was a central issue in debates about Jewish emancipation in the eighteenth century, especially in Germany. Critics of Jewish emancipation often held that the Jews were in some way biologically averse to such work. Their physical distance from the soil was also said to bespeak a more profound spiritual detachment, one that disqualified them from full participation in the life of the nation. In the minds of non-Jewish commentators, such participation was predicated upon the belief in a rootedness to the earth, a type of literal and figurative anchoring.[40]

Wolf himself tapped into this discursive vein in the context of a discussion about pregnant Jewish women. In his opinion, the esteem in which pregnant women were held among the Jews directly led to "harmful and disadvantageous excesses" on their part. Essentially, they led too pampered an existence. This sedentary lifestyle adversely affected the nourishment of mother and baby, hindered healthy bowel movements, and caused the appearance of "impure blood, and poor circulation in the abdomen" (15). In the typical fashion of his day, Wolf suggested that the remedy for the physical inactivity of Jews, especially women, "the majority of whom pass their time . . . like Lot's brash wife in Sodom, like a quiet statue fettered to a chair," was to engage in agricultural work (16).

From the Haskalah of the late eighteenth century to Zionist ideologists of the late nineteenth, Jewish critics often pointed to the unhealthy life of the yeshiva scholar or the tailor, who for hours on end pored over sacred books or rolls of fabric, studying or sewing under inadequate light, and without fresh air. For Wolf, the absence of a farming class among the Jews resulted in their concentration in occupations that promoted ill health. Incessant study and trade had the same tragic result: "If I am to describe a Jewish youth to my readers, I must introduce you to a pitiable slave, [one] who is either chained to the most profound and mysterious interpretations of the Holy Book by the sternest moral education, or has to bear, already in his youth, the sufferings of a turbulent market. I must show you a young man whose bodily parts are not entirely developed, and whose health is weakened and severely damaged through both kinds of bondage" (23).

Wolf's metaphor of slavery should not be construed as mere hyperbole. Its proponents saw the German Haskalah as a liberation movement, its primary aim being to break the shackles of tradition. Were this achieved, the maskilim believed, Christian society would reward the Jews by displaying a more tolerant attitude toward them.

Bolstered by the prestige and authority that are among the rewards of having a medical degree, and displaying the hubris so typical of that generation of maskilim, Wolf sought to cure his fellow German Jews of all that prevented them from fulfilling their destiny in their beneficent environment. He put it best when he said: "The health of the subjects of a state is an inexhaustible source of harmony for a state. A Jewish community that, through the benevolent decrees of a humanitarian ruler, is granted small civic privileges intended to keep them healthy, becomes like a productive mine, where the treasury department can exploit gold and silver from even the most unpromising strata" (90).

Wolf's sincerity is not to be doubted, nor is his desire to improve the health of the Jewish people to be dismissed. Nevertheless, his wish to make Jews more aesthetically sensitive, by encouraging them to take up the fine arts (92), and to be more aesthetically pleasing, by suggesting a change in lifestyle, was predicated upon a transformation of the Jewish body. It was the physical nature of Jewishness that needed correction. Wolf's main message was one in which the onus for the regeneration of the Jews was placed on their own shoulders. He was not blind to institutionalized antisemitism, lamenting that Jews had been excluded from guilds and prohibited from the purchase of land, but he remained characteristically optimistic that history was leading the Jews toward better days.

In a different context, the physician Moishe Marcuze echoed many of Wolf's views in his *Seyfer Refues* (Book of remedies) (1790), regarded as the first scientific medical text in the Yiddish language.[41] It is a very long treatise, divided into eighteen chapters and further organized into two hundred separate sections, with an appendix in which the recipes for scores of medications appear. It is certain that Marcuze used as a source for his own book the popular *Avis au peuple sur sa santé* (Advice to the people with regard to their health) (1761), by the Swiss hygienist and pioneer of preventative medicine, Simon-André Tissot (1728–1797). Without openly acknowledging it, Marcuze relied heavily on the German translation of Tissot's book. He was most likely also acquainted with the Hebrew translation thereof, entitled, *Refuot ha-Am*, by the Eastern European *maskil*, Mendel Lefin. Lefin's translation, prepared at the behest of Moses Mendelssohn, had been given approbation by Marcuze's fellow doctor and one-time classmate at Königsberg, Marcus Herz.[42] In commissioning and sanctioning such works, representatives of the Berlin Haskalah were clearly responding to broader bourgeois trends, leading them to tacitly voice their deep concern with the health and well-being of their fellow Jews, regarding their promotion as one of the reformative goals of the Jewish Enlightenment.

Although Marcuze shared the same goals as his counterparts in Berlin, his location in Poland required that for the mission to succeed, a different tactic needed to be employed. To this end, he wrote his book in Yiddish. Ironically, this most maskilic of medical projects, the writing of a popular medical treatise in the vernacular, was strongly encouraged by Raphael Kohen, the vehemently anti-maskilic rabbi of the combined north German communities of Altona, Hamburg, and Wandsbeck. Kohen was fiercely opposed to the Haskalah and in particular was a bitter critic of Mendelssohn's German translation of the Bible. Yet he approved of the book's production, and in stark contrast to the encouragement Lefin received from the Berlin maskilim to translate Tissot into Hebrew, it was Kohen, according to Marcuze, who strenuously urged him to write his medical treatise in Yiddish, so as to make it accessible to as many Jews as possible (57b).

In the choice of many of his clinical examples, Marcuze supplied anecdotes from Tissot that also appear in Lefin's work. Thus, structurally and intellectually, Marcuze's book resembles that of his Swiss and Galician predecessors. But *Seyfer Refues* was far more than a mere rendering into Yiddish of a French text that had recently been translated into Hebrew. It was a stunningly original work of abiding linguistic and ethnographic interest. A biting social commentary in which the author gave full expression to his secular and traditional erudition and linguistic dexterity—he moved easily from Yiddish to Hebrew, and was clearly fluent in German and Polish. Replete with midrashic homilies and pious declarations, Marcuze's *Book of Remedies* was an intimate portrait of the desperate social and sanitary conditions of Polish Jewry, and a diatribe aimed at the vast array of traditional healers whom Marcuze took to be charlatans.

Writing the book in the Jewish vernacular, Marcuze directed himself specifically at a Polish Jewish readership, noting on the title page his own credentials and purpose in writing his book: "*Sefer Refuot ha-nikra Ezer Yisrael* (*Book of Remedies that is called the Help of Israel*), for those who dwell in the land of Poland. Written in Poylish-Taytsh [Yiddish] by the distinguished Rabbi Moses, well known to many [and] who is called Marcuze Doctor, a government-paid physician appointed by the king and by the commission. He wishes to benefit the people with his book, so that each person might be able to help him or herself when no learned doctor is available. And whomsoever holds to the course of conduct prescribed will not become sick. Printed here in the holy community of Poritsk in the year 5550."[43]

Before proceeding, we must note that Marcuze felt obliged to apologize for the fact that he wrote his book in Yiddish. This was a fairly conventional maskilic tactic adopted by both those who truly felt awkward using the language and those who were comfortable employing it but expressed unease in order to stave off anticipated criticism. True to the Italian tradition of the physician-rabbi, Marcuze was a Torah scholar and wanted to write his work in Hebrew, yet he elected to do so in Yiddish.[44] Explaining himself in Hebrew, he justified his choice of language, noting that even "Maimonides, and there is none greater, wrote most of his books on philosophy and science in Arabic [and not Hebrew] in order that all of his contemporaries should know and understand what he had written, as did the Gaon, Rabbenu Bahya, whose book *Hovot ha-Levavot* and the rest of his books were also written in Arabic. Also I, the humble one, follow in their footsteps" (6b). If this had been all there was to it, then there would be no need to mention it. But Marcuze noted that he "[wrote] the book for his friends, who should show it to the whole world" (6a). It is curious, then, that he would go on to claim that in order to write the treatise he had to learn Yiddish by "crippling" his German (57b). Throughout the text, Marcuze passed himself off as a Prussian maskil, bringing enlightenment to the Eastern European Jewish masses. But the truth of the matter is that Marcuze had no need to make a special effort to learn Yiddish—one glance at the text proves the author's fluency—because he came from the Lithuanian city of Slonim.[45] While he claims that he was born in Prussia and left as a teenager, this is thrown into doubt by the fact that according to the University of Königsberg, from which he graduated in 1766, his birthplace was Slonim.[46] Whatever the case, writing a book in such idiomatic Yiddish for his close friends meant that Poland, both physically and culturally, was not for him the terra incognita he made it out to be.[47] Moreover, it raises questions about his own discomfort with his origins—his sojourn in Germany having provided him with a "new" Jewish identity and a deeply caring yet impatient attitude toward Eastern Jews. This is but one key to explaining the vitriolic tone he adopts when speaking of the medical community in Jewish Poland.

Finally, if Marcuze did in fact arrive in Poland around 1774, that is only one year after that country's partition at the hands of Prussia, Austria, and Russia. Shortly thereafter, public discourse about the need for overall reform in Poland turned to the "Jewish Question," with the firm belief expressed that Poland's eventual resurrection was dependent upon the modernization and assimilation of its Jewish population.[48] *Seyfer Refues* is Marcuze's contribution to the debate. It is also what links him to Elcan Isaac Wolf and, as discussed later in this chapter, Marcus Herz. In a sense, maskilic physicians shared similar thoughts on the relation of the Jews to the respective states in which they lived. Both Jews and their doctors tended to exaggerate the importance of the Jews in terms of national development. It is clear from Marcuze's program that just as Wolf had viewed the welfare of the German state as bound up with the improved health of the Jews, so did Marcuze share the sentiment of many Poles that the health and improvement of the Jews would be to Poland's overall post-partition benefit. This national or cameralist element of eighteenth-century Jewish medical literature distinguished it sharply from its predecessors.

Although Marcuze's etatist slant may have been innovative, the idea of writing a medical self-help manual for Jews in a Jewish language was not new.[49] During the seventeenth and early part of the eighteenth century, these texts, often a mixture of folk medicine, Kabbalah, and contemporary scientific medical practice had already become common and widespread.[50]

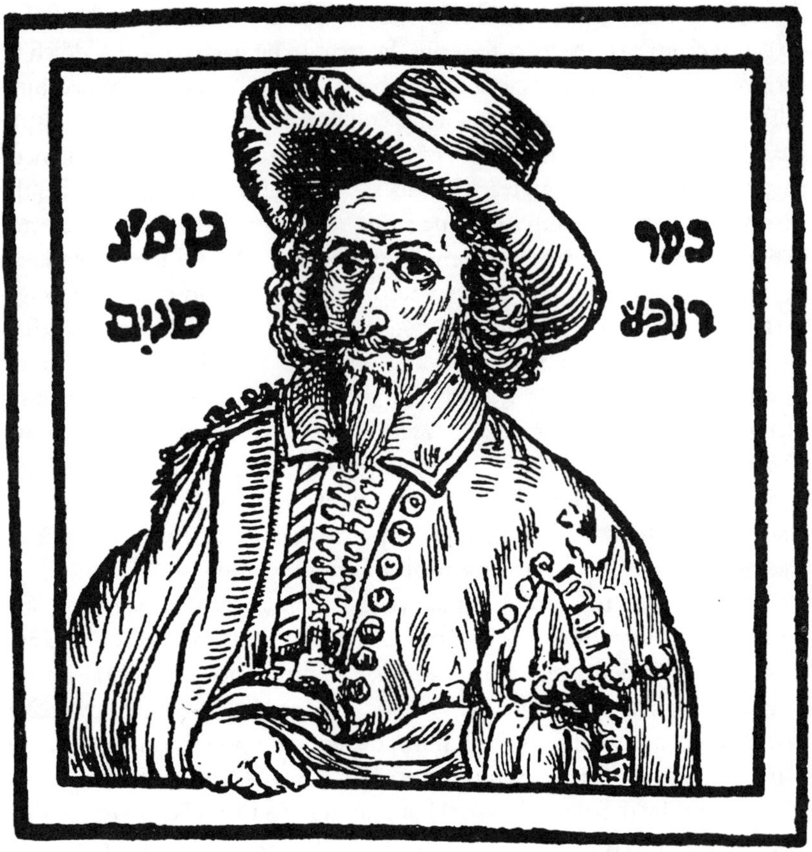

FIGURE 4. A picture of forty-three-year-old Issacher bär Teller, author of *Be'er Mayim Khayyim* (The wellspring of living waters), published in Prague around 1650. Describing his medical self-help manual, the author tells readers: "It is written in *loshn Ashkenazi* [Yiddish], so that every woman and man can understand this good little book with ease." Source: Georg Hermann Theodor Liebe, *Das Judentum in der deutschen Vergangenheit* (Leipzig, 1903).

Such books appeared in great numbers all over Europe, with nearly all the author-physicians stating that the principal motivation for their publication was to offer assistance to Jews who lived in towns with few or no competent medical personnel.

It would appear that there was a real shortage of qualified medical practitioners, particularly in more isolated areas, and hence the need for such guides was genuine. In one of the most widely used such books, *Be'er Mayim*

*Khayyim* (The wellspring of living waters), published in Prague around 1650, the author, Issacher bär Teller, told his readers: "Every son of Israel should buy [this book] for his home, so that in case of need he does not have to run far for doctors. Someone who already has some knowledge of medicine will read this book with more desire. With expert knowledge and things that have been tried, you will be taught how anyone can make medications on his own. It is written in *loshn Ashkenazi* [Yiddish], so that every woman and man can understand this good little book with ease. All the things [of which I write] have been tried out for many years. It is surely known that practice makes perfect."[51]

Teller had been a student of the luminary from Crete, Joseph Delmedigo, himself a staunch proponent of the dissemination of medical and scientific knowledge among Jews.[52] Their contemporary, the Italian Jewish physician Jacob Zahalon, published his *Otsar ha-Khayyim* in Venice in 1683, precisely to assist Jews who had only limited access to physicians. Like Teller before him, Zahalon encouraged his readers to be confident that the art of healing could be mastered by anyone, especially if they were in possession of a reputable self-help book.[53]

In Germany, with its restrictions against Jews studying medicine at the universities, the demand for such books seems to have been particularly acute. In 1677 and 1679, respectively, two Yiddish self-help medical manuals from Poland written by Moshe ben Benjamin Ze'ev of Kalish came on the market. *Yerushat Moshe* and *Yarom Moshe* both bore imprimaturs from leading Jewish physicians in Padua, Venice, and Verona, as well as medical opinions and prescriptions from various Italian doctors. According to Kalish, who had studied medicine in Rome, both books had been penned with the intention of providing medical advice to the isolated poor, for whom the cost of a trip to the doctor was prohibitive.[54]

Kalish's fellow Polish Jew, and the first Jewish entrant to a German medical faculty, Tobias Cohen, was the author of the widely circulated medical and science compendium *Ma'aseh Tuviyyah* (1707). By no means as popular in style and content as other Jewish self-help manuals, Cohen's book is nevertheless a classic, republished many times down into the present era. It is divided into two distinct parts, the first dealing with religion, and the second with medicine. *Ma'aseh Tuviyyah* is the work of an erudite, rationalist thinker who sought to battle against the superstitiousness that characterized the popular medical treatment of his day.[55] Drawing inspiration for his own project from Cohen, Moishe Marcuze referred approvingly to *Ma'aseh Tuviyyah* in his *Seyfer Refues*.[56]

From the heavily populated Frankfurt ghetto, Abraham Wallich, a member of one of European Jewry's most distinguished medical dynasties, practiced medicine and penned his popular Hebrew medical treatise, *Sefer Dimyon ha-Refuot* (1700). Like the others, it too was written expressly for the purpose of providing medical information to Jews who were without access to professional care.[57]

A final example of such medical guides is an anonymous work written in Judeo-German entitled *Sefer ha-Refues* (1722). Like Kalish, the author, who appears to have hailed from the town of Floss in Oberpfalz, touted the cost-effectiveness of having a medical self-help book such as his or, as he generously put it, "even someone else's in the house."[58]

In addition to the few representative texts mentioned here, scores of books offering herbal remedies appeared in Yiddish and Hebrew, constituting a genuine genre of literature. The vast popularity of such books also indicates the receptivity to such knowledge on the part of the Jewish public.

One hundred and forty years separated Teller's contribution from the appearance of *Seyfer Refues*, and although Marcuze's intentions do parallel those of his predecessors, they do not entirely duplicate the same motivations. Marcuze's aim was to call attention to the fact that only a trained physician was qualified to administer treatment to the sick. If such an individual could not be found, then scrupulously following the doctor's prescriptions, rather than seeing a quack—he claimed this to be the norm among Polish Jews—would ensure the patient's well-being.

What drove Marcuze to think this way was his personal sense of incipient professionalization. In *The Social Transformation of American Medicine*, Paul Starr has defined a profession as "an occupation that regulates itself through systematic, required training and collegial discipline; that has a base in technical, specialized knowledge; and that has a service rather than profit orientation, enshrined in its code of ethics."[59] This arrangement cannot be said to have begun in earnest in Germany until the beginning of the nineteenth century, and even after that in Poland. Yet it is highly likely that precisely because of his Jewishness, his sense of himself as having emerged from a traditional society, and his feeling of superiority toward his fellow Eastern European Jews, gained by his having received a German university education, Marcuze would have felt the need to distance himself in a professional way from the vast array of informally trained caregivers.[60]

Marcuze's was the sentiment of someone who, coming from a vilified out-group, displayed far greater personal and social insecurity than, for example, the sons of the nobility and the commercial bourgeoisie who flocked to the popular faculties of law. Those individuals recognized that their professional futures were assured precisely because their personal and collective pasts had been so established. The marginal character of Marcuze's pedigree offers a stark contrast to that of the confident members of the ruling class. The homogenizing role of the university in German society, exposing provincials in a relatively unsophisticated country to cosmopolitan manners and lifestyles helped bridge the disparate regional, cultural, linguistic, and class backgrounds of the students.[61] This led to the development of a certain esprit de corps and fed the desire of Marcuze and other maskilic physicians to see themselves as part of an elite professional group, an ersatz Jewish nobility.[62] As members of this learned estate, or *Gelehrtenstand,* Jewish physicians sought to enjoy the privileges of exclusiveness and authority in both Jewish society, and the larger world as well.[63]

Like Wolf's *Von den Krankheiten der Juden,* Marcuze's *Seyfer Refues* offered an uncompromising critique of traditional Jewish life. And like Wolf—whom it can be safely assumed he read—Marcuze led an attack on Jewish education, speaking to the debilitating physical side effects of traditional modes of study. In a chapter on the care of children, Marcuze also employed the metaphor of bondage to describe the young Torah scholar's lot. Reminiscent of the description of the heder provided by his Polish, maskilic contemporary, Solomon Maimon, who also made his reputation among the representatives of the Haskalah in Germany, Marcuze wrote:

> Also, we men, the fathers, have in Poland a lovely custom with our dear little boys. When they turn four years old, we already send them to prison, to the elementary school teacher. They must sit as prisoners over the aleph-beys the whole day, and early in the morning, when it is the best time for children to sleep and thereby grow, the assistant teacher comes and drags them to the *heder,* to the synagogue.
>
> And when the child has already been imprisoned for a year with his *aleph-beys* teacher, they release him from the *siddur* and he must go to prison with the *gemara* teacher. Here he no longer has time to pray, let alone study the Bible—but only *gemara* and more *gemara*. He must, at the age of five, know the law that in the case of "damage caused by pebbles in a public domain, half the damage is to be paid." . . . He must become a scholar. . . . You make your children pale, yellow, green. They cannot sleep well. Hence they do not grow, and many common men are afterwards mistaken about their children: they think they are already scholars because they have pale faces.[64]

When it came to child-related issues, Marcuze was above all concerned with childbirth. However, unlike Wolf, who tended to blame Jewish mothers for their own ill health and that of their children, Marcuze took the opportunity to rail against midwives. It was they, he believed, who were the source of so many medical complaints:

> How many thousands of women have I seen and spoken with? They became weak, sick, and crippled at the hands of the midwives, because of our many sins. How many men have had to divorce their wives, though before their confinement they loved them much? . . . How many during childbirth or thereafter became insane, melancholic? . . . How many became ill with epilepsy? How many became ill with tuberculosis, blood poisoning, growths in the womb? How many became ill with jaundice, swellings, hernia? . . . Can you imagine, dear women, how many thousands of women and children had to die at the hands of the midwives? Why do you make so many new weddings for your husbands? Why do you leave us so many orphans in the hands of other women? (76a-b)

Marcuze's passion was overstated and unsupported by fact. Certainly, both pregnancy and childbirth were indeed perilous undertakings in Marcuze's day. One need only read the account of the delivery room by Charles White, one of the founders of the Manchester Lying-In Hospital. Like Marcuze's book, White's description dates from 1790: "When the woman is in labour, she is often attended by a number of friends in a small room, with a large fire, which, together with her own pains throw her into profuse sweats; by the heat of the chamber, and the breath of so many people, the whole air is rendered foul, and unfit for respiration."[65] Certainly the description applies to the labor process in Poland as well as Western Europe. Filth, sepsis, and puerperal fever, a form of blood poisoning associated with childbirth and miscarriage, were prevalent before the modern period and were the principal causes of parturition-related fatalities. Marcuze also urged that standards of hygiene be improved by, for example, imploring women to dispose of the afterbirth properly "neither leaving it, God-forbid, in the bed nor in the house"(136). He issued his calls for improved obstetric conditions in the larger context of his diatribe, which he entitled "More Against Grandmothers and Witches." The essence of his complaint was that the superstitious advice of various "stupid" and "dumb" women involved in the birth of a child brought about unsanitary birthing conditions. Marcuze did not mention men, the general culture, or the conditions that obtained among

Christians as being responsible for or parallel to Jewish society. Rather, he placed blame squarely on the shoulders of Jewish midwives.

Generally speaking, the practice of midwifery in Jewish society was similar to that which existed in the Gentile world. In most decent-sized communities, midwives were employed by the *kehillah,* who paid their full salary or sometimes merely subsidized what the woman earned from private practice, through tax exemptions or free rent. Gifts and tips from patients also contributed to the midwife's earnings. As for privileges, these often had a religious basis. For example, among Christians, midwives were given special permission to baptize stillborn children. Jewish midwives were sometimes accorded special honors such as exemptions from certain sumptuary laws or, as was the case in Mannheim, were relieved of the necessity of providing a dowry if they wished to marry. Also patterned on the Christian model, Jewish midwives were examined before being hired, and in a city like Posen, they were employed for a probationary trial period.[66] The bulk of midwives' incomes derived from fees earned in private practice, the communities setting no limits on what could be charged, leaving such decisions to the marketplace and local custom.

Marcuze's hostility toward midwives reflects a larger cultural transformation. By the end of the eighteenth century, attitudes toward childbirth underwent radical change. For the first time in history, it was no longer seen merely as a natural event but primarily as a medical matter and thus best left to physicians. Thus, one result of the assault on midwives was the founding of the first European institutions for the teaching of obstetrics. Claims that doctors had greater competency than midwives because of their theoretical training were constantly invoked in the dispute between the two groups.[67]

Marcuze's stance toward the Jewish midwives in Poland was informed by the models he knew of and had observed in his travels through Northern Europe. He had been in England, where midwifery had gone into recent decline. This was partly due to the fact that midwives, who had previously come from the upper classes but had withdrawn to a world of respectability and affluence by the middle of the eighteenth century, had abandoned the profession. Consequently, women who lived in cities sought the services of the doctor rather than those of the less skilled village midwife.[68] In eighteenth-century Germany, very strict regulation and control of midwives resulted in obstetric authority passing on to the university-trained physician. Impressed with Northern European models, Marcuze seemed to favor a gradual approach for Poland, one akin to the situation he had observed in Holland, where the very tight system of control offered a short-term solution to the problem of midwife incompetency.⁶⁹ To implement his program, Marcuze beseeched his female readers: "Why do you not persuade your husbands to let the midwives study from learned doctors. . . . It will not cost you much. Let one from each town or townlet study, and twenty will learn and know. These twenty trained midwives will teach a hundred others, and the hundred in turn will teach a thousand others. . . . For your sake, let me bring it about that in every town or *shtetl* all should read about their health from my book, that you might have some knowledge—the men what pertains to men and the women what pertains to women, in case, God forbid, you should become sick."⁷⁰ Marcuze's pedagogic remedy betrays his goal and highlights his paternalism and professional anxiety—the former engendered by his sense of superiority, the latter by his faith in science and the physician's possession of privileged information.

Obviously, as part of their Enlightenment project, Jewish doctors were engaged in promoting a professional agenda. They were proud of their physician's credentials, gained, as Marcuze noted, in the "schools of the gentile sages"—a phrase similarly used by his predecessor from Frankfurt, Tobias Cohen, in his *Ma'aseh Tuviyyah*.⁷¹ Moreover, the widespread faith of the Jews in their own folk medicine, as Marcuze himself recognized, constituted both commercial competition—he chastises Polish Jews for being too "stingy" to pay for a real doctor—and even more important, a rivalry of authority (122b). He is particularly scornful of the public's trust in "our dear doctors or healers, who are called among us in Poland *rofim* and feldshers. I call them public, well-known specialists in killing [*bravitene memitim*], not doctors" (81b).

In addition to midwives, Marcuze's professional biases led him to turn his attention to the healing abilities of the most ubiquitous of medical caregivers in Jewish Poland, the feldshers. According to a recent study, feldshers were "persons with practical and theoretical training in medicine and surgery below the standard university level, licensed to exercise the medical profession under specific conditions and restrictions in certain countries."⁷² The term derives from the German word *Feldscherer*, or literally, "military man with shears." Appearing in the fifteenth and sixteenth centuries, these men cut the hair and shaved the beards of soldiers in the field, and eventually expanded their activities to include the administration of first aid and later bleeding, a most popular form of medical therapy. The feldshers, or barber-surgeons as they were known in Western Europe, continued to exist in Eastern Europe into the twentieth century. Marcuze, who viewed feldshers with suspicion and fear, claimed that they were completely unqualified and whatever medical knowledge they did possess had been acquired from reading smatterings of *Ma'aseh Tuviyyah*.

It appears that the first documented Jewish feldsher in Poland was David Ilin, who served with the Polish and Swedish forces during the wars of 1648 and 1656. Later, in 1683, Jewish feldshers were to be found in the army of king Jan Sobieski. This tradition of Jewish military medical service in Poland continued unabated through the following century and also helped establish the good name and reputation of the feldshers among the Jewish masses.[73]

From the start, Jewish and Christian feldshers were occupied differently because of religious proscriptions. Jewish practitioners rarely came to feldsherism via the barbershop. Jewish legal prohibitions against males shaving meant that few clients among Jews existed for these services, and so the Jewish feldsher limited his activities by and large to surgery and the treatment of wounds. It is possible that such focused clinical treatment made for a more medically skilled practitioner. However, this was not always the case. In one of the very few descriptions of medical care among Jews of the early modern period, we read about the slow death in the winter of 1689 of Hayyim Hamel. In this poignant Yiddish account by his wife, Glikl bas Judah Leib, better known as Glückel of Hameln, we learn that her husband insisted that a Sephardic physician and barber-surgeon be called. Feldsher Abraham Lopez, and the feldshers that Lopez in turn summoned for consultation, were all unable to effect a cure. For four days Hayyim lay in great pain, having suffered severe abdominal injuries in a heavy fall. In addition to the repeated applications of poultices and invasive surgery, the family called in a Dr. Fonseca, yet another Sephardic physician, and still yet another from Berlin. All proved ineffective. Seeking solace in his religious books, Hayyim studied for the last half hour of his life, silently recited the Shema, and passed away on Sunday, January 16.[74]

Unfortunately, we know very little about the activities of Jewish feldshers in the eighteenth century, our principal era of inquiry. However, we are well informed about the nineteenth century, and it is possible, with this information, to reflect backward 100 years to Marcuze's time and make some careful assumptions about feldsherism in his day. With the partitioning of Poland—1773, 1793, and 1795—the country was divided between Austria, Russia, and Prussia, with the eventual creation in 1815 of the Kingdom of Poland, also called Congress Poland. Absorbed into Russia, the Kingdom of Poland was granted a constitution, an elected lower house called the Diet, which enjoyed limited authority, and a reasonably autonomous army.[75]

## HASKALAH AND HEALING

This was the situation until the European revolutions of 1830 when Polish nationalists, emboldened by the collapse of the Bourbon regime in France, seized the opportunity to overthrow the Russians. Alone, divided among itself, and surrounded by superior Russian forces, the Polish revolution was easily crushed. Among the many repressive measures that followed was the dissolution of the once semi-autonomous Polish army. This meant that many, if not most of the military's feldshers had to seek employment in civilian society.

One result of the above-mentioned events was that under Russian rule, the number of Jewish feldshers by the end of the nineteenth century was staggering. Official statistics for 1887 indicate that there were 1,971 Jewish feldshers in Russia. Of these, over 90 percent resided in either the Kingdom of Poland or the Pale of Settlement. While Jews constituted only approximately 4 percent of the total population, 28 percent of all feldshers were Jews. Perhaps most important, there were fewer Jewish doctors — 1,077, to be precise. Just over 6 percent of all Russian physicians were Jews. Only Jewish dentists and midwives formed percentages comparable to that of the feldshers; roughly 20 percent and 19 percent, respectively.[76]

Although we cannot be as numerically precise about the population of feldshers in 1790, we can be certain that given the situation in 1890, at the very least, the number of feldshers and midwives in Poland significantly outweighed the number of university-trained physicians. In fact, it is safe to assume that the percentage differences may have been even greater in Marcuze's day, for the secularizing tendency of the Eastern European Haskalah, which eventually resulted in young Russian Jews flocking to medical faculties in Western Europe in unprecedented numbers was still a long way off.

Finally, one of the steps taken by Tsar Alexander I, who had orchestrated the creation of the Kingdom of Poland, was to establish professional schools for feldshers and midwives, modeled on the Prussian hospital, the Charité.[77] Although the two-year course of instruction was not of especially high standard, the formal training it provided combined with the extensive clinical experience of its teachers resulted in the graduation of fairly competent health care professionals. They were, in short, not as untrained and given to butchery and malpractice as Marcuze would have had his readers believe.

Nonetheless, Marcuze adopted an almost hysterical tone when discussing the damage done by those he regarded as charlatans:

> And I say again today: May those who publicly kill people, and no one prevents them from doing so, have their names wiped out. They are

given food, drink, and a few gold coins for expenses, so that they may travel further and again make dead men out of living ones. It is high time, dear people, for you to open your eyes for once and not let killings take place in your house, in your city. Place trustees and guards on such vile persons and transfer them into the hands of another people; let them be killed for all of you. Take a lesson from the whole world. One does not hear of such debauched characters dragging themselves about and openly killing people with no one to prevent them. Unfortunately many clothe themselves, because of our sins, in the garments of rabbis and have a bit of learning; these kill even more people. Punish them. . . . May their names be blotted out and may they be condemned to death by burning [*zoll zey alle in srayfe gevorfn verdn*].[78]

It is evident from this passage that Marcuze was concerned with the control and regulation of those he deemed unqualified to administer health care. In lieu of a state apparatus, he insisted that the Jewish community undertake the task itself, monitoring, prosecuting, and punishing the alleged offenders. In essence, Marcuze and other maskilic doctors sought to deny the masses access to traditional forms of medical care, no matter how efficacious or, indeed, similar to the type they would have offered. Marcuze's admission that he had himself bled several times a year—a common procedure generally performed by barber-surgeons—is an example of the similarity between certain medical practices offered by both "popular" and university-trained caregivers.[79] But as an interested party, Marcuze refused to accept and acknowledge that society sponsored the intimate proximity of medical orthodoxy and fringe practice.[80]

In suggesting the adoption of stringent measures, Marcuze was giving expression to contemporary notions about state control of (unlicensed) doctors and, by extension, patients. Although it was not until 1794 that the Prussian *Allgemeines Landrecht* prohibited the practice of medicine by unlicensed practitioners—a law honored mostly in the breach—the desire for such legislation had already been expressed for some time. In fact, Germany, where Marcuze had studied medicine, tended to lead the way in the eighteenth century in establishing the degree to which state intervention worked to control the learned professions.[81]

In seeking to impart their knowledge about medicine to the lay public, doctors of the eighteenth century were also making the claim that they could exercise control over disease. Through the dissemination of information about hygiene, medical manuals such as Wolf's and Marcuze's were part of a larger Enlightenment-inspired effort to rationally instruct and engineer society for the purposes of achieving the greater good. This in turn led to the creation of a field of specialty now called public health, the guiding principle of which was preventative medicine. Its origins lie in seventeenth-century England and are most closely associated with Thomas Sydenham and John Arbuthnot, whose chief concerns lay with effective disease treatment. On the Continent, under such figures as Friedrich Hoffmann in Germany, Bernadino Ramazzini in Italy, and François Bossier de Sauvages in France, the emphasis shifted to an investigation of the principal environmental factors that caused disease. The eighteenth century's classic expression of this "medical environmentalism," or what Michel Foucault has called a "medicine of climates" and a "medicine of places," was Johann Peter Frank's (1745–1821) tract "The People's Misery: Mother of Diseases," which appeared in 1790, the same year as Marcuze's book.[82] In it Frank identified poverty as the chief cause of disease, and demanded that the state implement social reforms in order to pave the way for the physical well-being of its citizens.[83]

Most significantly for maskilic physicians, who had been deeply influenced by these general trends, "medical geography," or the writing of a medical profile or case history of a particular locale, was especially well developed in Germany. There, the practitioners of the genre sought to enlist the resources of the centralized governments to push their programs of hygienic and sanitation improvement. Hence the Germans referred to the administration of such reforms as *"medizinische Polizey,"* or medical policing.[84] Wolf, Marcuze, and Marcus Herz were inspired by the possibilities offered by the teachings and practical implementation of Enlightenment medicine. Their goal as physicians was to assist their fellow Jews undergo environmental change, cultural adaptation, and behavioral transformation.

The cultural and intellectual universe in which maskilic physicians operated was shaped by Enlightenment medicine, with its stress on care of the body here on earth as opposed to preparation of the soul for the world to come.[85] To be sure, the secularization of medicine was a process further advanced among Christian physicians than among Jews in the eighteenth century. Marcuze, for example, expressed the traditional Jewish view of the physician as instrument of God when he exhorted his readers not to "believe in old women. Trust in God, blessed is He and blessed is His great name, and in His wisdom, of which he has given us so much, so that you can help me help you with the blessing of His aid" (136). It is noteworthy that this fundamentally Jewish teaching was ultimately compatible with the increasingly mechanistic and utilitarian trends in European medicine. Taken together, Jewish and Enlightenment medical outlooks helped foster the active and preventative medicine preached by the Jewish doctors of the Haskalah.

Finally, it is important to note that despite the prevalence of "medical geography" in Germany, neither Wolf nor Marcuze ever made reference to central figures in the campaign to improve urban conditions such as the above-mentioned Hoffmann and Frank, or to Johann Phillip Burggrave and Johann Adolph Behrends and their respective studies of Frankfurt, the largest Jewish city in Germany. Haskalah physicians were clearly aware of the writings of these people, their own works belonging very much to the genre. Nevertheless, their refusal to mention them could only have left Jewish readers with the impression that the deplorable conditions they described were particular to Jews alone. The texts were designed to shame as much as they were to educate their readers. Admitting that Christians also lived under despicable hygienic conditions — a fact the Jews could see for themselves — would have blunted the polemical force of the arguments of Jewish doctors.

Similarly, Marcuze's reformist project to promote the bourgeois sensibility of moderation among the Jews also led him to isolate another of their "vices," one that he conveniently failed to mention was a greater affliction among Poles. In the 1780s Marcuze settled in Volhynia, the cradle of Hasidism. Hostile to the growing movement, he went to great pains to denigrate members of the sect, including chastising them for excessive alcohol consumption. In addition to his criticism of the intemperance of the Hasidim, Marcuze virulently decried the practice of popular medicine and folk cures among the Jewish masses, especially that provided by Hasidim. It is little wonder, then, that the Hasidim were angered by this attack on folk medicine, given that Israel ben Eliezer Baal Shem-Tov (1700–1760), the founder of Hasidism, was in fact a faith healer and amulet writer, whose first followers in the 1730s and 1740s were patients who had come to him to be cured.[86] Moreover, some Hasidic leaders, such as Nachman of Bratslav, specifically instructed their dutiful followers to avoid doctors.[87] Finally, as a vigorous adversary of Hasidism, Marcuze was either influenced by or simply at one with Raphael Kohen, who not only enjoyed a reputation as a fighter against the Haskalah but also was a prominent *mitnaged,* or opponent of Hasidism. In response to Marcuze's attack on them, Hasidim bought up nearly every copy of his book and consigned them all to the flames. As a consequence, copies of *Seyfer Refues* are extremely rare.

The link between Marcuze's own enlightened Prussian origins — he stressed the fact that he sported no beard — and his antipathy for the Hasidim and most other Eastern European folkways is palpable throughout

*Seyfer Refues*. The author regarded popular medicine not only as bad in and of itself, but also more generally as representative of the backwardness of Eastern European Jewish culture. For Marcuze, folk medicine was symptomatic of that "primitive" culture. As he saw it, it was not only incapable of helping the ill recover, but could also actually worsen the condition of the Jewish patient. And, as stated above, the practice of folk medicine also challenged his own authority as a professionally trained scientist. In explaining why he penned *Seyfer Refues,* Marcuze provided a Chaucerian parade of Jewish characters who, with their own folk remedies, were integral to the popular Jewish medical and, indeed religious culture of late eighteenth-century Poland.[88] It was a culture that Marcuze, the Königsberg-educated physician, desperately wanted to eradicate: "I wished to benefit many thousands of people with my book . . . [to save them from] such defectives as, for instance, old women, bad midwives, exorcisors of the evil eye, . . . ignorant miracle workers [*baalei shemot*], and terribly wicked people; from pourers of wax [for magical purposes], from fortunetellers who diagnose all diseases, from bad preachers who offer remedies for sale, or for a good supper, or for the sake of a small contribution, and from little "doctors" who have made themselves doctors, or who have been made such by foolish old women" (6a-b).

Lest the impression be gained that it was only in Poland that this type of folk medicine was widely practiced by the Jews, in 1789 in Berlin the famous doctor and Kantian philosopher, Marcus Herz (1747–1803), felt obliged to write the following in defense of the medical profession in his "Tefilla La-Rofe" (The physician's prayer): "Oh God of faithfulness, place in the heart of the sick trust in me and my work, and an ear to listen to my advice. Remove from their bedside every quack doctor, every large entourage, [and all] heralds and saviors, who come forth regularly, like sages and councilors, to scheme together; also the gaggle of care-taking women, who pretend to know, *who dare to rise up and criticize the work of a doctor*. For they are a vile people. In their haughtiness, they hinder the good effect of medicine, and bring men down from Your health-giving and healing to the chambers of death" [emphasis added].[89]

Marcus Herz was born in Berlin and, like his mentor, Moses Mendelssohn, was the son of a Torah scribe. When he turned fifteen, Herz moved to Königsberg and, again like the sage from Dessau, worked as a commercial clerk after having begun study for the rabbinate. Not long after the teenager was welcomed into the home of the prominent Friedländer family, where he met the future community leader and advocate of religious reform, David Friedländer, Herz forsook his desire to become a businessman. The Friedländers were not only powerful but also thoroughly steeped in European culture. The taste of it, which Herz acquired in his hosts' company, changed him forever.[90]

Seeking to broaden his intellectual horizons, Herz attended lectures at the University of Königsberg from 1766 to 1770, but financially strapped, he had to abandon his studies. Nevertheless, Herz's experience at the university was of seminal importance to his intellectual development. From this time on, his interests developed principally in the areas of medicine and philosophy.[91] In addition, the impression he made on others while at Königsberg was significant. In August 1770, the philosopher Immanuel Kant defended his dissertation after having named Herz as his "advocate," despite the strenuous opposition of other faculty members.[92] In 1774 Herz graduated from the University of Halle with a medical degree, having been supported in that undertaking by David Friedländer.[93] Under the influence of the Enlightenment and Kantian philosophy, and perhaps especially Kant's negative views on biblical Judaism, Herz became an arch rationalist and eschewed traditional practice and ritual observance.[94]

Herz and his brilliant, beautiful wife, Henriette, led a glittering life in Berlin. Their house was one of the first of the celebrated Jewish salons, which arose in the capital in the 1780s. There, members of different estates and occupational groups gathered to socialize and exchange ideas.[95] The Jewish hosts entertained Gentile representatives of the Enlightenment and nobility in an extraordinary atmosphere of social conviviality that knew no precedents in modern times and marked the limited yet important exposure of upperclass Jews to the intellectual and social mores of the dominant society. The Herzs' open salon was one where she with her Romanticist sensibilities entertained guests in one room by expounding on the latest works of literature and art, while he, the classic Enlightenment rationalist, lectured on natural science, medicine, and philosophy in another.[96] In addition, he frequently demonstrated science experiments with his wife's assistance for the edification and amusement of their guests. Together, the two made an arresting couple. The manner in which they complemented each other and the social benefits they accrued from combining their respective qualities was not lost on Henriette. Recalling that time, she wrote: "Through his intellect and as a famous doctor Herz attracted people, and I attracted them through my beauty and through the understanding I had for all kinds of scholarship."[97]

The very different Jewish experiences the couple enjoyed respectively also had a major impact on Herz. They were married in 1779 when he was thirty-two, and she a mere fifteen. Henriette came from a wealthy family of Portuguese origin, having migrated to Berlin in the seventeenth century from Amsterdam, that refuge and safe haven for so many Iberian Jews. With her moneyed and culturally open background—she had command of French, English, Latin, Hebrew, Italian, Portuguese, and Danish, as well as familiarity with Turkish, Malay, and Sanskrit—this unusually precocious and gifted person exerted a profound impact upon her husband's sensibilities. The cultural and social avenues that became open to him via his marriage further challenged Herz's traditional and parochial background, already severely undermined during his sojourn in Königsberg. His material circumstances also contributed to the transformation. With the handsome income he now earned as a physician, Herz became a worldly, cultivated man, at home in European civilization, increasingly detached from his observant Jewish roots. Notably, many Jews with backgrounds similar to that of Herz had their faith sorely challenged after attending his lectures. As Wolf Davidson, a physician and radical proponent of Christian-Jewish union, remarked in a treatise on the civil amelioration of the Jews, "I know many an orthodox Jew who after leaving Herz's lectures on physics began to doubt the teachings on miracles."[98]

Yet Herz's abandonment of ritual was accompanied by neither a departure from the Jewish community nor a neglect of pressing issues of Jewish concern. He was an active and tireless community worker who enjoyed a stellar reputation as a communal doctor, and in 1782 became director of the Jewish Hospital in Berlin, a position previously held by his father-in-law, Benjamin de Lemos.[99] In fact, Herz was the quintessential modern, secular Jew. He remained within the fold and expressed communal solidarity and activism, yet ritual for him now more often than not entailed the performance of laboratory experiments rather than time-honored Jewish customs. The source of his authority within Jewish society was also new. It derived from an intricate combination of social standing, wealth, Jewish literacy, and his status as respected physician.

Herz's intellectual and religious development as well as his deeply held sense of responsibility to the community formed a cluster of sensibilities that made him the Haskalah's most celebrated Jewish doctor. His nonchalant attitude toward Jewish ritual and his passion for medicine and reason later served to place him at the center of one of the Haskalah's most important discussions of the Jewish body. It is to that which we now turn our attention.

Emblematic of the new attitude of Jewish physicians during the Haskalah, wherein they challenged the lifestyle of the Jewish masses as unhealthy and sought to assume the mantle of the sole protectors of the health of the Jewish people, was their stance in the "burial controversy" of the late eighteenth century. The most important doctor to become ensnared in the debate was Marcus Herz. Although Jewish historians have traditionally pictured the terms of the debate as a battle between religious reformers and traditionalists, it must also be seen as a chapter in the modern discourse about the Jewish body.[100]

Just as with life, ancient laws and customs stringently regulate the death of the individual Jew. Previously the singular domain of rabbis, the regulations concerning Jewish death became, in this period, subject to political and scientific discussion, just as they did among contemporary non-Jews. Beginning in the sixteenth century, but firmly in place by the eighteenth, the traditional European culture of death had been deeply and permanently affected by the uncertainty of the fate of the deceased, a concern spawned by the increasing secularization of society in the wake of the Enlightenment. According to Ingrid Stoessel, medieval consciousness was spared the angst that accompanies the reality of inevitable death by the religious "certainty of resurrection," or the possibility of there being an even "better life" to be enjoyed after death.[101]

With the Enlightenment doctrine that death was the absolute end of life, the fear of Hell and the promise of Paradise were cast aside. Within this new cultural climate of certainty, a sudden death could be accepted and understood. But apparent death—for example, a death-like coma that led to a premature burial and a prolonged, agonizing death in the grave itself—would underscore the ambiguous state in which the so-called deceased existed and thus could not be intellectually, let alone practicably, assimilated into the worldview of the rationalist eighteenth century. Premature burial and the resultant death in the grave itself would validate the belief in the existence of Hell. For Martin Patak, apparent death (*Scheintod*) was, therefore, the product of a clash between rational Enlightenment tendencies on the one hand and the hidden yet still prevalent power of irrationality and sentiment on the other.[102]

The emergence of the idea of Scheintod was given further impetus by changes in the artistic representation of the human body in anatomical dissections. In the sixteenth century, the body in such renderings continued to appear as though it were alive, only still. In the seventeenth century, the depiction of individual dissected and dismembered organs made it difficult if not impossible for viewers to recognize their own bodies in the artistic rendering.[103] These drawings also placed beyond the grasp of viewers the possibility of imagining bodily resurrection. This contrasted sharply with the dominant medieval worldview in the Christian West, for as Carolyn Walker Bynum has noted, "resurrection [in the Middle Ages] is victory over partition and putrefaction."[104]

By the second half of the eighteenth century, much had changed, although the desire for the security offered by resurrection remained strong. Instead of a traditional fear of death mitigated by the hope of resurrection born of religious conviction, secularization, art, and science had turned death into a clinical affair, shorn of emotion. In place of the old culture of death, the phenomenon of what was called "apparent-death" came to the fore. Said to be the condition of still being alive, while displaying no vital signs, such as respiration or pulse, Scheintod as a belief offered the possibility of a feeling or sense of immortality, and thus the hope that death had not really occurred, but had only appeared to have taken place. On the other hand, and of immediate impact, the "discovery" of the condition of Scheintod provoked a veritable craze throughout Europe in the eighteenth and nineteenth centuries, a fear of being buried alive.[105] Ingrid Stoessel has called Scheintod a "pathological form of angst," while Philippe Ariès has described the fear as "a vast anxiety [which took] hold of the collective consciousness." In attempting to explain why the issue had become so important to the medical profession, Ariès opines that the profound concern that modern medicine expressed over determining with exactitude the signs of death, in order to prevent premature inhumation, was most likely promoted by its particular quest for establishing scientific certainty. In the face of death, a most ambiguous condition, physicians were adamant that the body should not be permitted to linger in an ill-defined state—that is, hovering between life and death.[106]

The increasingly scientific, post-Galenic medicine that emerged in the eighteenth century bred a demand for greater exactitude and precision when both diagnosing disease and determining death. Most contemporary authors who addressed the topic asserted that reliable scientific evidence to prove that death had in fact occurred was difficult to come by. On this subject, considerable disagreement existed within the medical community. While most physicians still relied on traditional signs of death such as absence of pulse, cessation of breathing, skin pallor, and rigor mortis, others maintained that the only certain sign of death was the onset of putrefaction.[107] The first successful resuscitations of the drowned took place in the eighteenth century, only further fueling medical uncertainty about what constituted accurate signs of death.[108]

The belief in Scheintod, therefore, led to myriad proposals and measures, many of which involved gruesome surgical, electrical, and galvanic experiments designed to counter a misdiagnosis of death and its consequence, premature burial.[109] Moreover, within a ten-year period, beginning with Amsterdam in 1767, societies dedicated to the preservation and resuscitation of life were established all over Europe. The largest and most important of such institutions was the Royal Humane Society in London, established in 1774.[110]

But despite the widespread and sometimes exotic measures for revivification—tobacco enemas or the blowing of smoke into the intestines—and the development of an extensive scientific literature, most physicians and other interested parties remained uncertain and confused about the nature of death. Consequently, death would no longer merely be a medical or religious problem, but a political one. It would be the State's concern. In lieu of a medical consensus, it was widely held that the best solution was to establish mortuaries where the bodies would be watched over for a few days before proceeding with burial.[111] The social and cultural consequences of such a recommendation were negligible for the overwhelming majority of European Christians, who tended to forestall burial anyway—but not so for the Jews, who were and are obliged to bury their dead within twenty-four hours.[112]

In Germany in 1772, the Jewish community of Schwerin was the first on the Continent to face the practical consequences of broader European concerns about premature burial. In order to avoid the ghastly error of burying someone alive, the Duke of Mecklenburg-Schwerin, upon the recommendation of the missionary and Orientalist Oluf Gerhard Tychsen (1734–1815), suggested that the Jews be forced to wait three days before burying their dead.[113] Aghast at the prospect of violating the time-honored practice of speedy burial, the community turned to the eminent Rabbi Jacob Emden of Altona for support. He confirmed the correctness of the community's opposition and, moreover, requested that the philosopher, and spiritual leader of German Jewry, Moses Mendelssohn (1729–1786), write on behalf of the community to the duke in order to dissuade the latter from implementing a decree that defied Jewish tradition and law. Mendelssohn's appeal to the duke contained the suggestion that a physician should bury no Jew without prior certification of death. The duke accepted the proposal, and the matter was resolved. But in a cover letter to the Jewish community accompanying a draft of the memorandum he sent to the duke, Mendelssohn stated that he did not believe that following the ducal decree constituted a violation of any religious laws. The community was furious, and a major rift formed between Mendelssohn and Emden.[114]

There the issue lay until Isaac Euchel (1756–1804), a Danish-born maskil and the first editor of the Haskalah journal, *Ha-Meassef,* resurrected it in 1785.[115] Euchel, who had written the above-mentioned play, *Reb Henekh,* had migrated from Copenhagen to Königsberg in 1773, where, like Herz, he also later attended the lectures of Immanuel Kant, soon establishing himself as an uncompromising rationalist and radical maskil.[116] The links between Herz and Euchel were further cemented by virtue of the fact that just as Herz had been taken into the Friedländer home, Euchel also served as a tutor in the same house after settling in Königsberg. Additionally, both men were deeply attached to Moses Mendelssohn, with Euchel becoming his first biographer. Finally, like Herz, Euchel had become estranged from ritual, refusing to acknowledge rabbinic authority. Testimony for this comes from the Berlin rabbi Tsvi Hirsch Levin, who caustically remarked that: "Indeed, truly a world turned upside down. Once pigs used to eat acorns (*Eichel*), and now Euchel eats pig."[117]

In 1785, Euchel launched a campaign in *Ha-Meassef,* in which he argued against traditional Jewish burial customs.[118] In preparing the series of articles for publication, Euchel had sought the expertise of Marcus Herz, whose opinions in favor of delaying burial eventually appeared in his pamphlet entitled *Über die frühe Beerdigung der Juden* (1787) (On the premature burial of the Jews). A second, expanded edition appeared the following year.

Herz, the rationalist physician, philosopher, and learned Jew, resorted to a defense based not only on the most modern advances of medical science, but also on references drawn from relevant discussions in the Talmud. Written in a tone described by Ludwig Geiger as one of "beautiful irony" and "mordant sarcasm," Herz's position on early burial was directly related to the contemporary fear of premature interment.[119] His melodramatic description of being buried alive—inspired by his own near-death illness in 1780, which lasted for three weeks and from which he miraculously recovered almost overnight—clearly illustrates the horror with which a person of the eighteenth century beheld the prospect of such a ghastly occurrence. The description is worthy of being quoted at length because it constituted a broadside against his own fellow Jews who, he felt, remained wedded to practices that endangered the health and, indeed, the life of the Jewish people:

> My brothers, you simply can never have imagined the true horror of what it must be like for someone to awake in the grave! . . . Follow me into that musty grave, which only yesterday received its incumbent, not dead but slumbering. Only now he rouses from his slumber,

his energies revive, his heart regains its beat, his face its color and his soul returns to consciousness. The first thought which rises from the darkness is heartfelt gratitude to the gracious Creator who has called him back to the joys of life. Now a thousand ecstatic thoughts crisscross his mind: of good deeds in the future to render him worthy of such divine grace; of the happiness of his spouse who had almost died of grief at her loss; the leaping for joy of his children who had been so nearly orphaned. . . .

Now his recovery has progressed still further. He opens his eyes; around him everything is dark and desolate. . . . He groans, cries, pleads with all the powers that he has struggled so hard to regain: to no avail, he languishes unheard. He touches his bed and grasps, not the soft down of a bedspread, but instead a clod of damp, wormy earth.[120]

Herz framed his discussion of Jewish burial around four principal questions: First, he asked, "Are there unambiguous signs, by which one can distinguish in every case those who are truly dead from those who only appear to be so, within four hours (our usual waiting period [before burial])?" Second, "If there are, do the people working in the burial society know them, and if they claim to, on what do they base their certainty?" Third, "If there are none, are there religious, moral, or political reasons of such importance that they move us to bury the dead in this speedy manner; are such reasons so bound up with our welfare that we must follow them, heedless of the danger of burying a person alive?" And finally, asked Herz, "If there are no reasons of this type, would it not be advisable to discontinue this practice and follow the example of our ethical and enlightened neighbors, who watch over their dead for at least several days before burial?" (6–7).

As to the first question, Herz stated that, since ancient times, doctors had had tremendous difficulty in determining the signs of death. In fact, he related that he personally knew a twenty-year-old woman who, when she was four years old, was paralyzed by an apoplectic stroke and was thought to have died. Her family went into mourning and prepared for the funeral, but because the girl lived in a village and she "expired" on a Friday afternoon (and Jews are not permitted to perform a burial on the Sabbath), it was necessary to wait until Sunday before she could be transported to the nearest cemetery. The forty-hour wait saved her because en route to her own funeral she regained consciousness and was carried home in her father's arms (8). Herz corroborated this story with a similar example from the Talmud. Bas-

# Marcus Herz
## über
# die frühe Beerdigung
## der Juden.

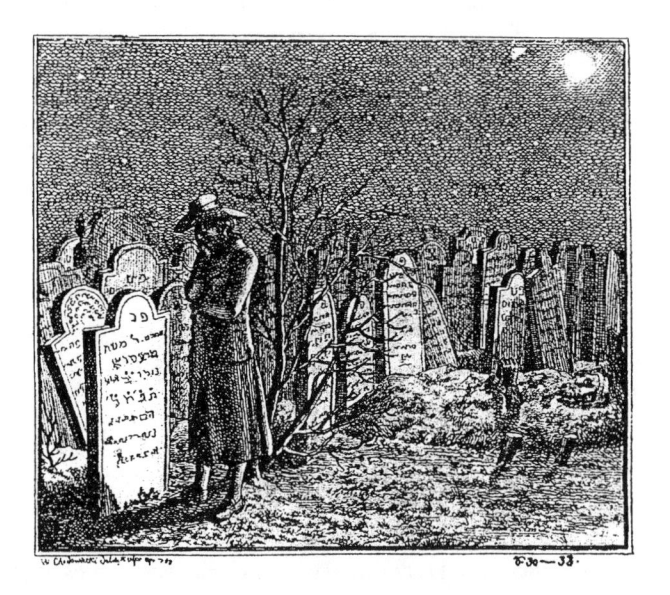

An die Herausgeber des hebräischen Sammlers.

Zweyte verbesserte und vermehrte Auflage.

Berlin, 1788.
Bey Christian Friedrich Voß und Sohn.

ing an argument on a reference such as the Talmud was intended to display his Jewish erudition and to lend substance, tinged with piety, to his remarks. It was also an opportunity to definitively distinguish the "close-minded" rabbis like Jacob Emden in Altona and Ezekiel Landau in Prague, "zealots who would banish Reason from the face of the earth," from the "wise" rabbis of the Talmud, whom Herz applauded for recognizing the limits of their own wisdom.[121]

With the second question, concerning the qualifications of Jewish burial society functionaries to determine the signs of death, we return to the crucial issue at the heart of maskilic medical texts: the battle to wrest control of the Jewish body from traditional Judaism and its representatives, and to place control in the hands of the scientifically trained and socially superior. To this end, Herz questioned the abilities of the men of the burial society, stating that: "in general, the criteria of death upon which the men of the sick-care and burial society rely are dilated pupils and the absence of pulse and respiration. They certify the last-named of these criteria if a candle flame held in front of the mouth burns quietly or if a feather held before the nose remains unmoving. No sooner are the examinations done than they declare the person dead, remove him from his bed, lay him on straw, and bury him after four hours. However, all of these examinations prove at most that circulation of the blood and respiration have ceased. In no way do they demonstrate that the inner cause of life is completely destroyed" (19–20).

For Herz, the answer was quite clear. The men of the burial society were unqualified to pass judgment on whether someone had or had not expired.[122] In this respect, he was correct. Membership in a *Hevra Kadisha*, or burial society, was not dependent on medical knowledge of any sort.[123] In fact, there were almost as many requirements for membership as there were brotherhoods. Sometimes all that was needed was proof of one's orthodoxy

---

FIGURE 5. The title page of Marcus Herz's *Über die frühe Beerdigung der Juden* (Berlin, 1788) (On the premature burial of the Jews), an engraving by Wilhelm Chodwiecki (1765–1805). In this Gothic scene at a Jewish cemetery, the mourner visits the grave of Moses Mendelssohn in Berlin. In semi-darkness, and lost in thought, he faces the headstone, oblivious to the fact that behind him, in the moonlight, a hand rises in the air from a man presumed to be dead. The fear of premature burial was widespread in the eighteenth century, and Herz, who wanted to emulate the Christian practice of delaying burial, found himself in the midst of a communal storm when he advocated that his co-religionists wait a period of three days before burying their dead. He lost the battle.

and sound character. In Amsterdam in 1742, Breslau in 1761, and Königsberg in 1779, membership was open only to Jewish men who wore beards—a telling comment about lapsing traditionalism and incipient modernity. Almost everywhere, admission fees had to be paid. Occasionally these took the form of monetary payments, and in other cases a Torah scroll, wine, and even pewter plates were accepted either as payment, or as supplements to cash. As a respected physician in Berlin's Jewish Hospital, Herz was clearly aware of all this.[124] It rankled him that some men of the Hevra Kadisha occupied the position because they had defrayed the costs of a banquet for the entire brotherhood membership, or that a minor, under the age of thirteen, could be admitted because his father was in the society. For Herz, the importance of the position demanded that doctors and not well-heeled community members be given authority to pronounce death.

In response to the third question, Herz saw absolutely no religious, moral, or political reasons inherent in Judaism that would oblige people to bury their dead so quickly. On the contrary, a religion so dedicated to the idea of "brotherly love, life, and blissfulness" would never ordain such dangerous practices. The "source" of the current dilemma was contemporary rabbinic authority, a force "bedecked in dark mystical expressions, enveloped in verbose and meaningless phrases." The moral problem was the rejection of reason as a guiding principle for human conduct. And politically, Herz was in complete agreement with Elcan Isaac Wolf. He, too, believed wholeheartedly that the Jews no longer lived under the yoke of arbitrary rule. Rather, living under benevolent laws in a state whose duty it was to protect its subjects, it was incumbent upon Jews to dispense with dangerous practices whose specifics emanated from "petty tyrants" (22–52).

Finally, to rectify the situation, Herz proposed that Jews wait two or three days before burying their dead in order to ascertain the cessation of all vital signs. Moreover, he recommended that the individual be brought to a mortuary that was roomy, ventilated, and heated in winter. Significantly, a physician was to visit the deceased to examine for any signs of life.[125] Herz also encouraged a delay in the onset of preparations for burial: they were not to begin until the waiting period was over. Finally, he addressed the case of pregnant women who had died, insisting that they were not to be removed from their homes until an obstetrician had examined them and determined whether and how the child's life might be saved. Above all, Herz insisted that a body was not to be considered a corpse, but merely as one suspected of having died, until the cessation of life could be indisputably confirmed (57–59).

Herz met with stiff opposition from an unlikely and interesting source, Jacob Marx. Unlikely, because Marx was a physician and a representative of the Haskalah; interesting, because the burial controversy was not just a pitched battle between reformers and traditionalists. The road to Jewish modernization was not a straight path. Rather, there were twists, sudden turns, and, in the case of radical changes to Jewish ritual such as prolonging burial, genuine cul-de-sacs. Although Marx was very similar to Herz in many ways, they disagreed violently on this matter, for although he was a maskil, Marx represented the conservative wing of the movement. And unlike Herz, Marx was sure that the order for Jews to expedite the burial of their dead was an order that proceeded from prejudice rather than out of enlightened concern. According to Marx, ghoulish stories about Jews burying people alive were told in fairy tales, written down, codified, and then passed on. But the truth was that cases of premature burial had occurred among non-Jews, despite their delaying burial, and that such cases were nearly impossible among Jews because of the close supervision and observation of the deceased by the members of the burial societies.[126] Qualifications did not concern Marx as they did Herz. Rather, practical experience and the loving-kindness Herz accorded Christian practice was what actually explained the judiciousness of Jewish burial customs.

Like Herz, Marx agreed that the surest sign of death was decomposition, stressing that reason dictated one need only forestall burial for twenty-four hours—the time within which putrefaction sets in. However, bodily decay was only one sign of death. Other measures, such as candle, mirror, and feather tests, were to be considered of equal worth. Marx also reminded Herz that the burial societies had physicians pronounce death (4–16, 40–41).

Marx, in what would become a common theme of future defenses of Jewish ritual in Germany, sought to establish the hygienic value of early burial. According to him, there were certain diseases that could be transmitted to living persons via the corpse of the deceased, and therefore rapid burial was a necessity. The source of Marx's authority on this subject was no less than Berlin's College of Medicine, which had reported that the bodies of victims of smallpox and other contagious diseases should not be left unburied, and that the gravediggers were to dig graves deeper than usual, and the carpenters were to cover the joins of coffins with tar. To Marx's satisfaction, the college also noted that Germans did not maintain a sufficient distance between cemeteries and dwellings, while "Mosaic law ordered that a distance of 50 ells be maintained." Marx also noted that in many places Germans ignored many beneficial laws that were on the books, while Jews carried out their laws to the letter (*"gründlich und recht"*) and were therefore beyond reproach (24–28, 33). This latter point was a direct response to Herz's claim that Jews should take a leaf from the book of their more enlightened German neighbors. For Marx, there were indeed lessons to be learned about hygiene and responsible burial practice, but it was the Germans who could stand to learn them from the Jews. After all, it was they who were practicing an ancient custom that the representatives of modern science honored with the stamp of approval. It was not dark mysticism but enlightened practice based on rabbinic wisdom grounded in reason that informed Jewish behavior.

In one sense, the issue of delayed burial in Mecklenburg-Schwerin can be seen as yet another chapter in the history of religious coercion. But it was not so much an act of religious intolerance by the duke as it was a discussion of Jewish corporeality. It went to the heart of contemporary discussions concerning the physical nature and meaning of Jewishness. Sometimes this meant the resuscitation of the medieval charge that the Jews were repulsive, or that they exuded a foul odor, as one eighteenth-century encyclopedia entry for "Jews" claimed.[127] A different claim in yet another encyclopedia held that the Jews suffered from "nervous hypochondria"—or, put another way—that the Jews did not know, indeed, could not know what was best for their own bodies.[128] It was with the burial ordinance of 1772 that the German state attempted to wrest control of the Jewish body from the Jews. And as it would turn out, the Haskalah, whether in Central, or (later) in Eastern Europe, was generally able to provide Jewish support for government initiatives. The three physicians discussed here were among such supporters.

In essence, Wolf, Marcuze, and Herz all shared a similar view of the condition of the Jews' body: the sorry state in which Jews found themselves was directly attributable to traditional Jewish social and religious culture. Certainly, they were also of the opinion that antisemitism was partially responsible for the Jews' social and physical condition. But for these physicians—critics from the inside, as it were—the retreat of folk culture in the wake of acculturation would lead not only to the amelioration of the civil status of the Jews but also to what the French advocate of emancipation, the Abbé Grégoire, called their "physical regeneration."[129]

CHAPTER 4

# THE JEWISH BODY DEGENERATE?

While the Haskalah formally ushered in the modern discursive critique of the Jews' body, such sensibilities continued to enjoy wide currency long after the Age of Enlightenment had passed. What began in the eighteenth century as an internal assessment by a handful of Central European Jewish doctors about the pathological condition of Jews developed into a widespread theme in European and American culture in the modern period.

In the nineteenth century, the age of empire, robustness and virility were seen as the true hallmarks of national greatness. Yet bereft of the normative and most basic attributes of nationhood—a common language, a defined territory, a flag, a national anthem, and a standing army—Jews represented the antithesis of European nations. Their own languages were perceived as either dead (Hebrew) or bastardized (Yiddish). Crowded into cities, Jews were seen as rootless, homeless, and devoid of martial values and spirit. All of this amounted to a picture of a corrupt, urban group, a countertype to a healthy peasantry with a noble agricultural tradition, or a knightly warrior class—further signifiers of European rootedness.

The modern era has seen the construction of an enduring Jewish type— the sickly Jew. He was first created, golem-like, by a host of unlikely ideological bedfellows: anti-emancipationist Christians and *maskilim* of the eighteenth century, then Zionists, assimilationists, and antisemites in the following two centuries. To a great extent, what allowed the burgeoning of such discourse was the idea of race and the determinative and pivotal role it came to play in all aspects of late nineteenth century culture.[1] Central to that culture was medicine, and the Jews constituted an especially arresting object of intensive examination. Their very otherness—the essence of what lay behind the fascination they had held for so many Christian thinkers for so long—was now the topic of much study in the medical world. The underlying and often unspoken assumption of such research was that perhaps evidence of Jewish biological difference could help explain the Jews' cultural and psychological apartness.

The result of the examination was that nineteenth-century medicine painted a picture of Jews as *extraordinarily healthy*. If there was such a thing as a particular Jewish pathology, then it appeared, at first blush, to be a positive attribute. Statistics the world over showed that Jews lived longer than non-Jews, had a significantly lower infant mortality rate, had a lower death rate, and seemed to be far less subject to the most common diseases of the day, particularly childhood illnesses such as measles, scarlet fever, diphtheria, and croup.[2]

These findings reveal a stunning paradox. In spite of all the contemporary evidence indicating that the diaspora produced healthy, virile, and vibrant Jews, it suited the political agendas of a host of antisemites and ideologues (physicians among them) from across the Jewish political and cultural spectrum to create a counterimage to the healthy Jew of social reality. How did this cognitive dissonance emerge, and how and by what means was medicine (and the other discourses it co-opted) able to ignore its own findings about Jews and portray them as a group at risk? This intricate process has profound implications beyond the immediately medical, going to the heart of how Jews and non-Jews have seen (and perhaps still see) Jews and their place in the modern world.

Although the medical discourse on Jewish pathology was universal in scope, the country at the heart of discussions concerning the Jewish body was Germany. Even though the evidence to be presented here includes data on comparative Jewish pathology based on studies of Jewish communities the world over, most of the research was either initiated in Germany or inspired by German medical research projects involving Jews. Alternatively, many of the non-German investigations of Jews and disease were published in the German language, even when German Jewry was not the focus of the undertaking. That is due to the fact that Germany was the world leader in medicine at the fin-de-siècle. Its prestige and dominance meant that what it considered important research was taken up by other medical traditions. And in Germany, the Jews were considered central to the resolution of larger medical, biological, and anthropological discussions of nature versus nurture, the connection between race and disease, and, above all, the pathological differences, if any, between Germans and Jews, or, as contemporaries were fond of saying, between Aryans and Semites. Put differently, medical discussions about Jews in Wilhelmine Germany were as much about German identity as they were about Jewish identity, and therefore they were central to the nationalist project of German self-definition.

Impetus to the discourse on the pathology of the Jews was provided by fin-de-siècle antisemitism and nationalism. The language of medicine and biological determinism bolstered antisemitism by providing it with the type of authority that could be garnered only from science. Because racism is a "scavenger ideology," to use George Mosse's term, the process entailed the "low" culture of the antisemitic gutter press picking over, ingesting, and regurgitating the language of the "high" culture of the medical and biological sciences. Both the scientific and the hate literature fed off each other. While obviously more temperate in tone, medicine was not immune to the common prejudices of the day. And the way Central European culture at the fin-de-siècle viewed and represented Jews became deeply embedded in the contemporary language of medical science.

Jews, too, were deeply influenced and swept along by these intellectual currents, for among them, racialized medical models proved seductive, having a decisive impact on Jewish self-representation. The degree to which some Jewish ideologues internalized many of the negative Gentile assessments of Jews should not be underestimated. It is a lesson in the malleability of the discourse of race and the corrosive impact of majority group prejudice on the psyche of the minority. Zionist thinkers regularly employed metaphors of illness and disease to describe the Jews' social and pathological condition in order to help forge an awakened national consciousness among European Jewry, one based on physical and spiritual regeneration.

Proponents of assimilation also encouraged Jews to improve their health, their appearance, and their psyches in order to assume their place as citizens of Europe. The pan-Jewish search for a cure for the condition that was "Jewishness" was incisively and disturbingly sketched out by Israeli novelist Aharon Appelfeld. In his novella, *The Retreat,* Appelfeld's characters meet at a mountaintop hotel outside of Vienna on the eve of the Shoah. The patrons are all assimilated Jews, attending this "Institute for Advanced Studies" in order to take lessons in "becoming" Gentile. The course involves unlearning all the physical gestures and ridding themselves of the various pathologies that supposedly make them Jews. One of the long-time residents of the retreat, Bruno Rauch, recounts to a recent arrival, Lotte Schloss, his longing for the good old days at the retreat, "the bracing, disciplined days when they got up early and went to bed early, ate peasant bread and yogurt for breakfast and worked on their accents. . . . They were days with a purpose. Once a man realizes that his body is weak and ugly, his nerves destroyed, his soul corrupt, that he bears within him a decayed inheritance, in short, that he is sick, and what is worse, that he is passing his sickness on to his children, what can he desire more deeply than reform?"[3] The sentiment that Appelfeld so brilliantly captures here was widely accepted. Explicating the social and cultural context in which it emerged and was contested is the business of this chapter.

In late nineteenth-century German-speaking Europe in particular, Jews as both patients and doctors came under close scrutiny and heavy criticism for their supposed defects.[4] In fact, one of the defining characteristics of anti-Jewish prejudice was its medicalization. Antisemitism, which took as its fundamental premise the racial or biological otherness of the Jews, became the standard fare and dominant trope of anti-Jewish expressions.[5] More insidiously, because it was less explicit, determinist and innatist depictions of Jews also informed contemporary medicine.

In what follows, we look at the role Jews were assigned in contemporary medicine by examining four discourses on the pathology of the Jews: the relationship between Jews and alcohol abuse, the vital statistics of the Jewish people, their supposed immunity to tuberculosis, and by contrast, their alleged susceptibility to diabetes. Of course, many other categories of analysis can be chosen. However, alcoholism, tuberculosis, and diabetes were rampant and aroused deep-seated fears, and can therefore be considered three of the most important diseases of the age. The enormous literature that contemporary medicine generated on these topics is testament to the immediacy of these disorders to people at the turn of the century. Concomitantly, the demographic explosion among Jews in the nineteenth century was directly linked by physicians to how the Jews were supposed to have fared vis-à-vis the above-mentioned diseases. Therefore, their vital statistics were seen as an important biological and cultural marker of the Jews' makeup. Any and all deviations from the Gentile norm were interpreted as indicative of Jewish differences that were racial or cultural or both. In Germany, such findings had profound implications concerning the successful integration of Jews into the nation. The discussions of Jewish vital statistics must also be seen in the larger context of concerns about demographic decline throughout Europe. The specter of Jews out-reproducing Christians only heightened an already acute anxiety about Jews.

## ALCOHOLISM

Of all the diseases studied by physicians and social critics in the nineteenth century, alcoholism was used as an object of reference and comparison among Jews more than any other group. For nearly all those who saw in the medical statistics evidence of the overall good health of the Jews, sobriety was hailed as the principal cause. Of widespread social and medical concern, alcoholism, while initially regarded as a sign of moral failure, was later viewed as a disease in and of itself. Moreover, it was (and is) held to be the cause of a host of other illnesses. Among these are peripheral neuropathy, various sorts of brain damage, diseases of the liver, gastritis, pancreatitis, a variety of heart and vascular diseases, and cancers of the upper respiratory and upper digestive tracts. Finally, chronic heavy drinkers face a substantially higher risk of premature death.[6] Therefore, susceptibility to alcoholism indicated an individual or group at great health risk.

The Jews played a central role in all the medical literature on alcoholism because almost singularly among Europeans, they were thought to be spared the disease.[7] The consistently low rate of drinking pathologies among Jews in both Europe and the United States applied equally to extreme forms related to chronic alcoholism, all the way to simple public drunkenness. One of the factors that most intrigued researchers studying the alcohol question as it related to the Jews was the fact that the absence of alcoholism among them would be easy to explain if Judaism, like Islam, preached total abstinence. However, it does not. Instead, alcohol occupies a special place in the life of Jews, to be imbibed principally for defined ceremonial purposes. Whether it is wine for the kiddush at the Sabbath table, or the prescribed four glasses at the Passover seder, or the drinking of high-proof distilled liquor on the festivals of Purim and Simchat Torah, and at celebratory, life cycle occasions, such as births, circumcisions, and weddings, observant Jews consume alcoholic drinks on a regular basis. Central to Jewish religious practice, alcohol is even given to children so that they may participate fully in the religious life of the family.

Nevertheless, the rabbinic sanctioning of drink did not translate into dispensation to drink at will. Judaism loathes the drunkard, and Jewish law warns repeatedly and without ambiguity of the consequences of overindulgence. In fact, according to one current alcoholism researcher, "Analysis of the hundreds of references to alcohol in the Old Testament reveals that it houses an extensive catalogue of the physical, psychological, social, religious, and economic effects of alcohol abuse. This rich harvest also yields a multiplicity of quasi-clinical observations which seem remarkably compatible with some modern descriptions of 'alcoholism.'"[8]

Striving desperately to explain Jewish sobriety, nearly all modern researchers have to one extent or another referred to the strictures against alcohol abuse in classical Jewish teachings. As one such student of the problem has remarked, "Continuities in style of drinking suggest clues to cultural stabilities."[9] But beyond this tenuous cultural explanation, science has still faced the conundrum of how to explain the fact that, as one modern researcher has put it, "the Jews as a group manage to drink extensively but in a pattern of moderation with few pathological consequences."[10]

Researchers at the turn of the nineteenth century pointed out over and over again that in their clinical experience they rarely came in contact with Jews who required treatment for alcohol abuse. For example, Hugo Hoppe, a Jewish psychiatrist from Königsberg and the author of an important study on Jews and alcohol, stated in the most declamatory manner that "in the great army of drinkers who fill our hospitals, our alcohol recovery centers, our mental asylums, our poor houses, our correctional institutions and prisons, one seldom meets a Jew. Delirium tremens, acute alcohol poisoning, and suicide as a result of drink is unheard of among Jews."[11]

The personal testimony given by the Anglo-Jewish physician William Feldman, before the Medical Society of London in a major address he delivered on alcoholism in 1923, corresponded to common medical experience. "In the course of some twenty years' professional practice among Jews of all classes, I have come across not more than two or three cases of alcoholism. I have a good many Jewish patients who are engaged in the sale of alcoholic liquors, but who are nevertheless perfectly sober."[12] Although Feldman was referring only to his London practice, the pattern of Jewish abstemiousness was universal, and statistics the world over tended to demonstrate that the sober Jew of popular imagination actually corresponded to statistical reality.[13]

Because of the widespread belief that alcohol was a causative agent in the onset of myriad illnesses, the oft-reported low level of alcohol use among Jews was cited in order to explain almost all the pathological advantages Jews seemed to display over non-Jews. These included an apparent immunity to plague, typhoid, smallpox, diphtheria, croup, measles, whooping cough, and cholera, and other infectious diseases, particularly respiratory ones such as pneumonia. Syphilis was also said to afflict Jews less than it did non-Jews because of their sobriety.[14] Psychiatrists, in particular, were almost unanimous in their opinion that alcoholism was the one *mental* disorder from which Jews did not suffer. In fact, they thought Jews to be free of all alcohol-related neuropsychoses, the most important of which contemporary medicine considered to be epilepsy.[15]

The reasons for the infinitesimally low rates of alcoholism among Jews are difficult to ascertain and that is not the task before us. However, over the past two centuries, various authors have tried their hand and in so doing provide us with a window onto Jewish-Christian social relations and the place of Jews in the majority culture. Long before the gathering of statistical data, Jewish sobriety had already been recognized. One of the first to formally comment on it was the German philosopher Immanuel Kant. In his *Anthropology from a Pragmatic Point of View* (1797), Kant remarked that, "as a rule, women, clerics and Jews do not get drunk — or at least carefully avoid any appearance of drunkenness — because their civil status is weak and they must be discreet (and hence sober)." In this statement, Kant did not distinguish the behavior of Jews from that of others who were subject to excessive scrutiny. But he continued, referring specifically to the Jews, offering a cultural and psychological explanation for Jewish behavior. In that era of heated debate in Germany over Jewish emancipation, Kant suggested that Jewish sobriety derived from the fact that the need to make a good outward impression on Gentile society determined whether or not the Jews got drunk, "for their worth in the eyes of others is based merely on others' *belief* in their chastity, their piety, and their observance of their separatist laws." But, according to Kant, the Jews themselves were intolerant of drunkenness: "As for [this] last point, all separatists — that is, people who submit not only to the public law of the land but also to a special (sectarian) one — are particularly exposed to a community's attention and rigorous criticism, insofar as they are oddities and allegedly chosen people; so they cannot relax their attention to themselves, since drunkenness, which does away with caution, is a *scandal* for them."[16]

To a certain extent, Kant's view concerning the social taboo of drunkenness in Jewish society was prescient, anticipating nearly all subsequent sociological, psychological, medical, and historical explanations for the absence of alcoholism among Jews.[17] Although, one must hasten to add that Kant painted an unreal picture of a Jewish community acting in unison and cold pragmatism. The Jews of eighteenth-century Prussia did not conspire to avoid drunkenness in order to win favor in the eyes of Gentile authorities, although they were certainly attuned to the fact that as Jews, their behavior was closely scrutinized. Perhaps more to the point is the fact that the greater level of excessive alcohol consumption among Christians made it a behavior that Jews associated almost exclusively with Gentiles, and therefore it became something for them to avoid. As one early twentieth-century Jewish physician noted, "It was the Jew of the Ghetto, isolated from his non-Jewish neighbour, who abhorred drunkenness as a sin, a disgrace, only fit for a Goi (Gentile) but not for the Chosen People."[18]

Into the nineteenth century, many physicians actually thought Jews to be racially immune to the effects of strong drink.[19] According to one Victorian expert, there was in operation among Jews "some inherited racial insusceptibility to narcotism, strengthened and confirmed by the practise of various hygienic habits." Norman Kerr, president of the Society for the Study of Inebriety, went on to note that "even among those Jews in whom there has been an unusual enjoyment of alcohol drinking, when (though they were not 'drunk') there has been a slight thickening of the speech, glibness of tongue, and unwanted exuberance of spirits, evidencing a certain amount of alcohol poisoning, I have rarely detected the existence of the disease inebriety. Of this strong impulse to alcoholic or other narcotism I have seen only one case among this distinctive people."[20]

Other commentators suggested that Jews were racially constituted in such a way that they could not tolerate liquor and therefore stayed clear of it. George Archdall Reid, the English authority on alcoholism, noted that Jews were not drunkards "because deep indulgence, so far from being delightful, is disagreeable to them." Applying a rather crude Darwinian model that he referred to as "alcoholic evolution," Reid maintained that alcoholism eliminated in a race those it afflicted, leaving only the sober types to perpetuate the racial stock.[21] Why alcoholism had not worked as an agent of selection among other groups, leading to its eradication, was not considered. Rather, and this is the curious feature about the representation of Jews in late nineteenth-century medical literature, even when they were being praised, as they surely were in discussions of alcohol abuse, their success heralded their abnormality. They resided isolated and alone, outside behavioral and pathological norms.

While the absence of alcoholism among Jews had definite pathological advantages, the majority of researchers nevertheless saw culture and not race as the key to Jewish sobriety. According to American sociologist William Ripley, "Conducive to longevity is the sobriety of the Jew, and his disinclination toward excessive indulgence in alcoholic liquors. Drunkenness among Jews is very rare. Temperate habits, a frugal diet, with a very moderate use of spirits, render the proportion of Bright's disease and affections of the liver comparatively very small."[22] According to renowned Australian-Jewish man of letters Joseph Jacobs, the low death rate among Jewish children and the greater longevity of Jews "can be attributed to the [fact that] *the Jewish nature does not require stimulants, and Jews are markedly free from alcoholism*. The tranquilising effects of Jewish family life, the joyous tone and complete rest of the Sabbath and other festivals, the unworrying character of the Jewish religion, are all important in the difficult art of keeping alive."[23] Likewise, the distinguished New York physician Maurice Fishberg noted that "the rarity of alcoholism" contributed to a low infant mortality among Jews.[24] As for their low death rate, Fishberg again returned to Jewish culture. Echoing Jacobs, he claimed that "one has only to recall that alcoholism is very rare and that the Sabbath is a day of rest among the orthodox Jews in Eastern Europe, and not of drink and dissipation."[25]

As with Kant, experts in the late nineteenth century saw the Jews' minority status and occupational structure as underlying causes of Jewish temperance. In Britain, James Samuelson declared that there were two main reasons for Jewish sobriety: "First, they are a small community; and their partial isolation from other religious denominations has a tendency to make them careful of their morals. The most important reason, however, is that they do not follow any avocations which necessitate great physical exertions.... [Thus] they are removed from the temptations to excessive drinking to which the great mass of our working-people are exposed.... [A]s a whole the Jews are a sober and exemplary race, whose habits in that respect are well worthy of universal imitation."[26]

Around World War I, the German socialist leader Karl Kautsky called attention to the fact "that the Jew — at least in the ghetto — is far less addicted to alcohol." Reiterating Kant, to some extent, Kautsky observed that in the contemporary campaign against alcoholism:

> the Jews have had a lead of centuries, not in the requirement of abstinence, but in their abhorrence of intoxication; not so much because of a scientific knowledge, as because of their social position.... The defenseless Jew was always far more exposed to danger than the non-Jew, and therefore sobriety was far more necessary to him. An intoxicated Jew who would transgress the laws would have brought great misfortune not only upon himself but upon the entire Jewry of his home town.... Although originally serving only to render the position of the Jews more secure, and perhaps practised as a habit handed down from their Oriental home, this abstinence has necessarily had an extremely favourable hygienic influence.[27]

And finally, according to a German Zionist lawyer and statistician, Arthur Ruppin, the Jews' "moderation is the more remarkable as total abstainers are rare among them — they drink, but are not drunkards, possibly because they are to a higher degree governed by reason."[28]

Precisely because all these explanations are culturally grounded, Jewish doctors at the turn of the nineteenth century began to express fears that with the gradual assimilation of the Jews, they would begin to mimic the drinking culture of their neighbors. Consequently, "many of the immunities which they enjoyed in former times, and which the Jews who live at present in the Ghetto atmosphere still enjoy, are bound to disappear with this change."[29] This cultural pessimism appeared in the work of scholars representing all points along the Jewish political and cultural spectrum, although it was enunciated most definitively by Zionist physicians.

Alarmed by what they regarded as the corrosive effects of post-emancipatory assimilation, Zionists feared that any biological advantages enjoyed by Jews as a result of specific cultural habits — sobriety, for example — were being undermined through increased fraternization between Jews and non-Jews. In the discussion of alcohol abuse and its consequences, the views of Jewish and Gentile physicians differed with regard to prognosis. In the far more static conceptions of the Jew held by non-Jewish doctors, there is no indication that Jews would ever become intemperate. For Christian commentators, the Jewish condition was cause for wonderment, even envy, while for Jews it was a source of both great pride and concern.

This anxiety among Jewish physicians was prompted by their unshakable belief in the power of the environment to effect change. In an important study on the connection between alcohol use and criminality among Jews undertaken in 1907, Hugo Hoppe sent a warning signal to his fellow Jews that things were changing. He maintained that increased criminality among Jews occurred as a result of their "assimilation to the drinking habits [of non-Jews]." Maintaining that the temperance of the Jews through many generations was the result of original religious proscriptions, Hoppe held that their innate aversion to alcohol had finally acquired the form of an inherited characteristic. But this acquired racial property was not indelible, he claimed, and just as the custom of abstention had developed, so too could that of alcoholism: "Their [the Jews'] ancient temperance, their immunity to alcoholism, is, unquestionably, in a slow process of decline. If no inner movement to counter it ensues and the general movement against alcohol cannot stop it, the time will soon appear when the Jews will be alcoholics like their neighbors and will not differ from them within one generation."[30] Hoppe thus becomes one of the first in a chorus of Jewish physicians with Zionist sympathies to boldly point out that not all the after-effects of emancipation and subsequent assimilation were to the Jews' benefit. But even non-Zionists such as Maurice Fishberg feared that "as soon as the barriers of the Ghetto are broken down and [the Jew] comes in more or less intimate contact with non-Jews, he learns much from them which is not always good for him. Drinking is one of those acquirements which is beginning to show itself among the Sons of Jacob in recent times."[31]

Fishberg's is a theory that owes much to the notion of ennui as developed by the French Jewish sociologist Emile Durkheim. According to him, modern society suffered breakdown when the ties of religion and custom that once bound small communities together began to disintegrate. This was facilitated by the movement of people to big cities. A tangible consequence of this development was a rise in the suicide rate, especially among Protestants, for whom suicide was related to the "spirit of free inquiry that animates this religion." When living under the watchful eye and moral code of a close-knit community, people dared not take their own lives. But living anonymously in large cities, freed from the restraints imposed by intimate living, desperate people were free — and, in fact, more inclined — to kill themselves. Durkheim explained the lower suicide rate among Jews as compared with that of Catholics and Protestants by arguing that despite their congregating in large cities, the Jews of fin-de-siècle Europe still constituted a close-knit moral community where approval and disapproval of certain behaviors was freely expressed. Moreover, antisemitism, which inhibited "the very possibility of free communication with the rest of the population," created an intense feeling of self-consciousness that likewise contributed to the low suicide rate among Jews.[32] For the time being, for Fishberg, the same sociological factors that explained lower Jewish suicide rates were at play in determining the Jewish disinclination to excessive drinking.

Not long afterward, a French alcohol researcher, L. Cheinisse, also applied the Durkheimian thesis to explain the low incidence of alcohol abuse among Jews. Once again, it was because they lived under the close scrutiny of the larger Jewish community. However, as the bonds of community atrophied under the pressure of modern, urban life, according to Cheinisse's theory, this would alter the Jews' historic relationship to alcohol. For Cheinisse, proof of this thesis was to be found in the increasing use of alcohol among the descendants of Jewish immigrants to Paris.[33] Despite this reported change in Jewish habits in France, the image of teetotaling Jews was an indelible one that could also have political repercussions. Well into the twentieth century, French antisemites scurrilously attacked the nation's two Jewish prime ministers by, among other things, highlighting their beverage preferences. Although they both represented constituencies "where alcohol was even more important a factor in sociability than in the rest of France,"

Léon Blum generally opted for water, while Pierre Mendès France regularly touted the health benefits of milk. For their enemies, their aversion to alcohol signified the wide and, indeed, unbridgeable cultural gulf that separated Jews from Frenchmen.[34]

Still, Jewish physicians and psychiatrists claimed that irreplaceable social mores and biological benefits were being lost in the wake of Jewish integration into the majority culture. Just as certain of the negative impact of alcoholism on human health as the rest of the contemporary medical establishment, they too were largely convinced that the increase in Jewish alcohol consumption could only mean that Jews would now acquire more pathological illnesses and become even more susceptible to the few psychopathological disorders to which they had hitherto been immune.

The fear that Jewish rates of alcoholism would rise as the process of assimilation gained speed was a reasonable one. Jews do tend to resemble the majority in myriad ways as they seek to become more like them. However — and this is the curious fact about alcohol use among Jews — the dire prognostications of fin-de-siècle Jewish physicians never came to pass. For example, patterns of morbidity that indicate alcohol abuse, such as carcinomas of the head, neck, and esophagus, alcoholic cardiomyopathy, cirrhosis, and alcohol-related traumatic injuries have made very few claims upon the Jews. Their warnings aside, Jewish physicians who raised alarm bells were only able to testify to the minuscule number of Jewish alcoholics, and, in fact, never witnessed a significant rise in the rate of alcohol abuse among Jews. They merely extrapolated from other behavioral patterns affected by acculturation and assimilation to claim that alcoholism would soon emerge as a problem among Jews, because it was one among Gentiles. It did not.

In a seminal article on alcoholism and the Jews published in 1952, Nathan Glazer reiterated the opinions of Kant and the German Zionist Arthur Ruppin, noting that "the Jews have been under siege for a long time . . . [and although] it is not the consciousness of the siege that prevents any individual Jew from taking one more drink . . . it is the consequences of the siege, passed down from generation to generation, and including such elements as the desire to hold on to one's senses and a distaste for the irrational, that sets a limit to Jewish drinking." But as Glazer points out, contrary to Kant, the Jew "is as temperate in all-Jewish company, or in an all-Jewish state. Rather, his restraint has become automatic."[35]

As a postscript to this discussion, it should be noted that nearly a century after the first medical studies appeared on the relation of Jews to alcohol, the most recent findings confirm what was initially believed. Jews suffer minimal, indeed numerically insignificant, levels of alcoholism.[36] Because of the near destruction of European Jewry in World War II, recent evidence by necessity has been drawn primarily from Israel and North America. Statistically minuscule increases of alcoholism have been detected among some Jewish communities, a scenario sarcastically commented upon by one American clinician: "There is an alarming problem with alcoholism in the Jewish community. I can name five alcoholics for you."[37]

A striking feature of the historical relationship between Jews and alcoholism is that alcohol, alone among all ingestibles, continues to be consumed in quantities that have remained relatively unchanged since the pre-emancipation period. Although a majority of world Jewry no longer adheres to the dietary laws, now eating what their neighbors do, Jews have universally resisted the emulation of Gentile drinking habits. Indeed, they do seem to enjoy what has been called a "cultural immunity." According to some experts, this has been built up over the ages by frequent ritualistic drinking in a most moderate fashion. This in turn has created a norm of sobriety in Jewish society and a concomitant negative sanction imposed on alcohol abuse. These features, plus the stigma attached to those members of the group who engage in excessive drinking, have historically functioned as powerful social controls.[38]

In defiance of the Jewish cultural pessimists at the fin-de-siècle, it would seem that the deeply ingrained taboo against alcohol abuse among Jews has survived the ravages of radical assimilation. In the United States, for example, where alcohol consumption has actually increased since the end of World War II and the intermarriage rate of Jews has risen to at least 52 percent, the incidence of alcoholism among Jews remains remarkably low.[39] Neither of these two factors has made an appreciable impact upon Jewish drinking habits. Rather, it would appear that sobriety has proven itself to be one of the most persistent and widely practiced cultural legacies that previous generations have managed to bequeath to contemporary Jews, irrespective of their level of Jewish identification and practice.

## JEWISH CULTURE AND VITAL STATISTICS

Temperance was but one component of Jewish culture that was believed to promote what were referred to at the fin-de-siècle as Jewish "biostatistical" advantages. There were other, deeply embedded and universally practiced ways of ordering the world that contributed to the overall picture of Jews as healthy and thriving. Above all, Jews appeared to live longer than non-Jews and enjoy lower mortality rates. One of the earliest Jewish researchers into this, Eduard Glatter, director of the Vienna Bureau of Statistics, made the bold pronouncement that as far as the physical tenacity of the Jews is concerned, "there is hardly an analogue in the entire history of humanity."[40]

Over the course of the nineteenth century, the Jews experienced a population explosion. While in its opening decades there were around 2.7 million Jews, constituting approximately 1.4 percent of the total European population, that number increased to a full 2 percent, or 8.5 million, by 1900. Their rate of growth was greater than that of any other European people.[41] This natural increase occasioned scores of statistical studies from all over the world relating to Jewish demography. The results of these surveys showed a remarkable uniformity in terms of birth and death rates, fertility, and life span. Everywhere, the Jews lived longer than their Gentile neighbors, had a significantly lower rate of infant mortality, and suffered fewer deaths per 1,000.

As for the longer life spans of Jews, research undertaken as early as the mid-nineteenth century showed that Jews in Frankfurt lived nearly forty-nine years, while Christians lived on average just under thirty-seven years. By 1900, the average life span in Budapest was twenty-six years for Christians and thirty-seven years for Jews. In London, the figures were thirty-six years and forty-nine years, respectively. In places as far-flung as Holland, Romania, and Algeria the Jews always outlived their non-Jewish neighbors, and according to the 1890 census bulletin of the United States, the "expectation of life" in America for Jews was fifty-seven years; it was forty-one for Christians.[42]

As opposed to life span, Jewish death rates the world over ran anywhere from 11 percent to 52 percent lower than they did for non-Jews. For example, of every 1,000 persons in New York in 1890, 45.18 Americans died. This statistic was divided up according to ethnicity: the figure for the Irish was 36.04, the Germans, 22.14, and Eastern European Jews, 16.71. In the period 1885 to 1893 in Hungary, the death rate figures were: Catholics, 72.2, Protestants, 55.0, and Jews, 37.6. In Germany's capital, Berlin, 15.7 percent of all Jews could expect to reach their fiftieth birthday, while only 12.4 percent of Christians could. Similarly, while 7.3 percent of Jews lived to turn sixty, only 5.5 percent of Christians did. Finally, 2.6 percent of Berlin's Jews reached the age of seventy, as opposed to 1.8 percent of Christians.[43]

There was also a staggering difference in infant mortality figures between Jews and Christians. While the nineteenth and twentieth centuries witnessed a decline in infant mortality as part of the larger reduction in mortality rates, the Jews of Europe heralded this improvement far in advance of other Europeans. With 60,000 Jews in 1900, Amsterdam was one of the largest Jewish communities in Western Europe. The death rate for Jewish children there under the age of five was 8.85 percent, while for Christians it was 11.52 percent. At the same time in London, 10 percent of Jewish children died between the ages of one and five, while 14 percent of Christian children in that age bracket succumbed. In Budapest, of 1,000 children, 32.39 Calvinists, 37.62 Lutherans, 41.43 Catholics, and only 14.42 Jews died under the age of five. Farther east, in Russia, the Jews lost 151 children under the age of one for every 1,000 born. Ethnic Russians, on the other hand, lost 284 offspring per 1,000 in the period, 1896 to 1897. When the infant mortality rate is calculated to include children up to the age of five, the figure for the Russian population is an astonishing 50 percent of children lost.[44] For the years 1855 to 1864 in the Italian city of Verona, 217 Jewish children out of 1,000 died under the age of seven. The figure for Catholics was more than double that, with 453 children out of 1,000 dying. Prussia in 1906 offers an instructive example. In that year, 53 percent of all deaths among Christians befell children under the age of fifteen, while for Jews, the figure was only 18.58 percent.[45]

So, irrespective of where Jews lived in Europe — whether they were middle-class Italians, proletarian Jews crowded into London's East End, tailors in the Russian Pale of Settlement, Hungarian professionals, or Prussian merchants — their common experience (borne out by contemporary statistics) was to see their children survive to adulthood in far greater proportion to those of their non-Jewish neighbors. It was, then, with considerable pride and not a little irony that a 1910 report in a Zionist periodical stated, "The death rate among Jewish children in the unhealthy, narrow confines of the Frankfurt ghetto is lower than the rate among the city's [Christian] patricians."[46] This situation throughout Europe led a French observer of the Jews, Anatole Leroy-Beaulieu, to remark that "the Jews . . . have a twofold advantage over their fellow-countrymen of different religions: they multiply more rapidly and with less waste. They bring fewer children into the world, but they bring more of them to maturity. It would seem as if, with their characteristic cleverness at calculations, they had instinctively solved the difficult problem of population in the manner most advantageous to themselves and most satisfactory to the economists."[47]

Partially responsible for lower infant mortality rates among Jews was their lower birth rate. Even though the number of births among Jews per 1,000 was not uniform, being significantly higher in Eastern than Western Europe, both places registered lower numbers when compared to the Christian populations among whom they lived. By the turn of the twentieth century the rate of demographic growth among the Jews, especially in Western Europe, had slowed to a trickle. For example, in Germany the percentage of Jews in the overall population actually went into decline. In 1871, with the founding of the Second Reich, the Jewish population was 512,158, or 1.25 percent of the total population. By 1910, the number of Jews had increased to 615,021, but this now constituted only 0.95 percent of Germany's total population. Greater affluence, increased use of birth control, rising levels of apostasy and mixed marriage, emigration, and aging all took a tremendous demographic toll, threatening the future of the community. It was only the constant influx of Eastern European Jewish immigrants that served to demographically replenish German Jewry. Jewish birth rates declined not only in Western Europe, but also in Russia, Hungary, Poland, and Rumania.[48]

Despite this trend, there appeared to be immediate health advantages to the low birth rate among Jews. Contemporary physicians (and even current researchers) were of the opinion that the low birth rate ensured lower infant and child mortality statistics. So even though Jews had fewer children than Christians, those children tended to live to adulthood. Jewish physicians offered several reasons, most of them cultural, for this phenomenon.[49]

First, contemporaries noted that Jewish parents had to divide their material resources among a smaller number of children. Fewer mouths to feed made for a higher caloric intake per individual. Similarly, there were fewer bodies to clothe. Second, it was noted that Jewish mothers in both Eastern Europe and America breast-fed their children to a greater extent, and for a longer period of time than did non-Jews.[50]

Third, Jewish mothers, especially in Western Europe, tended not to work outside the home after marriage, thus being on hand to tend to their children.[51] Certainly, the grinding farmwork done by Eastern European women barely finds an analogue among Jewish women, even those in rural areas. A Viennese physician, Martin Engländer, stated that contributing to Jewish well-being were the household atmosphere that was characterized by "affection and care for wife and child, and *the early exemption of pregnant women from physical labor*" [emphasis added].[52]

Fourth, by 1925, more than a quarter of the world's Jews lived in a mere fourteen cities.[53] Just prior to the outbreak of World War II, one half of all Jews lived in cities with populations of over 100,000, leading the eminent Jewish historian Salo Baron to remark that "one may thus speak of the metropolitanization rather than the urbanization of the Jews."[54] This had a decided impact on the occupational choices of Jews, one result of which was that according to Joseph Jacobs, "Jews do not lead 'dangerous' lives in the insurance sense (sailors, soldiers, firemen, miners &c.)."[55] Therefore, the high concentration of Jews in urban areas where life was safer and lived predominantly indoors, and where medical care was more easily available and superior, was seen to have given Jews a decided advantage for survival.

Fifth, unanimous opinion at the fin-de-siècle ranked Jewish habits of hygiene, particularly regular hand washing, as a major contribution to stemming the spread of infectious disease.[56] Sixth, by the late nineteenth century, Jews, especially those in Western and Central Europe, were better educated, earned more, and, overall, enjoyed higher standards of living than did non-Jews.[57] The vast majority were firmly entrenched in the middle class and displayed a host of bourgeois customs and habits that in the areas of hygiene and nourishment worked to minimize infant mortality and improve and extend the life of adults.[58] This last point, however, does not apply to the bulk of Eastern European Jews and immigrants from that part of the world who settled in New York and London, and who were decidedly poor and working class. Yet there too, Jews lived longer and more healthfully than did non-Jews, and they had a significantly lower incidence of infant mortality.[59] Contemporary physicians thus rejected arguments based on class to explain away superior Jewish vital statistics. Rather, culture and not economic status was seen as the key to explaining these statistics.

Almost all researchers (Christian and Jewish alike) noted the supposedly greater care Jewish parents took of their children. The provability of such a claim is completely immaterial. Rather, it was the widespread belief in its truthfulness that counts when tracing the emergence of modern assumptions about the physical Jewish body. Instructive by stark comparison are the deadly ante- and neo-natal practices en vogue among Russians in the nineteenth century: forcing pregnant women to do heavy fieldwork, with no respite right up to the time of labor; wrapping newborns in the putrid clothes of the father in the hope they would make the child robust; performing baptisms in unheated rooms with ice water to simulate the conditions of a church in winter; flogging young children to make them tough; suspending the newborn from the rafters of a hut in a "fly-infested crib filled with dirty rags"; nurturing children preferentially, providing more for those deemed most likely to survive; and, finally, feeding the newborn with the *soska,* a cloth filled with bacon rind and flour that the grandmother chewed on and left in the child's mouth, where it generally rotted, leaving mold to grow around the mouth of the infant.[60]

These were brutal habits, far removed from what went on in Jewish homes, even though the two groups lived in very close proximity to one another and grinding poverty was the norm among Jews. Although characterized by an exaggerated idealism, the following ethnographic description of the first five years of a shtetl child's life indicates the stark contrast between Russian and Jewish child-rearing habits, or at the very least the way they were represented:

> The first months of a baby's life are a constant bath of warmth, attention and affection. . . . All its wants are attended to by the mother, or by female relatives.
>
> Wrapped and pillowed, the baby is carried around a great deal by grownups and by older brothers and sisters, for if it lies down too much its lungs will be weak. . . . [I]t is almost never allowed to remain still or unattended. . . .
>
> The baby who is welcomed so eagerly and sheltered so anxiously, is nevertheless hurried out of babyhood. For all the kissing and cooing, all the baby talk and coddling, there is no effort to keep him infantile. On the contrary, he is treasured as a potential adult, and the admiration of his audience is most evident when he shows signs of precocity. Early sitting, teething, creeping, crawling, standing, walking, and above all early talking, give tremendous satisfaction to parents and family. . . .
>
> Slow development is a cause of serious anxiety. If a baby is late in walking or talking the family tries to cover up his deficiencies but they grieve and worry in private.[61]

According to Samuel Weissenberg, a distinguished Russian Jewish physician and anthropologist who wrote extensively on Jewish child care practices, Jews performed a host of domestic habits that made sound hygienic sense. In addition, they were far more likely to retain the services of a physician than were non-Jews, and this was equally true for urban and rural Jews. Taken together, these behaviors were seen by nineteenth- and early twentieth-century physicians as having contributed substantially to the radically lower infant mortality rate among Russian Jews.[62]

Elsewhere too, Jewish parenting was said to make a difference in child mortality rates. Referring to the fact that in the United States between 1911 and 1916 the infant mortality rate per 1,000 was 94 for native-born white children and 54 for foreign-born Jewish children, the lowest of any ethnic group, Odin W. Anderson posited that the reason was not to be sought in general economic factors, but "a closer examination would probably reveal a pattern of infant care of a high order embedded in the Jewish culture."[63]

Different cultures manifest different behaviors in response to illness, particularly that of their children.[64] Ethnographic and sociological studies done in the second half of the twentieth century have much to teach us about nineteenth-century Jewish attitudes toward health and illness, for they tend to confirm the speculative assumptions of that earlier literature. For example, in the 1960s, a study of the link between ethnicity and response to illness led to the conclusion that Jewish mothers display "near-compulsive" concern about their children's well-being. That this could lead to psychological problems was pointed out by the author of the study, who concluded that "it is probable that the concern of Jewish mothers makes their children highly sensitive to 'abnormal symptoms' and may in fact induce a tendency to 'hypochondriasis.'"[65]

Another comparative study, focusing on Jewish, Italian, Irish, and "Old American" patients' reactions and attitudes toward pain, revealed something similar. The culturally determined responses to pain were inculcated from early childhood. Jewish and Italian mothers were zealously overprotective, constantly worrying aloud whether their child would catch cold, get hurt in fights, or be injured while participating in sporting activities. The investigator of the study claimed that this attitude had a deleterious impact on the children. Because of the ceaseless harping on such issues, the children developed a complaining and tearful manner. "In Jewish families, where not only a slight sensation of pain but also each deviation from the child's normal behavior is looked upon as a sign of illness, the child is prone to anxieties with regard to the meaning and significance of these manifestations."[66] There was, however, a positive side to all this. The children themselves became sensitive to illness, paying particular attention to pain, complaining about it and seeking sympathy and relief. According to researchers, thanks to the proverbial "Jewish mother," there was inculcated among Jewish children and adolescents a higher sensitivity to the abnormality of pain.

The seemingly excessive concern with health is best reflected in the relationship of the Jews to their physicians. An oft-repeated claim made by observers from the late nineteenth century on was that Jews had an abiding faith in doctors. They tended to go to them more readily and more often. If this tendency does indeed exist, factors such as urbanization, education level, and socioeconomic status would help explain why. But culture, too, played a role. The high proportion of Jewish doctors, especially in Central Europe, meant that there was a very good chance that the Jew who visited a doctor would be seeing a Jewish one.[67] The cultural affinity shared by doctor and patient, and the confidence of the patient in the treatment prescribed, a confidence born of ethnic affinity and the shared cultural outlook of healer and healed, had a decisive impact on Jewish behavior in the face of illness.

On the other hand, Jewish faith in doctors should not be read as Jewish subservience to their word and opinion. Paradoxically, the familiarity between the two parties, and the nonhierarchical or stratified nature of Jewish society, often translated into the oft-attested-to willingness of Jews to challenge their doctors and seek second and third opinions. The culture of questioning, the need for confirmation, and the desire to make themselves educated medical consumers were common to Jews in Eastern and Western Europe.

Thus, while respected, the physician was not regarded as infallible. Recourse to medical science notwithstanding, the Jews of Eastern Europe, for example, always hedged their medical bets. Faith and trust in the physician did not preclude the use of more traditional cures. As Samuel Weissenberg wrote, "The almost pathological concern with his health is for the Jew, in chronic cases, even responsible for his not only seeking out expensive medical care, but for his taking refuge behind various superstitions [folk cures]."[68]

Among Russian Jews, many of the practices involved superstitions such as placing amulets around the neck of the child or renaming children so as to fool the "angel of death." In addition to folk remedies employed by Jews, the Yiddish expression *freg nit dem royfe, freg dem khoyle* (Don't ask the doctor, ask the patient) indicates as much as anything the great confidence Jewish patients had in *themselves* as diagnosticians. It also points to the fact that Jewish patients could rarely be satisfied with one expert opinion, especially if that diagnosis did not concur with their own assessment. This would lead the patient on a search for the "right" diagnosis, driven by what Weissenberg called the Jews' "nosophilia and nosophobia."[69] For Munich psychiatrist Johannes Lange, who studied manic-depression among Bavarian Jews, the latter suffered from, among other things, "a well known physician-neediness."[70]

An American observer who studied the different attitudes of some 1,300 university students in the United States in the early 1960s found that Jewish students were far more likely to miss class and to visit a physician when feeling unwell than were either Protestant or Catholic students. That a culture of medical concern had been passed on to the Jewish students is without doubt. Personal religiosity played almost no role in what sociologists call "illness behavior," for while the majority of Christian students in the sample attended church regularly, only 6 percent of the Jewish respondents attended synagogue on a regular basis. Thus, when confronted with illness, residual and older patterns of Jewish behavior make themselves manifest, even in those Jews who have moved furthest away from traditional Jewish religious culture.[71] One doctor in the 1940s assessed the long-term consequences of the Jewish eagerness to seek medical care when he wrote, "Increased visits to physicians and clinics, and reliance upon their directions results not only in an increase in the diagnosis of less readily diagnosed conditions, but also to the decrease in other conditions through the widespread adoption among Jews of effective prophylactic measures such as vaccination against smallpox, diphtheria, etc."[72] As anthropologist Raphael Patai observed, "Attitudes toward health are inculcated by Jewish mothers into their children from the earliest age on. By the time a young Jew reaches college, or even high-school, age, these attitudes have long been internalized to an extent which renders him practically immune to influences emanating from the peer group."[73] Here a similarity can be detected with the situation as it pertains to alcohol abuse. Whatever the extent of remove from Jewish religious tradition, individual and group attitudes manifest latent yet deeply ingrained patterns of behavior when it comes to health care.

A combination of factors, almost all cultural, served to promote the generally superior health enjoyed by Jews in the nineteenth century. A lower birth rate led to a lower infant mortality rate, and thus Jews had a significantly higher percentage of children surviving past the age of five than did non-Jews. Moreover, according to ethnographic and anecdotal accounts by both Jews and Christians, these children were inducted into warm and nurturing environments where the extended kinship group saw it as its primary task to care for and shepherd the child through the risky first years of life. Also, the occupational structure of Jewish life and the internal value system conspired to relieve pregnant Jewish women and new mothers of the onerous work responsibilities that were the lot of Christian mothers in both Central and Eastern Europe. A high regard for the efficacy of breast-feeding and the comparatively longer periods it was employed also served the nutritional interests of the Jewish child, and more frequent washing kept pathogens at bay. Finally, the extreme concern that Jews displayed for their health, which both Jewish and Gentile commentators have described as a near-compulsive behavior, did mean that Jews were more likely to be under the constant, professional care of a trained physician, and very often a Jewish one, with whom they had a shared code of cultural values. This extreme concern also meant that Jews practiced a sort of prophylactic health care regimen, wherein even the slightest manifestation out of the ordinary was treated with the utmost seriousness and attended to immediately. All these features, along with the absence of alcohol abuse, help account for the extraordinarily strong biostatistics displayed by a vital world Jewry as it entered the twentieth century.

## TUBERCULOSIS

Tuberculosis was the most widespread and feared illness of the nineteenth century. It was a global killer of enormous dimensions, wreaking devastation on individuals, families, and entire communities.[74] Not only did it grip the popular imagination because of the terror it instilled, it even came to play a leading role in high culture, featured, for example, by such artists as Giuseppe Verdi in his operas, *La Boheme* and *La Traviata,* and Thomas Mann in his classic novel, *Magic Mountain*.[75]

Despite what appeared to be the indiscriminate ravages of the disease, many scientists posited that some groups were at greater risk than others. It was held that susceptibility to the illness could be determined by bodily shape and other forms of phenotypical organization.[76] By the medical standards of the day, Jews presented themselves as ideal candidates for contracting the dreaded disease. According to one scientific description written in 1911, Jews were in possession of a certain body type that was conducive to contracting tuberculosis. Known as the *habitus phthisicus,* it: "is to-day found in a large proportion of Jews. Indeed, that frail, undersized, emaciated body, with a long, narrow, flat chest, in which the ribs stick out prominently, the chest-bone is depressed, and the shoulder blades project in the back like two wings, may be considered characteristic of a large number of Jews. . . . The Jew's chest is usually less than one half his height, while among others it is almost invariably more than one-half the height in healthy persons. Physically, the Jews can, under the circumstances, be considered predisposed to pulmonary diseases, especially consumption."[77]

In addition, the social and economic conditions under which most Jews lived, particularly in Eastern Europe, made them especially vulnerable to tuberculosis. In his 1904 study of diseases among Jews, the German physician Heinrich Singer noted that because of their "small chest cavity, weak bodily development, inadequate living conditions, irrational choice of occupations which badly neglect physical activity in the open air, the frequent absence of cleanliness and not least, the incessant moral pressure under which the majority of Jews live," they were very susceptible to contracting tuberculosis.[78] Just exactly which Jews Singer was referring to was never made clear. Certainly not the Jews of his Germany, but inherent in the racialized medical practice of the day was the urge to generalize and stereotype.

## THE JEWISH BODY DEGENERATE?

A similar assessment was made by Maurice Fishberg. As clinical professor of medicine at New York University and Bellevue Hospital Medical College, and as medical examiner to the United Hebrew Charities of New York City, Fishberg spent a lifetime caring for, studying, and writing about the health and physical aspects of the Jewish people. On the social conditions propitious for the spread of consumption among Jews, Fishberg succinctly described the situation thus:

> everything favourable for the development and spread of tuberculosis is found among them. They are pre-eminently town dwellers, and in cities the bulk of the Jews reside usually in the most densely overcrowded sections of the city; and lacking proper ventilation, fresh air, and sunshine, they are thus in an atmosphere favourable for infection with tubercle bacilli. Their occupations, which are usually of the indoor variety, such as tailoring, shoemaking, fur, etc., also enjoy the evil distinction of supplying a greater number of consumptives than outdoor occupations. When to this are added poverty, grief, anxiety, and excessive mental exertion, want of proper exercise, fresh air and sunshine, conditions under which the majority of Jews live in various parts of the world, it would be expected that they should be attacked more often by this disease than others; indeed, *a priori* they should actually be decimated by the White Plague.[79]

Yet, medical science was presented with a dilemma, for irrespective of where they lived, Jews apparently had a mortality rate from the disease that was markedly lower than that of non-Jews.[80] This despite the widespread belief of physicians that the social environments of Jews were breeding grounds for tuberculosis bacilli. Evidence garnered from Eastern Europe, Russia, Hungary, Rumania, Austria, New York, Tunis, and New South Wales (neither of the latter two places lacking sunshine) showed a lower number of Jews succumbing to tuberculosis than non-Jews.[81] To take but two examples, detailed evidence was gathered for the imperial capitals of Vienna and Budapest. In the former, from 1901 to 1903, victims of all forms of the disease per 100,000 of the population were Catholics, 496; Protestants, 328; and Jews, 179. When considering pulmonary tuberculosis on its own, there were, per 100,000 of the population, 388 Catholics, 246 Protestants, and only 131 Jews. In Budapest from 1901 to 1905, for every 100,000 of the population, the mortality rate from pulmonary tuberculosis was 441 among Catholics, 392 among members of other religions, and 200 among Jews.[82]

Because there was a seeming paradox in the fact that Jews presented all the hallmarks of a group at particular risk but did not suffer inordinately, this group became the focus of considerable scientific attention. Prior to World War I, medical science had put forth a variety of explanations to account for the relative immunity of Jews to tuberculosis. As they had been in other medical and anthropological discourses, Jews served as the litmus test in the literature on tuberculosis for larger discussions of nature versus nurture.

Especially because those Jews who lived in extreme poverty and unhygienic conditions had low mortality rates, some leading researchers concluded that race was the primary explanation.[83] Conversely, other observers, most of them Jewish, opted for an environmental explanation of the disease. The Italian Jewish physician Cesare Lombroso (1835–1909) turned common knowledge and prejudice on its head and claimed that by being engaged in indoor occupations, Jews had actually been shielded from exposure to tuberculosis, which he claimed was promoted in adverse weather conditions.[84] There was also the Darwinian explanation propounded by Maurice Fishberg: "The Jew, living for centuries in the Ghetto, could under the circumstances have adapted his organism to an adverse milieu, to overcrowding, to dark and ill-ventilated dwellings, etc. Those Jews who could not adapt themselves to a confined atmosphere succumbed to various diseases which thrive in such a milieu, chief among which is tuberculosis, and they were eliminated from their midst, having had slight chances to perpetuate their kind."[85]

Natural selection was also on the mind of Alfred von Sokolowski. In his 1912 study of Polish Jews and their susceptibility to contracting tuberculosis, this Warsaw physician maintained, in similar fashion to Fishberg, that because Jews had for centuries lived in cities, the focal points of tubercular infection, and had engaged in endogamous marriage, they had, in effect, successfully bred resistance to the disease among themselves. By contrast, Sokolowski cited the extent to which Gentile rural migrants to urban areas had succumbed easily to infection, precisely because they had not had the luxury of centuries of selective urban breeding.[86]

Although Sokolowski's findings confirmed the lower incidence of tuberculosis among Jews, he was not of the opinion that the statistical difference was as significant as other authors maintained. Rather, into the discourse on Jews and tuberculosis Sokolowski injected a most important new dimension. His study was based on the contents of his own patient files accumulated over a thirty-year period. In his private and hospital practice,

Sokolowski had treated approximately five thousand Jews and five thousand Christians. While he claimed he was unable to detect any prominent differences in the symptoms and appearance of the disease and the way it ran its course between the two groups, he went on to catalogue one crucial difference in the form tuberculosis took in Jews. The determining factor involved the respective mental state of Jews and Gentiles. Of the Jews, he noted, "Just as the entire symptomatology of the Jewish race is characterized by the influence of the neurasthenic predisposition, so too does the over-excitement of the nervous system account for the divergent appearance of tuberculosis among Jews." What Sokolowski meant was that in the early phase of the illness, Jews displayed physical symptoms such as "chest pains, a tenacious cough, especially among women, vomiting, sleeplessness, appetite loss, which among women often manifests itself in complete anorexia, [and] the expectoration of blood brought on by panic."[87] In the later stages, Jews experienced a host of debilitating gastrointestinal disorders.

There is, perhaps, an ironically positive dimension to what Sokolowski called the Jews' "hyper-nervousness." He noted that Jews tended to have boundless faith in the capacity of medicine to cure them. "To the last blink of the eye, Jews, both rich and poor, energetically seek [medical] help, for they firmly believe what the Talmud teaches—one should seek out only a qualified physician who, inspired by the help of God, will prescribe a suitable medicament and thus will the patient be saved."[88]

Such a view was echoed by the Polish Jewish physician Schamschen Kreinermann. In 1915, he accounted for the lower mortality rate from tuberculosis among Jews by suggesting that in addition to *kashrut* and hygiene laws that demanded strict personal and household cleanliness, there was the ready willingness of Jews to seek early medical treatment. This, Kreinermann added, was mandated by the Jewish religion itself. The value Judaism placed on medicine was patently manifest by the fact that when rabbis wrote responsa, practical legal decisions on fine points of law, and the issue pertained to matters of a religious-medical nature, they sought the advice of physicians. This, claimed Kreinermann, cemented the much vaunted position of the doctor in Jewish society and in turn assured the superior health of the Jews.[89]

An explanation for the lower incidence of tuberculosis among Jews was offered by William Moses Feldman, who owed a debt of intellectual gratitude to the French naturalist Jean-Baptiste Antoine de Lamarck (1744–1829). According to Feldman, the acquired immunity of Jewish children to the illness was due to "frequent exposure to mild doses of tuberculosis." Apparently, the poor conditions under which they lived led to a greater frequency of the disease among Jews. However, the form it took was milder than that among Gentiles for two reasons: first, "the great care which Jewish mothers bestow upon their children gives them a stronger constitution to fight the disease," and second was their "great sobriety."[90] Together, these factors worked in perfect harmony to reduce the risk of tuberculosis among Jews.

Other, peculiar cultural explanations also made their way into the respectable medical literature of the day. In attempting to account for the lower level of tuberculosis among Jews in Tunis as compared to their Arab neighbors whose crowded, dank, and unhygienic surroundings they shared, the French military physicians Tostivint and Remlinger opined that the Jews' aversion to dusting their homes, as opposed to wiping surfaces with a damp cloth, meant a reduction in the amount of tubercle-infected air circulating in their midst.[91] Even if this claim had been true for Tunisian Jews, it was obviously not valid for Western European Jews, whose habits and methods of domestic hygiene were identical to those of their Christian neighbors.

Others believed that Jewish ritual dietary laws warded off contagion. Writing in the journal *Nineteenth Century,* Henry Behrend held that the close inspection to which animals killed ritually were subjected meant that bovine tuberculosis was prevented from spreading among the Jews.[92] Although the disease could be transmitted from animals to humans, this explanation based on *kashrut* would have worked only for the conservative Jewish communities of Eastern Europe and the Middle East. The lower rate of tuberculosis among Western European, British, and American Jews, who had increasingly abandoned the dietary laws, demanded an explanation of disease immunity based on something other than observance of the dietary laws.

In 1908, a more universally applicable explanation was offered by the expert on Jewish pathologies, Hugo Hoppe. Among his list of reasons for the lower incidence of tuberculosis among Jews were "the stronger sense of family, even among poor Jews, the great worry over providing for children's education, adequate nourishment and clothing, the dietary laws, meat inspection," and their ability to allocate scarce financial resources, which was superior to that of their equally poor, yet "alcohol-consuming," Christian neighbors. Hoppe, studying the situation in London, rejected race as an etiological factor. Nevertheless, he had to account for the fact that tuberculosis rates among English Jews, while less than those among Christians, had risen dramatically between 1901 and 1906. In that time span, tuberculosis among Jews in London rose from 5.2 percent of all Jewish deaths to 13.3 percent. Certainly the conditions that Hoppe deemed to have earlier afforded protection to Jews were still in operation.

What had happened to so drastically alter the picture? According to Hoppe, the gradual assimilation of Jewish youth, especially to the drinking habits of Gentiles, while still minimal in comparison, had changed enough to affect the overall susceptibility of Jews to the disease. But most important, according to Hoppe, during the Russian pogroms, which had occasioned the massive influx of Jews into London and New York, Jews were arriving desperate, robbed of their possessions, and without any material resources. The strain placed on Jewish welfare institutions was enormous, and they were unable to meet the demand. "Herein," declared Hoppe, "was perhaps the principal cause for the increase of tuberculosis among Jews."[93] Hoppe's analysis is compelling in that his environmentalism led him to identify Jewish vulnerability to tuberculosis as the result of Christian violence and Jewish behavior. Physical terror as a result of the pogroms, while the main cause of the problem, was aided and abetted by moral breakdown in the form of Jewish assimilation. Here the modern world was a threat to Jews. Whether in the hostile political climate of Tsarist Russia or in the more beneficent environments of New York and London, Jews were under physical threat.

The association of Jews with tuberculosis at the fin-de-siècle had a cultural dimension that was of equal significance to the pathological one, and therefore a seemingly straightforward question of etiology and nosology becomes significantly complicated. While the bulk of fin-de-siècle medical literature asserted that Jews were at less risk for contracting tuberculosis than were their non-Jewish neighbors, one strain of medical discourse offered a contrary view, and one that had a uniquely Jewish twist. Some physicians posited that Jews were especially prone to tuberculosis because it was spread by the *mohel* during the ceremony of ritual circumcision, the *brit milah*. Together with syphilis, pulmonary tuberculosis was regarded as the number one medical consequence of the ritual of *metsitsah,* the sucking of blood from the circumcised male member in order to staunch the bleeding.[94]

In his study of Franz Kafka, Central Europe's most famous tubercular Jew, Sander Gilman has indicated that like syphilis, tuberculosis was understood to be a "disease caused by immoral or intemperate habits."[95] Certainly for its detractors, metsitsah would thus qualify. But for Kafka, as Gilman shows, the ceremony of metsitsah as performed in Eastern Europe was presented as one that encouraged rapid healing rather than promoting disease. The retention of metsitsah in the East was interpreted by Kafka as a sign of both individual and communal Jewish well-being, because it was a marker of authenticity. Just as he considered Hebrew and Yiddish the authentic and therefore healthy modes of Jewish expression, so too did Kafka regard the authenticity with which Eastern Jews performed the ceremony of brit milah, to be a prophylactic against the acquisition of the "social diseases" of tuberculosis and syphilis.[96]

To further demonstrate the complicated nature of this problem, Kafka did not establish binary categories of healthy Eastern versus sick Western Jews. Despite the deracination and de-ethnicization that characterized the more "hygienic" brit milah ceremony in the West, those Jews too remained protected against the ravages of assimilation because of the kernel of authenticity that remained in the very performance of even their own culturally "sterile" version of the circumcision ceremony.

For authors like Kafka and the scientists mentioned above, there is a link between culture and wellness. Whether they were protected by their inclination to readily seek medical care, their occupational structure, their development of an immunity to tuberculosis because of regular exposure to it in the ghettos, their consumption of kosher meat, or their performance of ritual circumcision, Jews were believed capable of warding off the greatest killer disease of the day. But as with alcoholism, relinquishing aspects of traditional culture threatened to place the Jews at risk, making them as pathologically vulnerable as their Gentile neighbors. Culture could protect. Its absence could kill.

## DIABETES

In contrast to alcoholism and tuberculosis, Jews were believed to have suffered so inordinately from diabetes that the disease was known colloquially in the German language as the *Judenkrankheit* (Jews' disease). German Jews even made jokes about the high incidence of diabetes among them, such as: "Nebbech, we Jews get it from all sides. When a Goy is thirsty he has a couple of pints of beer. But when a Jew is thirsty he goes and has himself checked for sugar."[97] With remarkable uniformity of opinion at the fin-de-siècle, medicine identified the Jews as being at particular risk for contracting diabetes.

That consensus stands in sharp contrast to the first studies of the disease that began to appear in the seventeenth century. Take, for example, the work of the Englishman Thomas Willis, published in 1674. He did not once mention the Jews.[98] The same is true for the studies of John Rollo and Robert Watt, two pioneers of British diabetes research.[99] Two centuries later, that picture had altered completely. The Jews were not only mentioned in the medical literature on diabetes, they were the focal point of all discussions that sought to identify links between ethnicity and the disease.

In 1870, the University of Vienna professor of medicine and Carlsbad sanitorium physician, Joseph Seegen, was the first researcher in the modern period to "establish" the predisposition of the Jews to diabetes. Based on a case study of 140 patients he saw in private practice, Seegen identified 36 as Jews—or over 25 percent. This percentage was confirmed fourteen years later by the German physician Friedrich Theodor von Frerichs. One important study that analyzed mortality rates from diabetes in the city of Frankfurt from 1872 to 1890 found that of 171 people who had died from the disease, 33.3 percent were Jews. As a proportion of the total population, this meant that Jews succumbed to the deadly illness at a rate of six times that of the non-Jewish population. In Prussia, Heinrich Singer found an even slightly higher disproportion between Jewish and non-Jewish deaths from diabetes, with Jews dying at a rate of six and a half times that of Gentiles. In Marburg, Rudolf Külz found that among the 692 diabetics he had treated, 123, or nearly 18 percent, were Jews. Considering that the Jews made up only 1.2 percent of the total population of the German Reich, Külz professed his astonishment at the "extraordinary disposition of Israelites to diabetes." Similarly, Georg Heimann found that of the 100 Prussians who had died from diabetes in 1897, the number of Jews among them was six times higher than their percentage in the population.[100]

Elsewhere in Europe, in 1891, the French Academy of Medicine took up a discussion of illnesses among Jews. At their Paris meeting, most of the physicians who attacked the problem were struck by the seeming predisposition of Jews to diabetes.[101] New York also provided an important setting for comparative studies of diabetes among ethnic groups. Based on his study of 136,761 patients over an eleven year span (1890–1900) in five city hospitals—Mount Sinai and four non-Jewish institutions—Julius Rudisch calculated that of the 196 treated for diabetes, 86 were Jews, and thus "we find that diabetes is nearly three times as prevalent among Hebrews as among any other race or creed."[102]

Just as the nineteenth century came to a close, Heinrich Stern, also in New York, reported that in 1899, 54 of the 202 people who had died from diabetes that year were Jews. Although the Jews made up approximately 10 percent of the city's population, they constituted 25 percent of all deaths from diabetes. Farther north, in Boston, H. Morrison studied statistics on mortality from diabetes between the years 1895 and 1913 and found that "the ratio of the number of deaths due to this disease to the total number of deaths from all causes is .018 among Jews and .007 among non-Jews."[103]

What could explain this situation? The apparent uniformity of the findings led several researchers to conclude that the Jews had a unique, racial predisposition for contracting diabetes. While he admitted to being unsure as to why this was so, German physician Carl von Noorden was, nevertheless, absolutely convinced that race was the determining factor among the Jews. "Surely," he wrote, "certain races show a preference for diabetes. The Semites are particularly prone to the disease. This fact can be asserted with absolute certainty for all of European Jewry. . . . In my private clinic in Frankfurt, where patients from all over the world visit, 1,487 diabetics came for treatment over an eleven year period [1895–1906]; of them 31.5% were Jewish."[104] And in a classic example of racialized medical speculation, typical of the late nineteenth century, von Noorden suggested that the increasingly frequent intermixture of Jewish with "Indo-Germanic blood had greatly contributed to the spreading of the disease among the Jews."[105] Just what the mechanism was for the increase of the disease through racial mixing the author does not say. And if it is indeed true that fewer Christians than Jews suffered from the disease, as all the data indicated, how was it that such mixing served to increase diabetes among Jews, when the opposite effect, following such logic, could have reasonably been expected? Clearly, von Noorden was more concerned about the increasing rate of intermarriage than about the rising rate of diabetes among Jews. Simply put, race-mixing was for him a sin against natural pathology.

For Felix Buschan, a noted anthropologist and physician in private practice from Stettin, there was "convincing proof" that the higher degree of diabetes among Jews was caused by "an inherited weakness of the central nervous system of the Jewish race."[106] According to the American physician H. Morrison, history had created the pathological conditions that explain the Jews' predisposition to diabetes. That is, "a severe environment during many centuries has developed a nervous type easily thrown out of balance."[107] Or as Joseph Seegen observed, "Over the course of their long history of suffering . . . the Jewish people have [developed] an unstable nervous system, and I see in this a confirmation of the experience of others, that diabetes, in so many cases, is brought on by psychological disturbances."[108]

In similar fashion, the renowned Strasbourg specialist Bernhard Naunyn found that a staggering 38.8 percent of his diabetic patients were Jews. While he attributed much to the role of environment, citing factors such as "a richer life-style, and inbreeding," he also resorted to an organic explanation, stating that these and other influences promoted the development of a "neuropathic disposition."[109] By citing "inbreeding" as a cause of diabetes among Jews, Naunyn made reference to one of the most important debates among nineteenth-century physicians vis-à-vis the etiology of disease. Scientists were divided as to the pathological consequences of inbreeding versus crossbreeding. On this hotly debated topic, both camps appealed to the example of the Jews because of their unique marriage patterns. In this context, "inbreeding," meant either Jews marrying among themselves, as they had for centuries, or the institution of consanguineous marriage, which was permitted by Jewish law. Now it was the commonplace claim of scientists that such marriages among Jews led to either their susceptibility or their immunity to certain kinds of disease.[110] According to the Jewish physician Heinrich Stern, "The cardinal predisposing cause [of diabetes among Jews] . . . is the breeding in and in to which in very pronounced measure, the Jewish and the Irish race still adhere."[111] Hugo Hoppe went further and suggested that the two major causes of nervous and degenerative diseases among Jews were "city life" and "inbreeding." Of all hereditary and degenerative disorders, diabetes was especially pronounced. Through inbreeding it had been passed on from "generation to generation," afflicting Jews as a result of the accumulated effects on the nerves of "pressure, poverty, and persecution."[112]

Most often, the studies on Jewish pathology were conducted in major urban areas, but to test the "inbreeding" theory and the effects of inheritance, physicians sometimes studied the rate of diabetes among Jews in provincial locations. One such study of diabetics in the small Hungarian town of Nagy-Kanisza led the investigator, Arnold Lorand, to report that in this, his own hometown, there are "very few large families [among the Jews] who do not have members who are diabetics."[113] But when Lorand summarized his argument, he went beyond the narrow confines of Nagy-Kanisza to generalize that "inbreeding" or "marriage between relatives" was responsible for the high rate of diabetes among all Jews. Here the ill health of a few tainted the vast majority.

Although they were in a decided minority, there were also Jewish physicians who subscribed to a racial explanation for the seemingly higher prevalence of diabetes among Jews than among Gentiles. In 1903, a diabetes and digestive-system specialist in Berlin, Wilhelm Sternberg, insisted that only a theory grounded in sound scientific method could explain the discrepancy between Jewish and Christian rates of contracting the illness. In his own study of diabetics, he included not only those "legally" born of Jewish mothers, but also those who could be categorized as racially Jewish, by which he meant converts. Of his sample of 650, there were 252 Jews. Therefore, he concluded, "as physicians and scientists we must assume the only point of view that appears authoritative, that the universal difference does not, as the theologians of all faiths frequently wish it, lie in religious differences, but only in the different racial origins [of the two groups]." Sternberg went on to make a finer distinction. "Diabetes," he said, "was more prevalent among those of Semitic background, and if, in turn, these people were to be divided up into different categories, the disease would be shown to take its greatest toll among the Jews of Europe."[114] Similarly, one of the most important Jewish race scientists of the fin-de-siècle, the Zionist physician Felix Theilhaber, declared that "the decisive factor in the inclination of the Jews towards diabetes is to be found, perhaps, in their racial disposition."[115]

As diabetes came to be studied more and more, some specialists expressed their concern that perhaps something was amiss with the statistics. Perhaps it was merely a matter of sampling error. With justification, some physicians were alarmed by the fact that the majority of the comparative European figures showing the heightened predisposition of Jews toward diabetes were culled from German bathing resorts and sanitariums. Spas, with their fully trained medical personnel, were favorite vacation haunts of German-speaking Jews. It should be added that poor Russian, Polish, and Austrian Jews also flocked to these places. Attracted to these institutions in proportionately greater numbers than other ethnic groups, Jews went in search of the cures and treatments provided by the renowned specialists who practiced on the premises. It is this habit that made the claim that Jews suffered inordinately from diabetes so problematic for some researchers.

To Jewish physician Ottomar Rosenbach, who in clinical tests found little difference between Jewish and Gentile susceptibility to diabetes, it was obvious that "when a physician treated many well-to-do patients, and only few poor ones, and especially when such observations took place in spa-resorts populated by individuals or members of a specific class or religion [namely Jews], then the great, absolute, and relative number of diabetics should come as no surprise."[116]

In the famous resort of Carlsbad, Arnold Pollatschek showed that in the period from 1891 to 1900, he had treated 4,719 patients. Of these, 2,381 were Christians, 2,333 were Jews, and 5 were Muslims. Among them there were 653 diabetics — 289 Christians and 364, or 56 percent, Jews. But precisely because the clientele at Carlsbad was predominantly Jewish, the statistics were distorted, and as far as Pollatschek was concerned, the incidence of diabetes among them was more apparent than real.[117]

The subject of the Jews' excessive concern for their health reappears in the discussion on diabetes and the impact that had on the statistical studies. According to one author, "Relative to race, it appears as though the Jews possess a certain predisposition to diabetes. But as everybody knows, they are much more anxious about their health than the Teutons or the Latins and are in relatively better economic circumstances, and so there is much greater opportunity to observe and treat their illnesses."[118] According to Friedrich Frerichs, who Pollatschek paraphrases, "The well known anxiety and willingness to make sacrifices for the preservation of their health leads Jewish patients from all over the world to seek out the most famous clinics, because it is a well-known fact that the Jews prefer to consult with the most famous professors."[119]

Diabetes, like many other ailments, was open to wide cultural interpretation, and many sought to explain the seeming prevalence of diabetes among Jews as a consequence of identifiable social and cultural factors.[120] One of the first to claim that the Jews were not biologically predisposed to diabetes but were at risk because of certain lifestyle features was Joseph Jacobs. In addressing the alleged immunity and or susceptibility of the Jews to various diseases, Jacobs rejected the idea that diabetes and race were linked. Rather, he was of the opinion that "if we cannot claim for Jews any racial immunity from special disease, neither can it be asserted that they are liable as a race to any, such as haemorrhoids and diabetes. *So far as these are prevalent among Jews they are due to sedentary habits*" [emphasis added].[121]

With Jacobs there begins a definite trend, especially among Jewish researchers, to view the rate of diabetes among Jews as the result of their peculiar lifestyle rather than as a consequence of their biology. And here, Germany serves as the focal point of all discussions. It appeared to physicians that even if it were true that the general Jewish population suffered disproportionately from diabetes, then it was German Jewry specifically who seemed to be the most afflicted—hence the appellation *Judenkrankheit* (Jews' disease), the correlate of which was not to be found anywhere else. The reason for the focus on the Jews of Germany involved principally four discrete but related things: the highly racialized nature of German medical research; the fact that the Jews constituted Germany's most important "racial" minority; the concomitant fact of high Jewish participation in medicine, which served to drive research in certain directions; and the fact that the diabetes discourse was tied to the unique social circumstances of Wilhelmine Jewry.

Diabetes was considered to be a disease that struck the wealthier classes more than it did the poorer ones, and city dwellers to a greater degree than it did those in rural areas. According to late nineteenth-century medicine, the German Jewish population, overwhelmingly middle-class and urbanized, led lifestyles that placed them at risk. The sheer pace and nature of modern life led to the following observation made by one physician in 1897:

> All observers are agreed that Jews are specially liable to become diabetic. There is some reason to believe that modern life is in itself a cause of diabetes. . . . A person belonging to the richer classes in towns usually eats too much; spends a great part of his life indoors; takes too little bodily exercise, and overtakes his nervous system in the pursuit of knowledge, business or pleasure. . . . Such a description is a perfectly accurate account . . . of the well-to-do-Jew, who raises himself easily by his superior mental ability to a comfortable social position, and notoriously avoids all kinds of bodily exercise.[122]

In Budapest, where one of Central Europe's greatest concentration of Jews was to be found, a German Zionist physician, Elias Auerbach, conducted an important study on the causes of death among Jews in the Hungarian capital. He too detected a remarkably high incidence of diabetes among them. Between 1902 and 1905, Auerbach found that of 487 reported deaths from diabetes, 238, just over 50 percent, had been Jews. This when they constituted 23.6 percent of the total population. His calculated death rates from diabetes per 1,000 were 5.9 among Catholics, 7.2 among people of other faiths, and 21.4 among Jews. Now, given much of the prevailing opinion concerning the link between race and disease, it would have been easy for Auerbach to interpret his findings thus. Yet he resisted this temptation. Instead, he looked at those who died according to their occupational status and found that 1 out of every 296 artisans, 1 out of every 28 professionals, and 1 out of every 65 merchants succumbed to diabetes. Given the high proportion of Jews among the latter two groups, the link between diabetes and the stresses attendant to a professional and commercial life seemed to indicate that occupation, more than race, was a contributing factor.[123]

In what was a typical trope of medical discourse at the time, some physicians displayed an openly anti-capitalist bent when describing the etiology of diseases that Jews contracted. It was their opinion that many of the specific illnesses that afflicted Jews—diabetes preeminent among them—were brought on by or exacerbated by the stress of a commercial life. According to Hermann Eichhorst in Zurich, "It is without doubt that intense psychic excitement can call forth diabetes mellitus. . . . I have [also] learned that numerous, failed stock-exchange speculations are a direct cause of the disease, and one can even observe a correspondence between the rise and fall of the market and the improvement and the worsening of the disease."[124] As the entry on diabetes in the *Jewish Encyclopedia* of 1903 noted, "When stocks fall, diabetes rises in Wall Street."[125]

In his important work on the diseases of the Jews, Heinrich Singer identified both race and environment as the etiological factor of illness among Jews, and concluded that "the Jews are heavily predisposed toward diabetes because of the nervous systems which they have inherited, their occupational choice, and the restlessness of their activities." Echoing the prevailing anti-capitalist sentiment, Singer noted that "it is precisely the merchant class with its business worries and excitement that provides an undeniably greater proportion [of diabetics] than other classes."[126]

Similarly, Maurice Fishberg focused specifically on German Jews to explain the predisposition of the global Jewish population to diabetes. Taking that group to be paradigmatic insofar as the pathological consequences of modernity were concerned, Fishberg observed: "Persons of a nervous temperament are very often affected, and it is not uncommon to elicit a history of insanity, consumption, and gout among the blood relatives of diabetics. Sudden emotional excitement, grief, terror, worry, and anxiety may each and all be followed so closely by diabetes that there is no room to doubt as to their having been the cause of it. . . . It is also more frequent among the class that is given to high living, to overfeeding, lack of proper exercise, etc. All these etiological factors are found among the Jews in Germany owing to their superior economic status." And as if to underscore the point about the exceptional nature of German Jewish life in relation to the rest of world Jewry, Fishberg further asserted that "we know of no ethnic causes for the frequency of this disease, and among the class of Jews who live moderately, it is no more frequent than among others of the same class."[127] The value judgment passed here is an important one because it entails a transvaluation of lifestyle arrangements. Suddenly, it is Eastern European Jewry, poor and working class, that displays a sensible level of moderation, one that accrues to its pathological benefit. By contrast, German Jews, and Fishberg even includes German Jewish immigrants in the United States, lead lives so lavish that diabetes prevails among them as a form of punishment for their bourgeois delinquency.

For H. L. Eisenstadt, the sins of the German Jewish bourgeoisie were the principal cause of diabetes among them. As an explanation for the apparent high rate of diabetes among Jews, few were more novel than his. According to Eisenstadt, "Diabetes is a consequence of a disturbed sexual life. . . . Among Western European Jews seeking to attain economic improvement, a psychological victim [namely, the modern Jew] has come to the fore: regulating him is sexual abstinence, celibacy, late marriage, the two-children per marriage system, the disinclination of the widower to re-marry, and his associating with prostitutes." For Eisenstadt, diabetes was a psychosexual disorder. The Jews lead unsatisfied sexual lives and so, in order to compensate for the absence of a normal sex life, the Jews "regress to the feelings of childhood autoeroticism and take delight in that with which their mothers satisfied them during childhood — sweets."[128] As a consequence of being in the vanguard of modern, urban life, the relatively well-to-do German Jews consciously limited family size, and quite possibly the frequency of sexual relations. An infantilized sexuality and the desire for oral satisfaction caused the Jews to yearn for the foods of childhood, and thus did sweets become a substitute for sex and a cause of diabetes.

With these Freudian explanations we must turn to Vienna. There, in the Habsburg capital, Martin Engländer, a physician and staunch Zionist, sought to identify the many features of modern urban life that he believed were responsible for the alleged poor health of the Jews. He echoed many others in claiming that "diseases of the nervous system, exhausting intellectual work, psychological agitation — all these pre-dispositions we have found among the Jews in superabundant quantity. Therefore, it is no wonder to us that the Jews have a special share in the increasing [incidence] of diabetes *brought on by nerves*" [emphasis added].[129]

Engländer offered a series of concrete proposals to be put in place to counter the prevalence of diabetes among Jews. Among the measures he suggested were for the family physician to closely observe his patients for signs of the disease, given that it was inheritable. Those predisposed to diabetes were to be put on a strict diet and individually designed and effective nutrition programs. Regularly administered urine examinations were to be undertaken in order to track the course of the disorder and possibly highlight any attendant illnesses. Finally, as a Zionist activist, Engländer was concerned with social engineering. For him, culture rather than biology were in large part to blame for the diabetic state of German Jewry. He suggested that, to help solve the problem, "consideration be given to the education, occupation-selection, and the entire arrangement of one's life-style."[130]

Aside from the 125-year time span and scientific advances that Engländer had incorporated into his text, there was, in fact, little that separated the self-critique of Engländer from that of Elcan Isaac Wolf. Whether eighteenth-century maskil or twentieth-century Zionist, to be a physician and hold to either place on the spectrum of modern Jewish politics was to see something inherently wrong with the nature of the Jews' social and cultural organization. Moreover, in the West, their successful modernization and movement into the middle classes was seen to be compromised by the stressful occupations they chose, which in turn prejudiced the health of the Jews.

The time span of a century and a quarter also separated Elcan Isaac Wolf from Heinrich Singer. For that reason, it is astonishing to read an almost identical critique of the German Jews' diet in Singer's work. The three principal causes of diabetes among Jews, according to Singer, are "heredity, a neuropathological taint, and their unsuitable lifestyles." As part of the latter, Singer asks his readers to consider the "special liking of the Jews for sweets and pastries. The Jew is known as a gourmand (*Feinschmecker*), and as a lover of tidbits. His sense of taste has not been dulled by alcohol abuse and he takes pleasure in the joys of the table." For Singer, when this is taken into account, along with the fact that "the Jews steer clear of manual labor, and sporting activities (both necessary for the burning of sugars) and lead sedentary lives . . . [then] diabetes, gout, and corpulence . . . among Jews are facts, the correctness of which are not to be argued against."[131]

But above all, it was their shattered nerves that served as the major catalyst for diabetes among Jews. As one physician noted, "The only reasonable explanation of the frequency of [diabetes] among Jews is their extreme nervousness, the Jews being known as the most nervous of civilized peoples."[132] Nearly all doctors at the turn of the century mentioned the Jews' unbalanced mental state, while few ever explained what they meant by it. This is not surprising given the indefinable quality of words such as *neuropathy* and *neurasthenia,* or the words of one German doctor: "The Jews are the most nervous people on the face of the earth."[133] Physicians at the fin-de-siècle used such language with abandon, never bothering to provide a definition, precisely because nearly everyone understood what was meant by them. Such words were common linguistic currency, and physicians as well as laypeople, Jews as well as Gentiles, traded in it.

To observers of the late nineteenth century, nervousness epitomized the Jews. They appeared to be a harried and restless people, and indeed, this was an opinion formed, to some extent, by social reality. The approximately two million Jews who left Russia between 1881 and 1914 certainly helped reinforce that impression. The Jews of Eastern Europe were on the move, while Western and Central European Jewish aid agencies sought to assist the refugees with funds to keep them moving farther west. So whether ambulatory or sedentary, all Jews were in some way implicated in the process of a European Jewry in constant motion.

As we shall see in Chapter 5, the notion that nervousness was a defining attribute of the Jews led the medical profession in Central Europe to the deeply held conviction that Jews suffered inordinately from a variety of mental illnesses. Here, it will suffice to say that in order to demonstrate the predisposition of Jews toward diabetes, the medical community needed to paint a picture of the modern Jew that was the opposite of his idealized Gentile neighbor. While the latter was lithe, well-proportioned, athletic, calm, and self-possessed, medical science portrayed the Jew as corpulent, having a sweet-tooth, misshapen, decidedly unathletic, nervous, even hysterical. What is remarkable about this composite picture of the Jewish male is how closely the description resembles the common image of women at the fin-de-siècle. They too were supposedly given to hysteria, were physically vulnerable, and were too delicate for the great outdoors. These were not the traits ordinarily associated with European males. They were, however, peculiarities that the medical establishment identified as being shared by Jews and women alike.

## GENDER AND THE JEWISH BODY AT THE FIN-DE-SIÈCLE

The fin-de-siècle medical discourse on some of the more important pathologies and vital statistics as they pertained to Jews was influenced by the larger political and popular culture of modern Germany, the very culture in which the majority of physicians who studied the pathology of the Jews either lived in or were influenced by. It was from that multi-hued palette of representations of the Jews that medical commentators drew, enabling them to ignore or distort many of their own findings to paint a picture of Jews as weak and unhealthy.

We have, on the one hand, this rather typical late nineteenth-century description of the Jew: "There are, in every country, many Jews of poor build, stunted growth and weak constitution. There is a singular contrast between the Jew's persistent [inner] vitality and his bodily infirmity. His feebleness often gives him a somewhat unmanly appearance. He is of frail bodily structure; the skeleton and the muscular system lack strength. He is wanting in breadth and squareness; in many countries he is manifestly unfit for heavy work. The contrary is true of the Englishman, the Auvergnat, the Piedmontese, the Spanish Gallego, all of whom seem constructed for hard work. The Jew is, moreover, misshapen; few races have so many men who are deformed, disabled, or hunchbacked, so many who are blind, deaf-mutes, or congenital idiots."[134]

## THE JEWISH BODY DEGENERATE?

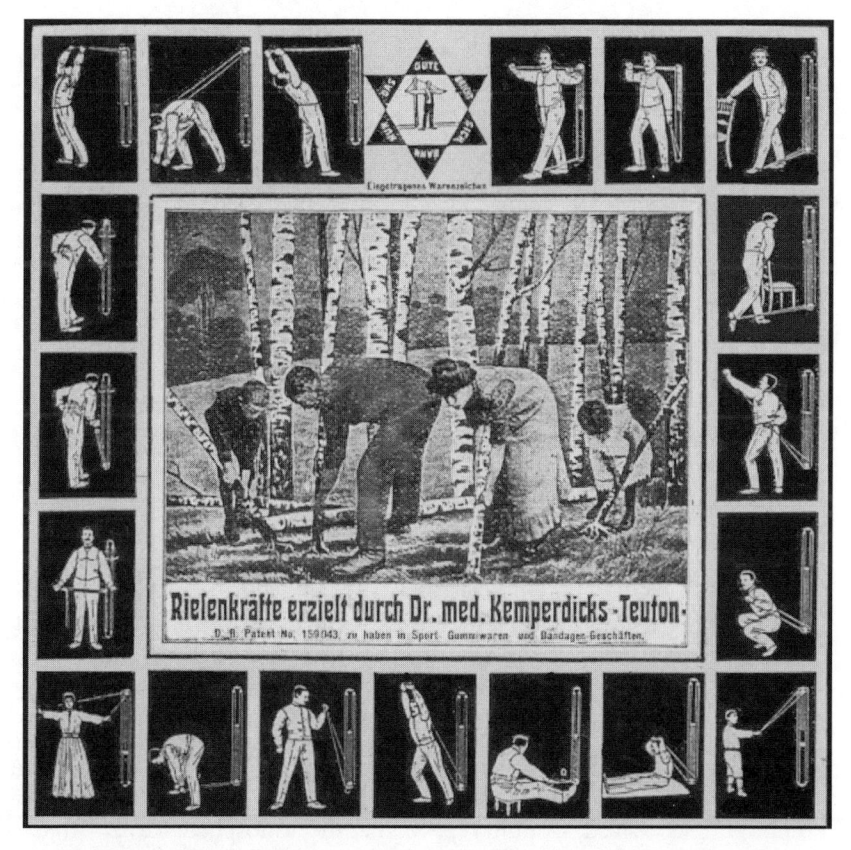

FIGURE 6. The normative representation of Jews in the nineteenth century was that they were physically weak and sickly. This advertisement for an exercise machine appeared in 1908, in the Zionist periodical *Die Welt*. It promises that: "Enormous strength can be attained with Dr. Kemperdick's Teuton." In addition to the revealing use of the word *Teuton* to name a piece of exercise equipment, and its being promoted in a Jewish periodical, note the Star of David and the sight of Jews literally uprooting trees with their bare hands, presumably after having worked out with the Teuton.

On the other hand, this view needs be contrasted with all the statistical evidence that showed the Jews to be a healthy and vigorous people. Yet medicine, and popular culture's view of the diaspora Jew was (and indeed still is) of someone who is frail, timid, weak, and sickly. How did this come about? How did the "unmanly" Jew described above become the normative Jew of scientific and popular imagination?

## THE JEWISH BODY DEGENERATE?

The key to the riddle is gender, for the particular diseases Jews were thought to be afflicted by or immune to were interpreted in deeply gendered ways. Alcoholism was mainly thought of as a man's disorder, because the act of imbibing was itself so much a part of Christian male culture. This point is illustrated by the reminiscence of Arthur Ruppin, a German Zionist lawyer, who detailed an experience concerning alcohol that serves as ample testimony to the fact that the culture of excessive drinking was foreign to young Jewish men in Wilhelmine Germany.[135] In his memoirs, Ruppin devotes ample space to telling the story of the peer pressure he experienced from fellow lawyers when he took up his first post as a *Referendar* (junior barrister) in the town of Klötze in 1902. At around 10 AM on his first day of work he was greeted upon arrival at the train station by the district judge, who immediately informed him that he and several dignitaries from the town met three times a day for drinks — morning, evening, and night. The morning drinking hour was fast approaching, so they went to the hotel where Ruppin was introduced to his new colleagues. "They gave me a warm welcome and were apparently satisfied with me and my drinking habits (I had learned the students' drinking ritual in Halle). I drank five to six glasses of beer to make the proper toasts to each one of them. Afterwards I had to drink wine with my lunch at the hotel, and my head was heavy at five o'clock, when I made my way to the court in order to take the oath." At this stage, Ruppin's colleagues were still unaware that he was Jewish. Soon after, when asked his religion, he made it known. When the time for early evening drinks arrived, Ruppin reports that the atmosphere turned "freezingly polite." Pretending not to notice, he proceeded to drink with them. By the nighttime round, a concerted vindictiveness had set in, and Ruppin noted that the others "intended to drink [me] under the table. In Halle I got used to drinking a few glasses of beer, but on this evening I was obliged to down a total of twenty-two glasses, and this had a devastating effect on my intestines. I felt terribly sick but did not let it show. I continued to sit up straight in my chair, apparently not at all drunk, and decided I would burst rather than give in. At one o'clock in the morning, the district judge left the pub, apparently reconciled to 'his' *Referendar,* who could hold his liquor."[136]

Ruppin's story is a most revealing one. That he made so many references to drink in his diaries, including this one unforgettable episode, tells us much about the different recreational habits of Germans and Jews at the turn of the century. We are informed about the extent to which Jewish accommodation to Gentile practices was necessary to ensure social harmony.

We are also witness to the central role played by alcohol in the lubrication of social interactions. It is clear that if the coercive drinking habits of Germans demanded much of Ruppin, much the same would have applied to other German Jews. Drinking, as this anecdote makes clear, was a fundamental expression of German masculinity. Ruppin had to learn the behavior, mimic the dominant values, and feign a fondness for drink so as to avoid being thought of as anything less than a worthy German man.

Unfortunately, we do not know how many others were unlike Ruppin and refused to play the game. Perhaps the majority. When Aharon Appelfeld's character Bruno Rauch considers the "defects" of the Jews — he tallies up two hundred — he concedes that others, too, have defects, but quickly counters that "their defects are healthy. People say the Austrians are heavy drinkers. Of course they are, but that, if it can be called a defect at all, is a healthy defect. A man forgets himself for an hour, which is healthy for him and everyone else. If only the Jews knew how to drink, and relax, they would surely be different — stronger, braver, perhaps even more honest."[137] The common perception of Jews as very moderate drinkers, amply supported by statistical evidence and anecdote, should also be seen as an implicit comment on the perceived otherness of Jewish masculine behavior.

That very otherness also manifested itself in the domestic sphere. One physician after another commented on the nurturing and tender atmosphere that was to be found in Jewish homes. How accurate such a sweeping generalization may be is unimportant. What counts is the medical perception of such behavior. Moreover, it indicates that according to nineteenth-century norms, it was the maternal qualities of nurturing and tenderness that dominated and characterized the atmosphere in the Jewish home. Almost all commentators saw this as one of the main reasons for the lower infant mortality rates among Jews. Moreover, the excessive concern Jews exhibited for their health, their "physician-neediness," was also regarded as a hysterically and — thus by definition — feminine form of behavior.

With their *habitus phthisicus,* "that frail, undersized, body," the Jews should have been more susceptible to tuberculosis than they were. But despite their feminine bodies, the Jews were supposedly immune to the disease. Late nineteenth-century medicine dealt with this anomaly by claiming that the Jews were at greatest risk for contracting consumption precisely at that moment when they were transformed into Jewish males — at the ceremony of brit milah. On the eighth day after being born, Jewish boys were rendered physically distinguishable from German boys. The respective maleness of the two groups was differentiated by an act that Christians saw as emasculating and thus feminizing, while for Jews it was the single most important ceremony designating entrance into the fold of Jewish manhood.

Finally, even certain diabetes symptoms were thought to be gender specific. Carl von Noorden expressed his astonishment at the extent to which many Jewish patients lived on for years with glycosuria, finally succumbing not to diabetes but to heart failure. According to him, however, this form of diabetes was most frequently observed in women and almost exclusively among Jews.[138] Maurice Fishberg, commenting on this phenomenon, noted that "this peculiarity may be explained by the rarity of alcoholism among the Jews [and women] . . . [for] it is well known that diabetes in alcoholics is much more severe, and the course is more rapid than among those who abstain from the abuse of alcoholic drinks."[139] Thus it would appear that to the medical community at the turn of the century, the symptomatology of diabetes was similar between Gentile women and Jews, while among Christian men it took a different course as a result of the drinking rituals of European males.

Women of all religious affiliations attracted the attention of medical science in the nineteenth century, and in Germany, medicine's and popular culture's assessment of women often necessitated confronting the Jewish question, which in turn meant acknowledging the biological dimension of Jewishness. Just as medicine contributed novel features to antisemitism, so too did it assist in the construction of an elaborate stereotype of women by scientizing misogyny. As Cynthia Russett has shown, Victorian medicine pathologized women, seeking to scientifically demonstrate their moral, intellectual, and physical inferiority to men.[140] Sometimes both projects overlapped. According to one recent observation, "What antisemitism and misogyny have in common in the nineteenth century are many small points of connection in the dreary landscape of biologically fortified prejudice."[141] In fact, the establishment of scientifically grounded bigotry was a hallmark of the oppositional or "anti" discourse of groups who wielded power in fin-de-siècle Europe.[142]

Biological racists and misogynists posited the inferiority of Jews and women on the basis of a blend of anthropometry and stereotype. With the former reinforcing the latter, ancient prejudices were confirmed not merely on a consensual, and thus subjective, basis, but supposedly on the unassailable grounds of "objective" statistics—the principal methodology of the quantitative enterprise of anthropometry. It is this that made biological determinism—an act of science in the service of bias—so consoling and reassuring to its practitioners and purveyors.[143]

## THE JEWISH BODY DEGENERATE?

The category of gender is of critical importance for understanding the place of the Jews in fin-de-siècle Central European culture. In particular, in both the antisemitic and medical imaginations of the era (not necessarily distinct from one another), Jews—and this generally meant males—were metaphorically likened to women.[144] Such an evaluation resided not only in the physical realm, with descriptions of frail, delicate, and vulnerable Jewish bodies, but in the psychological arena as well. As Carl Jung said when distinguishing Jewish from Aryan psychology: "[Jewish men] have this peculiarity in common with women; being physically weaker they have to aim at the chinks in the armor of their adversary, and thanks to this technique which has been forced on them through the centuries, the Jews themselves are best protected where others are most vulnerable."[145]

So powerful and all pervasive was the notion of the feminized Jew that even committed Jews espoused such beliefs. As early as 1869, a Viennese rabbi, Adolf Jellinek, published an ethnographic study entitled *The Jewish Tribe*. It was Jellinek's opinion that Jews shared several traits in common with women. In a chapter on "The Femininity of the Jewish Tribe," Jellinek noted that both groups were unsystematic thinkers, yet possessed of lively and sharp intellects. In both groups, actions were determined by emotion rather than by reason, and both were especially susceptible to flattery—women from men and Jews from Gentiles. The positive side of being like women was that Jews could use these "feminine" traits of adaptability and mimicry to more easily adopt the mores of the majority and assimilate into the dominant culture.[146] This was indeed a frequent complaint of the antisemites.

As a measure of the extent to which this peculiar brand of antisemitic prejudice could be internalized in a place like Vienna, even the Jewish psychiatrist and member of Freud's inner circle, Otto Rank, called Jews "women among the people." Noting their outsider and feminized status, he implored Jews to "join themselves to the masculine life-source if they are to become productive."[147] No individual expressed all the sexual and racial anxieties of his age better than the Viennese Jew Otto Weininger, for whom a solution to the Jewish Question necessitated that "the Jew must first conquer Judaism."[148]

Weininger was vigorously opposed to the emergence into the public sphere of women and Jews, that is, to the respective emancipation of both groups. With his (in)famous and elaborate homology of women and Jews, *Sex and Character* (1903), Weininger produced the proof text of fin-de-siècle Central European misogynist-antisemitism.[149] Originally presented as his doctoral dissertation at the University of Vienna, this book, which appeared shortly before the young Weininger dramatically shot himself to death in Beethoven's house, had a profound influence on contemporary medical discourse as it related to women and Jews.[150]

In multiple areas of human endeavor, Weininger found that Jews and women shared certain moral characteristics. They were, of course, both tainted. Like the composer Richard Wagner, before him, Weininger declared tersely, "It is this want of depth which explains the absence of truly great Jews; like women, they are without any trace of genius."[151] According to Weininger, both groups were perfidious. They lacked humility and a sense of humor, they needed to be ruled, and they were morally flawed, for: "Greatness is absent from the nature of the woman and the Jew, the greatness of morality, or the greatness of evil. In the Aryan man, the good and bad principles of Kant's religious philosophy are ever present, ever in strife. In the Jew and the woman, good and evil are not distinct from one another."[152]

As extreme as his ideas were, Weininger was very much a reflection of his times, for effeminacy was the dominant image of Jewish male sexuality in fin-de-siècle Central Europe, and medicine was deeply influenced by and contributed to such representations.[153] Disease, and especially the representation of the diseased body, are not objective categories, suspended in an imaginary state of pure science.[154] Together with the patient and the medical practitioner, they lie subjectively and deeply embedded in the cultures from which they originate.[155] In the case of Central European Jewry, this meant that the medical community saw Jews as the prevailing culture did: effeminate, weak, degenerate, hysterical, and at risk.

The association of Jews with certain medical disorders in Germany underscored and highlighted their physical otherness. And at the fin-de-siècle, that very otherness was inscribed on the Jews' body in two distinct yet related ways: through circumcision, and through disease. In Central Europe, circumcision was the defining and distinguishing physical characteristic of the Jew. Living in a culture where Gentile circumcision was extremely rare, and in the midst of a people whom, through acculturation, they came more and more to resemble, at least superficially, Jews were distinctive for having been circumcised. As much as circumcision in the form of brit milah may have been invented by the Jews, so, too, was the Jew invented by brit milah. As a signifying marker of tribal membership, inscribed directly onto the body, circumcision affirmed Jewish separateness by corporeally abetting abstract or theological ideas of difference between Jews and Gentiles. But by the end of the nineteenth century, "the fantasy of the difference of the male genitalia was displaced upward—onto the visible parts of the body."[156]

This displacement manifested itself by ascribing to Jews various pathological peculiarities, such as have been detailed in this chapter. In so doing, medical science transposed the hidden marker of the Jewish male onto the exposed body in the form of pathological uniqueness. By association, Jewish women, too, could now be identified as bearers of distinct "Jewish" illnesses. What can thus be observed is actually an insidious and lethal democratizing of the antisemitic medical rhetoric about Jews. By transferring the invisible marker of Jewish difference—the circumcised penis—to the visible parts of the body in the form of disease precisely at that historical juncture when Jewish assimilation was well advanced in Germany, medicine, with its own categories of patient identification and stigmatization, reinscribed upon *all* Jews a new symbol of their physical difference.

No matter how long they lived, how many of their children survived past the age of five, how little they drank, and how apparently infrequently they succumbed to tuberculosis, Jews were depicted by many in the political and medical worlds as a sickly people. In the value system of the late nineteenth century, well-being was predicated upon masculinity and vigor. Yet the Jews, for all their relative good health, were, largely because they did not possess their own nation-state, represented as feminine and frail, a point underscored by their supposedly principal pathological trait—nervousness. Real men were not hysterics. So despite myriad indications that the Jews were a healthy people, they enjoyed the wrong kind of health, for it was without honor. It was womanly. John Hoberman has perceptively called attention to the "Jewish male predicament," wherein fin-de-siècle Jewish men were represented as ugly, deformed, weak, and unheroic—the exact opposite of genuine, healthy masculinity, that being the Germanic ideal.[157] In response, Zionist physician Max Nordau called for Jews to "once again become deep-chested, taut-limbed, steely-eyed men." Through having Jews participate in sporting activities, he hoped, a "muscular Jewry" would be created. The subsequent establishment in Central Europe of Jewish sports associations around the turn of the twentieth century that sought to masculinize and invigorate the Jews was a direct response to this prevailing negative image.[158]

Like their Gentile colleagues, Jewish physicians, both those with and without Zionist sympathies, employed the dominant cultural categories of masculinity and femininity to describe the Jewish body, and central to such discourse was the claim that the Jews were predisposed to mental illness, for nervousness and hysteria were seen as disorders that struck women more than men, and Jews more than any other group. Pinpointing just what the causes were informed the work of many researchers in German-speaking Europe. At the turn of the nineteenth century, some of the most important debates concerning the intersection of medicine and Jewish identity took place among Jewish psychiatrists, and it is to that Jewish conversation that we now turn.

CHAPTER 5

# THE PSYCHOPATHOLOGY OF EVERYDAY JEWISH LIFE

Karl Kraus, the Viennese Jewish satirist and cultural critic, once quipped, "Psycho-analysis is the disease of emancipated Jews; the religious ones are satisfied with diabetes." Kraus' biting remark, which implies that religiosity and ritual observance are incompatible with political and civic freedom, goes to the heart of much of the fin-de-siècle's medical representations of Jews. Whether implicit or explicit, that discourse established firm links between ethnicity and disease, between varieties of Judaism and various pathological states. So, as surprising as Kraus' remark may appear today, it would have resonated with familiarity to his contemporaries, for such notions were commonplace expressions within the fin-de-siècle discourse about the Jewish body.

Conversely, what would have been most strange and perplexing to Kraus, a self-hating Jew and convert to Catholicism, is that his own diagnosis of the Jewish condition, simultaneously intended to dismiss Eastern Jews and deride Western ones, was largely echoed by Jewish physicians of the day and, moreover, by individuals most unlike himself—that is, those who were secure in and proud of their Jewish identities.

According to Kraus, Eastern European Jews merely suffered from a physical ailment that may or may not have been hereditary. However, much more complicated was his diagnosis of Central European Jews. In one of his many withering attacks on Viennese Jewry (he once declared, "They have the press, they have the stock exchange, now they also have the subconscious!") Kraus identified the course of treatment, psychoanalysis, as a disease in and of itself, elevating it to the level of the killer diabetes.[1]

Most important, the true implication of Kraus' remarks about the Jews of the Habsburg capital is that they seek psychoanalysis because they are mentally ill. Ironically, he links that psychological disturbance to their assimilation, a stance he both advocated and held in the extreme. Indeed, in the European psychiatric literature pertaining to Jews, it was widely believed that while assimilated Jews suffered from a host of mental illnesses, the rigorously Orthodox were afflicted primarily with physical ailments.

By the turn of the twentieth century, the pathological isolation of the Jews was expanded to include their mental state. In one branch of medicine, psychiatry, there was widespread belief that Jews had a higher incidence of insanity than non-Jews. By *insanity* we mean here a group of disparate psychopathologies that were regarded at the time as indicators of mental illness. These ranged from the clinically diagnosable schizophrenia to the more subjective and commonly referred to fin-de-siècle condition of neurasthenia.

Already by the mid-nineteenth century enough statistical data had been collected from various parts of Europe and even America to support the thesis that Jews were more prone to mental illness than their neighbors. In 1855 in the Lower Rhine, the researcher Henri Dagonet found there to be one mentally ill person for every 349 Jews, compared to 414 Protestants and 471 Catholics.[2] In 1858, Joseph Czermak published such figures for Freud's native Moravia, as well as Silesia. He found that per 100,000 inhabitants, 220 Jews were mentally ill as compared to only 80 Protestants and 70 Catholics.[3] Figures tabulated for Italy in 1879 indicated that the incidence of mental illness among Jews was 4.5 times higher than that among Christians.[4] According to Württemberg's 1880 census, the locale's 13,331 Jews constituted a mere 0.67 percent of the total population.[5] Yet for every 100,000 inhabitants, the mentally ill population consisted of 159 Jews and only 59 Catholics and 65 Protestants. The disparity was also glaring in Bavaria: per 100,000, 98 Christians as against 252 Jews.[6] The figures from Prussia, with its large Jewish population located primarily in the Imperial capital, Berlin, are the most comprehensive. Taken over a twenty-year period, 1881–1900, and based on admissions to mental institutions among 100,000 inhabitants, the following numbers throw into stark relief the problem at hand.[7] The comparative figures for Christians and Jews, respectively, read as follows: 1881—29.7:92.9; 1890—39.7:120.4; 1895—58.0:145.6; and 1900—68.3:163.1.[8] In 1890 in Hungary, Jews constituted 4.18 percent of the total population and a full 7 percent of the mentally ill population. Conversely, in countries with tiny Jewish populations, the figures were consistent with those found in other, more densely Jewish parts of Europe. For example, in Denmark, 5.8 Jews as compared to 3.4 Christians per 1,000 inhabitants suffered from mental illness.[9] Finally, Eastern Europe displayed a pattern similar to that in Western Europe. A study undertaken of Tsarist soldiers stationed in Kiev in

1895 to 1896 found that among 10,000 troops, 219 Jews, 106 Muslims, 92 Poles, and 91 Russians had been treated for mental illness.[10]

It is possible that the Christian medical perception that Jews had a higher incidence of mental illness was based in an element of truth. But rather than resulting from any Jewish biological or racial deficiencies, as many Gentile psychiatrists suggested, it is far more likely that the explanation involves Jewish sociological attributes and cultural expressions. In that age of overall heightened mental anxiety, Jews—especially those who had been forced to leave Eastern Europe as a result of poverty, pogroms, or civic disabilities, or those in Western Europe who had witnessed the rise of modern antisemitism as well as wild commercial fluctuations of boom and bust business cycles—may well have experienced inordinate mental stress.

Over and above this, Jews resided primarily in big cities, where psychopathologies caused by or irritated by the pressures of urban life may have taken a disproportionate toll on them. In addition, there was the ready availability of medical, especially psychiatric, care in large urban centers. And because Jews attended spa resorts in great numbers, they made disproportionate use of the vast array of Jewish specialists who provided them with an intimate and safe setting for frank discussions of health matters, especially those of a psychological nature.[11] Hence a symbiotic environment was created wherein large populations of Jewish patients and physicians encountered one another. Sigmund Freud's own roster of Jewish patients is testament to this.[12]

But what caused Jews to suffer so inordinately from mental illness? According to many Christian diagnosticians, Jewish psychopathologies often stemmed from the intricate interplay of racial predisposition and moral perfidy. As the Elberfeld physician Heinrich Singer noted: "Already in the childhood of racial development the number of mentally ill among the Jews was great. The Old Testament already mentioned this condition. . . . [And] whomever has paid attention to the further history of the Jews and their ideas up until our day—and has not closed their mind to the facts—surely cannot be surprised [to find] that the modern Jew must atone for the suffering and sins of his fathers—and we want to be fair—also for his own sins."[13]

Such views of Jewish immorality were tenacious. In the early years of the Weimar Republic, Johannes Lange, who had conducted research on Jewish manic-depressives at his clinic in Munich, addressed the annual conference of the Bavarian Psychiatric Association. Lange affirmed the higher incidence of mental illness among Jews on the flimsy logic that while Jews constituted 3 percent of his practice, they accounted for only 2 percent of the total population. Lange also maintained that Jews became sicker at a younger age than did non-Jews, and remained ill for longer. Moreover, he declared that "atypical profiles of sickness (*Krankheitsbilder*) [among Jews] which defy all attempts at diagnosis are manifest daily." According to Lange, Jewish melancholics displayed hypochondria to an inordinate extent. He also complained that his Jewish patients exhibited brooding, grumbling, and unhappy countenances seldom seen to the same extent among his non-Jewish patients. Most important, he echoed Heinrich Singer by stating that twice as many Jews as non-Jews professed the idea that impoverishment (*Verarmungsideen*) leads to hysteria. Thus, implied Lange, insanity among Jews was triggered by their lust for Mammon. Mental illness as a result of the idea that one is committing a sin is "almost completely absent as a religious idea [among Jews], while among Christians, it is of the greatest significance."[14] In contrast to the insanity diagnosed among the Christian population, insanity among Jews was rarely attributable to pangs of morality and conscience, for Judaism, claimed Lange, failed to make such demands on its adherents.

In his *Psychiatrie: Ein Lehrbuch*—which was first published in 1883 and went through nine editions by 1927, thereby making it one of the single most important and widely used medical texts of the day—Emil Kraepelin (1856–1926) noted that a multiplicity of biological and environmental factors was responsible for causing mental illness. Among these were the various influences of race, lifelong habits, climate, diet, and general conditions of health. But when turning to the Jews, Kraepelin privileged race above all other possible causes, maintaining that it was the most important etiological factor in producing insanity among them. He observed: "That the peculiarity of a people can play a role [in causing insanity] is proven by the case of the Jews who can be compared to the surrounding population without making great [statistical] errors. The comparison shows that at least in Germany, and likewise in England, the Jews are inclined to mental and nervous disease in considerably higher numbers than the Teutons. Certainly alcoholic forms of insanity are rare amongst them; on the other hand, we see extraordinary disturbances caused by hereditary degeneration. Perhaps the Jewish preference for consanguineous marriage plays a role."[15]

Like Kraepelin, Richard von Krafft-Ebing (1840–1902), one of the most influential psychiatrists and sexologists of the nineteenth century, charged that race was the principal cause of Jewish psychopathologies.[16] Yet in this strictly biological interpretation, he identified and linked certain Jewish cultural forms as bringing about the higher frequency of mental illness among Jews. In particular, he held that their religious fervor, derived from a racial predisposition to insanity, encouraged deviant sexual practices such as consanguineous marriage. In the nineteenth century, several Gentile psychiatrists held that such unions produced mentally ill offspring, leading to the malicious charge that the Jews were inbred. Linking Jewish religiosity and biology, Krafft-Ebing opined that: "Very often excessive religious inclination is itself a symptom of an originally abnormal character or actual disease, and, not infrequently, concealed under a veil of religious enthusiasm there is abnormally intensified sensuality and sexual excitement that lead to sexual errors that are of etiologic significance."[17]

Similarly, Heinrich Singer believed that several factors caused Jewish insanity, but according to him inbreeding was of the greatest import. The psychopathology of the Jews was caused by "the centuries-long continuation of inbreeding, frequent marriages with blood relations [who bear] a hereditary taint, big-city nervousness, indefatigable absorption in purely intellectual professions, the early attainment of puberty, and many other things. [These] form a fateful chain of unfavorable effects."[18]

In the nineteenth century, the terms *inbreeding* and *degenerate* appear with great frequency in the non-Jewish texts that discussed Jewish insanity. Strict Jewish taboos against marrying outside the fold led Gentile scientists to assume erroneously that millennial intramarriage—they referred to it as inbreeding—among a small population group explained the high incidence of mental illness among Jews.[19] The term *degenerate* was used to describe groups as varied as criminals, prostitutes, avant-garde artists, and members of foreign races. Perhaps, most frequently, the word was applied in popular and medical usage to describe the sexual deviant.[20] Again, Gentile psychiatrists who often questioned Jewish sexual practices such as intramarriage maintained that the etiology of Jewish insanity lay in the degenerate sexual practices of endogamous marriage. According to Krafft-Ebing: "This [inbreeding] is a phenomenon similar to that observed in certain highly aristocratic and wealthy families, whose members, whether from motives of honor or money, constantly intermarry, and thus have many insane relatives."[21] Emil Kraepelin suggested that hereditary degeneration among Jews was most likely caused by their preference for consanguineous marriage. A syllogism is operating here: The insane are degenerates; the Jews are insane; therefore the Jews are degenerate.

A younger generation of Jewish doctors was incensed by these claims. In Vienna, Martin Engländer stated that Jews had, for centuries, been aware that inbreeding led to generations of neuropathically burdened individuals, and as such, Mosaic law had forbidden it. "Is then," he asked with indignation, "the Jewish race of today one large family which sprung from the loins of Abraham and the womb of Sarah and can only continue to multiply from within itself?" Relying on the authority of historians and natural scientists who argued that the Jews had mixed with other nations, Engländer denied the existence of a Jewish race and, by extension, the possibility that mental illness among the Jews was based on racial factors. Rather than inbreeding, he claimed, it was business pressures and the general conditions of life that were responsible for the neuroses of the Jews.[22]

Max Sichel, an assistant psychiatrist at the Frankfurt am Main City Mental Asylum, stated that the purported connection between consanguineous marriage and insanity was not borne out by his clinical observations. "Of the 128 cases we observed, only two had parents who were blood relatives. Inbreeding as an etiological factor among our ill plays no demonstrable role and so it must be due to other important factors."[23] Thus, even while accepting that there was a considerable proportion of Jewish patients in his asylum, Sichel flatly rejected any theory that assigned the cause of their presence there to sexual promiscuity.

Leo Sofer in Vienna went even further than Sichel in claiming that there was no link between Jewish insanity and consanguineous marriage. Turning a common assumption on its head, he claimed that endogamous marriage actually bore a prophylactic property in combating physical and psychological disease. Sofer approvingly quoted a Dr. Reibmayer, who wrote of the Jews, "They can give up all their customs; as long as they don't give up inbreeding they will not lose their biostatistical advantage."[24] Another Jewish physician writing in a popular periodical noted that contrary to the widely held view that the Jews were a "degenerate people . . . our longer average lifespans and lower infant mortality rate are due to temperance and centuries of inbreeding and the natural selection of an acquired resistance-capacity against many infectious diseases such as tuberculosis and typhus." Similarly, the inbreeding had failed to create "a special Jewish nervousness."[25]

Elsewhere in Europe, too, Jews were believed to be disproportionately afflicted with mental illness, a disease they were said to pass on to their offspring. In Paris, Sigmund Freud's teacher Jean-Martin Charcot held this view. Under his direction, the Salpêtrière school promoted a theory of the inheritable nature of disease, which included a vast array of disorders affecting the central nervous system. The host of chronic illnesses, or diatheses, to which certain patients were presumed to be predisposed, often because of their race, was referred to as *la famille névropathique*.²⁶ As far as the racial predisposition of Jews to mental illness was concerned, Charcot's entry for October 27, 1888, in his *Tuesday Lessons* read simply: "Nervous illnesses of all types are innumerably more frequent among Jews than among other groups." Like Kraepelin, he attributed this condition to inbreeding.²⁷

Influenced during his sojourn in Paris, Freud, for whom Charcot became a father figure, also initially subscribed to the idea that Jews were especially prone to mental illness, and even suggested as much about members of his own family.²⁸ But by 1892, in the footnotes to his German translation of Charcot's *Tuesday Lessons,* and even in his 1893 obituary for Charcot, Freud expressed doubts about the idea — without entirely abandoning it — that heredity played a major role in the etiology of disease.²⁹ And instead of Charcot's racially deterministic view of heredity — on several occasions Charcot advised Freud to look specifically at Jewish families as examples par excellence of members of a racial group suffering from a host of inherited neuropathological diseases — Freud supplanted degeneration theory with a universalistic explanation of neuropathologies that stressed the role of environment and sexuality in their acquisition.³⁰ In highlighting Freud's departure from the teachings of Charcot, Toby Gelfand has aptly remarked that "for the French school, what was true for everybody was more true for certain subgroups such as Jews. For Freud, what was true for the Jew became true for everybody."³¹ The fundamental proposition, especially as it related to Jews, that external circumstances outranked organic reasons for psychological disorders became a canonical teaching among Freud's fellow Jewish psychiatrists.³² But, where the issue of "sexual identity" was of prime consideration to Freud in such matters, the nature of "Jewish identity" shaped the diagnostic and therapeutic discourse of his German Jewish colleagues.

I specify German-speaking Jews because although the debate on insanity among Jews was also alive in other parts of Europe, especially Paris, where it was guided largely by Jean-Martin Charcot and his student Henry Meige at Salpêtrière, the response of Jews in France was different from that of German Jews. The former were less engaged in the debates, and there are a number of reasons for this. First, there were, quite simply, far fewer Jewish psychiatrists in France than in Central Europe. The large numbers of such specialists in Germany and Austria set those countries apart and made possible vigorous responses by epistemologically conversant Jewish physicians. Second, the historically important encounter between Eastern and Western Jews at the intersection of the nineteenth and twentieth centuries, so central to the Jewish psychiatric discourse, was played out in German-speaking Europe. Third, and finally, there is the fact that Jewish self-defense was institutionalized in Germany with the founding of the *Centralverein* (Central Union of German Jews) in 1893. Lacking (perhaps not needing) a comparable institution such as this, the Jews in France at that time were absent the same spirit and culture of self-defense that animated German Jewry.[33] When all these factors are taken into account, the accuracy of Jan Goldstein's observation becomes evident: "French Jewry remained oddly phlegmatic and forbearing in the face of the Salpêtrière school's contribution to the new scientific lore about the Jews."[34] Such cannot be said of Jewish psychiatrists in German lands.

In Central Europe, psychiatry's marginalization of the Jews, its burdening them with a unique psychopathology, completed the attempt of the medical profession to represent Jews as biological others. In Germany, for example, whether it portrayed Jews as physically different (and this could even mean in a positive sense, such as possessing an immunity to this or that disease) or psychologically distinct from Germans (whose supposedly contemplative "nature" was more apt to result in chronic melancholia as opposed to the hot-blooded Semitic Jew who suffered more frequently from various manias), the authoritative and prestigious German medical community sought to return Jews to a theoretical ghetto of psychopathological difference.[35] Ironically, this process occurred at the very moment when acculturation had progressed to the point that by a host of outward measures, German Jews had become largely indistinguishable from their Christian neighbors.

But by its emphasis on the pathological differences, German medicine made certain the continued identifiability of the Jews. Despite having embraced the trappings of German culture after acquiring citizenship with the founding of the Second Reich in 1871, the Jews remained conspicuous outsiders.[36] Their incomplete integration bespoke a psychological divide that separated them from Germans. Here psychiatry played an important role, for only it was qualified as a scientific discipline to analyze the inner mind of the Jews, and thus perhaps provide a solution to the riddle of their continued separateness.

The medical and the political were never very far apart.[37] The former aided and abetted the latter when, after 1871, Germany began a protracted and what would turn out to be painful quest for national integration, state building, and identity formation.[38] Central to this large-scale project was defining who was part of and who was to be excluded from the national community. Medicine and race science were important tools for this undertaking, for the practitioners of both — they were often one and the same — provided the expertise to determine the biological nature of the "true" German. The exclusivist nationalism in Germany, predicated on race, meant that in the recently unified Kaiserreich, national integration in an ideal world meant the incorporation of similar-looking and like-minded peoples. By definition, it also meant the exclusion of traditional others, and the Jews were Germany's most conspicuous other.[39]

German psychiatry's diagnosis that the Jews were mentally ill, and in ways that distinguished them sharply from Germans, exacerbated the Jews' outsider status. As the Jews began to experience an increasingly hostile climate characterized by the growth of antisemitic political parties, psychiatry provided a new language and set of ideas to antisemites. While the Jews could outwardly change to make themselves resemble Germans, it was the inner mind of the Jew, his supposedly unique and, as his enemies claimed, "destructive spirit" that made him permanently different from the Germans.

Challenged by the claims of Gentile psychiatrists, Jewish psychiatrists throughout Europe began a debate on the mental illness of the Jews, producing a considerable corpus of literature on the subject. In tracing the dynamics of their response to mainstream psychiatry's depiction of the Jew, one can detect in Jewish psychiatric literature the adoption of clear political-ideological trends by these Jewish psychiatrists.

Jewish practitioners tended to delineate Eastern from Western European Jews, creating distinctions between what they believed were the different pathologies of the two groups. Eastern European Jews were initially represented as inclined toward psychological illness, while Western European Jews were believed to be more prone to physical ailments. However, over time, a paradigm shift took place within this construct. There was a change in the representations as to which Jew, the German or the Polish, best represented a model of Jewish insanity. The original image of the mentally sound Jew, the *Westjude*, which initially dominated the discourse and continued to do so throughout the nineteenth century, gave way by the fin-de-siècle to one that identified the *Ostjude* as typifying the psychologically healthy Jew. This shift was fully crystallized with the advent of "nationalist psychiatry," that is, psychiatry written from the Zionist perspective. The assimilated German Jew was portrayed by Zionist physicians as mentally unfit, a creature psychologically tormented by a crisis of identity, while the Eastern European Jew, secure in his cultural identity, was held up as the model of sound, Jewish mental health.

What made for the emergence of these men was a mixture of politics (the acceptance of Zionism as a panacea for the ills of Jewish diaspora existence), a generational conflict that saw them reject the political, religious, and acculturationist sensibilities of older, Jewish psychiatrists, and the application of non-Freudian explanations of neuroses to determine why mental illness among Jews seemed to be so widespread. Unlike their more famous Jewish contemporaries such as Sigmund Freud, Max Eitington, and Karl Abraham, the doctors whose work is examined here focused their research specifically on the mental illnesses of the Jews. Almost all were clinical psychiatrists practicing between 1900 and 1939 at famous clinics such as the Burghölzli in Zurich, large city institutions such as the Irrenanstalt zu Frankfurt am Main, or private Jewish mental hospitals in Eastern Europe. Their written findings, therefore, were based on close observation of Jewish patients in a hospital setting. This, plus the fact that Jewish psychiatrists sometimes undertook large-scale studies, allowed them to claim the objective-scientific high ground—a feature many of them felt was absent in the work of non-Jewish psychiatrists. Most of the psychiatrists also had a broader impact on Jewish life in that many of them published popular versions of their scientific papers in mass-circulation Jewish newspapers, periodicals, and even literary magazines. By the turn of the twentieth century, the issue of mental illness among Jews had become a common topic of discussion in Jewish communal life in both Eastern and Western Europe. As a consequence, absolutely none of the arguments presented below would have struck contemporary Jewish ears as unusual, or even idiosyncratic.

Two primary factors motivated the work of these men. First, Gentile psychiatrists' limited clinical experience with Jewish patients and Jewish life in general led Jewish psychiatrists to challenge what they claimed was a lack of objectivity in the work of their non-Jewish colleagues. In the work of the Jewish psychiatrists studied here, Jews were the major focus—not marginal, as they were in the writings of men such as Emil Kraepelin, Richard von Krafft-Ebing, and Eugen Bleuler. For unlike much of the medical and anthropological literature on Jews, which was often generated by hostile non-Jews, the psychiatric literature on Jews was produced mainly by Jewish psychiatrists. It was they who came to dominate the discourse, define its terms, and set its boundaries.

Second, many of the Jewish psychiatrists were in complete accord with the findings of the non-Jewish doctors, accepting the claims about the higher incidence of and predisposition toward nearly all forms of mental illness among Jews. For example, a review of a Gentile psychiatrist's findings on the subject was repeated without comment in the Zionist periodical, *Die Welt*, when the author wrote, "Jews fall prey to mental illness four to six times more than the other civilized nations [*Kulturnationen*] among whom they live."[40] What prompted them to carry on their work was inspired not so much by differences concerning the Jews and mental illness, but, rather, by their different prescriptions for a cure. Rejecting the pessimistic Kraepelinian-Charcotian paradigm of hereditary degeneration, they opted, instead, for one that held out the hope of psychological redemption and rehabilitation.

In the course of their work, Jewish psychiatrists tested hypotheses and challenged commonly held assumptions, and, far from achieving the desired objectivity, they were highly polemical. Their personal politics, class background, and geographic location, and the type of patient they treated came to determine the focus of their works, the questions they asked, and the solutions they offered. A partial list of the questions that formed the core of their enterprise reads as follows: Are Jews more frequently predisposed to mental illness than non-Jews? If so, which illnesses and why? Is there a specific *Psychosis judaica*? Is the predominance of a particular illness due to heredity or environment? If it is environment, what is it about Jewish life that promotes insanity? On the other hand, if Jews are immune to certain diseases or mental disorders, is this caused by something peculiar to the "race" or, rather, the conditions under which they live? Can it perhaps be due to the observance of endogamous marriage resulting in the development of an immunity? Or is the converse true? Is the sex life of European Jews detrimental to their physical and mental well-being? Is there any significant psychological difference between Eastern and Western European Jews? Above all, as men dedicated to healing, all the psychiatrists were occupied with the most important question: Is there a cure?

The image that Jewish doctors had of the mental health of Jews and one that was to last until the beginning of the twentieth century was established largely during the Berlin *Haskalah*. In Chapter 3 we discussed Elcan Isaac Wolf's diagnosis of the Jewish body. But in his *Von den Krankheiten der Juden*, Wolf also addressed the condition of the Jewish mind.[41]

According to Wolf, the Jews not only lived in a state of physical despair; they were mentally ill as well. Wolf's book thus was one of the first modern medical texts by either a Jewish or a Gentile physician to charge the Jew with mental illness. According to Wolf, it was a combination of the exigencies of daily life and the traditional Jewish way of worship that caused Jewish neuroses: "It is also not difficult to grasp why most of my brothers are thin, living skeletons and from where their tawny color and the extraordinary sensitivity of their nervous system derives. The incessant, corrosive grief caused by constant reflection on daily living expenses, the agonizing apparition of decreased vitality in the future, the loss of riches through withering capital and illegal exchange . . . is immensely disadvantageous for the nerves. It is also little wonder, therefore, that among us we observe so much hypochondria which little by little degenerates into irritability and melancholia. From thence there develops the constant disturbance of their mental powers, so that one observes in Jews a constant *Delirio* with all kinds of changes in appearance and conduct. This sensitivity of the nerves is caused by our mode of prayer."[42]

What we read in the work of Wolf, a *maskilic* physician, is that it was the traditionally observant, unenlightened Jew, or Eastern Jew, the one whose life revolved around the synagogue and the eking out of a miserly existence, who was in desperate need of rehabilitation in order to prevent his physical and mental deterioration.

However, even the path out of the ghetto could be fraught with psychological danger. In 1774, the Bavarian pastor and supervisor of the mint in Ansbach, Johann Jacob Spiess, sought biographical data on Moses Mendelssohn, in honor of whom a medal was to be struck. On March 1 of that year, Mendelssohn wrote to Spiess, and after telling him of his traditional Jewish background and education, he turned to the issue of his not having enjoyed a formal, secular education. Mendelssohn recounted how he had undertaken this task on his own, the consequences of which were that "I overdid it, and the overzealousness with which I pursued my studies brought on a nervous weakness that renders me all but incapable of any scholarly occupation."[43] Many years later, in his standard textbook on mental illness, German psychiatrist Johann August Schilling described Mendelssohn's breakdown as follows: "Convalescing in 1771, after a difficult sickness, Moses Mendelssohn was so [mentally] disturbed that everything he had heard all day long he heard again in an even louder voice in the evening. He was for a long time tormented by these aural phantoms."[44] A heavy price to pay for the attainment of secular knowledge.

Despite the sad consequences of Mendelssohn's own path to enlightenment, he and other maskilim — his friend Marcus Herz had referred to the traditional practice of burying Jews as quickly as possible as a "psychopathological illness" (*Seelenübel*) — would have concurred with Wolf's diagnosis of the problem, which called for a cure entailing a program of *Selbstbildung* (self-cultivation) and self-liberation.[45]

Although Mendelssohn tripped on the path to Europeanization, the need for Jews to become "civilized" occupied an important part in psychiatric assessments of Jewish patients by Gentile and acculturated Jewish psychiatrists into the twentieth century. In the early part of the nineteenth century, the frequently cited bad behavior of Jewish patients at mental asylums in Germany was most often held up as being a result of their Jewishness, rather than their being mentally ill. This stands in marked contrast to other hospitalized patients whose poor behavior, while notable, was rarely if ever referred to in the medical records as being the result of the inmate being "a Protestant" or "a peasant." Hardly anyone was ever said to exhibit "typically Catholic" behavior. The story was different for Jews. For example, in Germany's Eberbach asylum, a patient release report of 1831 could read that the patient's "allusions and bad jokes have their origin more from the peculiarity of the Jewish race than from madness or mental bondage."[46] The catalogue of imagined behavioral infractions attributed to Jewishness included scornfulness, filthiness, craftiness, roguishness, maliciousness, deceptiveness, cunning, curiosity, mistrust, satirical and obscure senses of humor, and an inclination to tease and mock.[47] Perhaps as a consequence, bad "Jewish" behavior at Eberbach was also treated more harshly than was the misbehavior of non-Jews. A report of 1821 sent by the asylum to the government stated that "punishment measures are only rarely used due to the especially manageable [*lenksam*] patient population. Exceptions are some lunatics from the line of Judas [*aus dem Stammen Juda*], against whom one must always proceed with the greatest severity."[48]

Later in the nineteenth century, when mental illness itself became designated as characteristic of Jews, accusations about their purportedly objectionable and unique behavior persisted. In 1900, an English psychiatrist, Cecil Beadles, claimed on the basis of 1,000 cases that the Jews were racially predisposed to mental illness.[49] In particular, he found that Jews displayed an "abnormally great predominance of general paralysis," accounting for approximately 21 percent of all admissions to the Colin Hatch asylum. Jewish women were afflicted in similar proportions to the men. For the general population, Beadles claimed that the comparable figure was between 10 and 13 percent. In summation, he described Jews as follows, drawing special attention to their behavior as mental patients: "Mental anxiety and worry [among Jews] are the most frequent causes of mental break down. They are all excitable and live excitable lives, being constantly under the high pressure of business in town. In all forms of mental disorder the prospect of recovery in Jews, both males and females, is less than with other patients.... The Jewish patients supply many of the noisy and troublesome patients in an asylum; they are all indolent, frequently faulty in habits, morally degraded, and are destructive of clothing."[50]

Cecil Beadles' findings were a topic of discussion at the annual meeting of the Medico-Psychological Association held in London in 1900. There, the appropriately named Dr. Savage stated that he agreed with Beadles' assessment, adding that "the forms of moral depravity common among Jews are very marked and disproportionate, and perhaps that is not altogether surprising, considering the history of the race."[51] Across the Atlantic, Beadles' findings were echoed by the American psychiatrist Frank Hyde, who noted that "the Hebrews as a race are hysterical and neurasthenic" as well as "ignorant, vicious, suspicious, complaining and frequently morally perverted."[52]

What was first observed and reported on in German mental institutions about Jewish behavior made its way into the findings of psychiatrists the world over. But in German-speaking Europe, the behavior of Jews who were mentally ill spoke to the larger and still unsatisfied concerns of those who doubted that the Jews, precisely because of the way they acted, could ever become German. Thus were the stakes higher in Central Europe, for the mental state of Jews went to the heart of whether their emancipation and integration were ever really possible.

The more urgent nature of the Jewish Question in Central Europe and the larger number of Jewish psychiatrists there saw the latter enter into debate with hostile non-Jewish practitioners from wherever they came. Cecil Beadles' scurrilous paper occasioned a formal response by Moritz Benedikt (1835–1920), the distinguished Jewish neurologist from Vienna. Benedikt's rebuttal, a description of the "mental and nervous qualities" of the Jews, contrasted starkly with Beadles' highly jaundiced judgment of their supposed immorality. Arguing for the Jews' intellectual and moral maturity, Benedikt maintained that it was the very possession of original Jewish character traits that prepared them to become the bearers of Mosaic teaching and act as the spiritual forebears of Christianity: "No nation in ancient times was so fit to receive abstract ideas on cosmogeny and the fundamental questions of metaphysics as the Jewish people were, fifteen centuries before Christ. Moses must have recognized this quality in his followers, for he made the bold experiment of imparting to them knowledge of the highest importance from Hamitic and Semitic philosophers.... The second psychical quality which was necessary in order that a people might bear this burden was, that high ethical predisposition to sacrifice their political, social, and economic interest to profound ideas and convictions."[53]

According to Benedikt, the Jews "are a very intellectual and neurotic nation," the former quality manifest in the development of Judaism itself, the latter, the consequence of dispersion and persecution. Having lost contact with nature, hard work, sport, and the arts, Jews became different from members of other nations who, having their own territory, "could find an outlet for their passions and emotions in outward action." The Jews, on the other hand, "found an outlet for them usually at the expense of [their] health, and so became more and more neurotic."[54]

The inner-directed nature of Jewish life meant, in Benedikt's view, that the Jews focused excessively on the family. This, however, had grave physical and mental consequences. Despite his earlier affirmation of the high moral standard of the Jewish people, Benedikt drew the line at extending those qualities to contemporary Eastern European Jews. Like Elcan Isaac Wolf before him (and many other Jewish physicians), Benedikt blamed the victim, charging that the development of an overly intimate family life led to lapsed ethical standards, which in turn were to blame for the psychopathologies of Eastern Jews. He was convinced that the unique sociology of Jewish family life, especially in the East, contributed to the high incidence of mental disorders among them. Cut off from the outside world, the Jews turned inward, developing a family life that "often resulted in excessive sexual intercourse, *inter matrimonium*."[55]

It is true that a number of non-Jewish psychiatrists had also charged the Jews with this inner directedness. However, their descriptions of Jews were static, undifferentiating and all-encompassing, including both Western and Eastern European Jews. But Benedikt was more selective. He was an acculturated Jew practicing in Vienna around 1900. It was Orthodox Jewry—specifically, the sexual life of Eastern European Orthodox Jews—that Benedikt called into question: "The females," he wrote, "chiefly suffered by these excesses, and even at the present day, among Orthodox Jews, every female is condemned from maturity till the menopause to an uninterrupted series of pregnancies, parturitions, and lactations. No wonder, then, that *hysteria gravis* is so frequent among Jewish women."[56]

While the Eastern European Jew remained for Benedikt a figure whose way of life and language promoted insanity, his prognosis was a hopeful one. He was convinced that although "the inherent qualities of the Jews have persisted for many centuries . . . they are endowed with a great aptitude for variation, both mentally and physically."[57] All that was required to stimulate the metamorphosis from traditional, afflicted Jew to modern, healthy one was a change of milieu. A contemporary education and the adoption of the ideas and sentiments of this new environment would ensure that the latent mental strength of the Jews—the prerequisite for the receipt of Mosaic law—would again surface.

Benedikt's studies of Orthodox Jews forced him to reevaluate the accepted causes of degenerative neuroses and general paralysis, a symptom of untreated syphilis, and other neurological disorders. Fin-de-siècle psychiatry had identified two of the principal causes as alcoholism and syphilis.[58] But while Jews suffered from the gamut of neuropathological disorders in numbers disproportionate to the population, the number of Jews afflicted with alcoholism or venereal disease was low. "From these facts," wrote Benedikt, "I am convinced *a priori,* that the modern etiological theory is erroneous." Because Benedict's idea of Jewish insanity was, specifically, Eastern European Jewish insanity, he concluded that the two major causes of general paralysis among Jews were persecution and ill treatment.[59] However, these two historical conditions were a feature of contemporary Russian Jewish, not German Jewish, life. It is clear from this fact that Benedikt dismissed any theory of hereditary insanity based on race. It was the Eastern European environment, both Jewish and Gentile, and nothing about the physical or psychological constitution of the Jews themselves that fostered mental illness. It is worth noting that such views were also expressed outside the European context. In a seminal study on the racial qualities of the Jews, Maurice Fishberg, a Russian-born American Jewish physician, wrote of Jewish mental illness: "Nearly all physicians who have practised among the Jews agree that derangements of the nervous system are very frequently met with among them." But specifically, he notes, "The Jewish population of [Warsaw] alone is almost exclusively the inexhaustible source for the supply of specimens of hysterical humanity, particularly hysteria in the male, for all the clinics of Europe."[60]

At the end of World War I, Benedikt contributed an article to the German literary monthly *Nord und Süd,* in which he continued to pursue and expand upon the theme of Eastern European Jewish mental illness.[61] After studying an epidemic of mental illness, accompanied by paralysis among Jewish tailors in London's East End that occurred in 1901, again rejecting the causative role of alcohol and venereal disease, Benedikt went on to discuss the etiology of Jewish insanity in historical rather than biological terms. In his view, the mental illness of Eastern European Jews had been caused by their specific mode of diaspora existence and the way they had adapted to it. Specifically, he referred to Jewish alienation from artistic and agricultural pursuits.

The key element responsible for the increase of insanity among these Russian Jews, according to Benedikt, was the persistence of traditional Jewish education. "From childhood years on, especially in religious circles, the dialectics of the Talmud are forced on capable and incapable brains, whereby paralysis is actually bred."[62] Here again, it was the Eastern European Jew who was the victim of mental illness. These psychopathologies were a direct result not only of external pressures, such as pogroms, but also of internal obscurantism. Benedikt's assessment bears a striking similarity to Wolf's diagnosis of 140 years earlier, which attributed the mental illness of the Jews to their "mode of prayer."[63]

To fully appreciate that for Benedikt the *"geisteskranke Jude"* (mentally ill Jew) was the Ostjude, it is important to be aware of the context in which his assessment took place. His discussion was not only an essay on the paralysis epidemic in London of 1901 but also a polemic aimed directly at the most important Zionist psychiatrist of the day, Dr. Rafael Becker, and a fierce denunciation of Ostjudentum in general. Benedikt was responding to the fact that by 1918, Zionist psychiatrists had made significant contributions to the diagnosis of both Western and Eastern European Jewish psychopathologies. Thus, the Zionists set the terms of the debate over Jewish insanity and, most important, prescribed cures in keeping with the nationalist Zeitgeist. It must also be noted that in the intellectual world of early German Zionism, the movement to repatriate the Jews to Palestine was undertaken as a solution to the plight of Eastern European Jewry only. It was never intended that the mass of German Jews should depart Europe forever.[64] Benedikt denunciated Becker's point that German Jewry stood to gain the most from the Zionist enterprise. Although he was no Zionist, Benedikt implicitly adopted the standard German Jewish line: that if Zionism was to be for any one group, then it was to be for the Jews of Eastern Europe.

Becker identified Western European Jewishness as the etiology of Jewish insanity, whereas Benedikt regarded Eastern European Jewishness as a pathological condition in itself, causing both physical and mental degeneration:

> Herr Dr. Becker . . . expects a racial-hygiene improvement through Zionism. [Zionism] is a bold posture, contributing much, and in place of the generally scatterbrained ideas [of Ostjudentum] generates a

healthy concept of discipline. [But] his goal of a national rebirth strikes great difficulty. This rebirth is chiefly an *ostjüdische* question. And there stands in the way, above all, the Yiddish language. It has stirred up much disaster. . . . In Italy, France, and the Anglo-Saxon world, just as in the Germanic and Scandinavian, and also in a part of the Slavic world, the Jews have adapted culturally, nationally, and politically, as well as amalgamated with the population. Rude bodily forms, especially posture, etc., disappear mostly in the next generation. [But] the Eastern European Jewish emigration to England and the United States sees the monstrous language [Yiddish] hang on. These countries, with their tolerance, have gone so far, that this so-called language has even been conferred with official status. . . . One wants a perfect national language, and one has come into being . . . and as far as can be evaluated by an outsider . . . [the newly developed Hebrew] is in as good a shape as modern Greek.[65]

Thus, according to Benedikt, a Hungarian-born Jew, Eastern European Jewishness in general, and the Yiddish language in particular, was both a sign of and contributor to the mental illness of the Jews. It was an impediment to the healthy integration of Jews such as had taken place in Central and Southern Europe.[66]

In the end, Benedikt held that insanity was caused not only by language but also by politics. Despite his gratuitous claim that it was a "bold posture," Benedikt claimed that Zionism was itself a sign of psychopathology. It appeared palatable only when compared to all other aspects of Eastern European Jewish culture. But as a political idea, it was a dangerous fantasy, symptomatic of disturbed minds. Tersely, he wrote, "But also the madness must disappear . . . that in Palestine, a kind of national state can be created."[67]

German Jewish psychiatrists of the older generation such as Benedikt never reconciled themselves to Eastern European Jewry, retaining an antipathy toward that group that resonated in their professional and personal lives. Unlike the younger generation of psychiatrists and other intellectuals in Germany who came of age between 1900 and 1918, they did not participate in the cult of the Eastern European Jew. Rather, they steadfastly clung to the belief that Western European Jewry, with its secularism, its *Kultur*, its *Deutschtum*, was the ideal symbol of modern Jewry, an ideal to which all Jews should aspire.[68] They identified the acclimatized and educated Western European Jews as being mentally healthy, while Eastern European Jews stuck in a quagmire of poverty and religious obscurantism, were afflicted with all forms of psychoses and neuroses.

No one expressed this view as strongly as the celebrated Berlin neurologist, Hermann Oppenheim (1858–1918). In 1908 he published an important article in the prestigious *Journal für Psychologie und Neurologie* entitled "On the Psychopathology and Nosology of the Russian-Jewish Population," in which he noted that "approximately three quarters of all Russian-Jewish patients are neuropaths and hypochondriacs."[69] According to Oppenheim, the high rate of mental illness among Russian Jews was directly attributable to their environment. He listed four main causes: the pogroms; the mental and physical strain of everyday life; the poor hygienic conditions that resulted from poverty and overcrowding [*Zusammenpferchung*]; and finally, the Eastern European Jewish obsession with study "(even after a full day's work) in enclosed, unventilated rooms."[70]

All these features of Jewish life in Russia were obviously rectifiable, in theory. However, under existing conditions in the East, the possibility of reform was very unlikely, and Jews would continue to leave, seeking better conditions in the West. In attempting to account for the inordinately large numbers of Eastern European Jews in Western Europe specifically seeking medical care, Oppenheim painted a picture that fit into his world view of the superiority of German science, and life in general, especially as it applied to Jews: "A further factor is the world-wide renown of our German spas, Austrian baths and mineral springs, and Tyrolean mountain health-resorts — the way to all of them leads through Berlin. When one further considers that Russia does not possess many such spas and that staying in [those that do exist] is off limits to Jews, then the rush of Russian Jews to our consulting hours is fully explained."[71]

In short, according to Oppenheim, Russia prior to the Great War was a bad place for Jews to be. Conveniently ignoring the scores of German spas that specifically advertised themselves as being closed to Jews, not to mention the general level of antisemitism in the *Kaiserreich,* Oppenheim identified Russia as offering Jews nothing but misery and torment. It was, therefore, also the cause of myriad mental disorders. All of this stood in marked contrast to the conditions that prevailed in the German-speaking lands, where reason, science, advanced medicine, a high living standard, and tolerance toward Jews were the hallmarks of a more civilized society—one where Jews had been allowed to integrate and had, as a consequence, become paragons of mental health.[72]

In comparing his Russian Jewish patients with those from Germany and other western countries, Oppenheim concluded that they were in possession of certain traits and characteristics that would be of special interest to the "psychologist and psychopathologist." The primary one that Oppenheim diagnosed was nosophobia, a morbid fear of disease. "The nosophobia," he wrote, "is either the illness itself, or only an appendage to the real suffering, covers it, and overlays it, and thus becomes the main source of the complaint. . . . The patient suffers much less from his illness, than by his reflections upon it, and sometimes these reflections are his only suffering."[73]

Oppenheim also identified distrust and suspiciousness as specifically Eastern European Jewish psychological traits. Refusing to believe the word of just one physician, Eastern European Jews consulted as many specialists as possible, in what Oppenheim referred to as a *"furor consultativus."* The progress of this ritual was impeded only by the fact that the Jew generally ran out of money.[74]

The etiology of the distrust itself lay with the low level of occupational structure of Russian Jews, most of whom were engaged in jobs that encouraged the deployment of cunning and deception. "It is no wonder that this gradually passed into the flesh and blood and became a fundamental characteristic."[75] Thus, Oppenheim's diagnoses of Eastern European Jewry's mental health problems were based on both the cultural and class distance he observed and, indeed, felt. For Oppenheim, the hypochondriacal Russian Jewish proletariat stood in marked contrast to the mentally fit, solidly bourgeois community of German Jewry.

Heirs to that stream in Haskalah ideology that encouraged the abandonment of traditional ritual and the acquisition of secular culture and Christian behavioral norms, Benedikt and Oppenheim perpetuated and elaborated upon the Wolfian stereotype of mentally ill Jews. While Wolf and other maskilim targeted all traditional Jews as ill in some way or another, stressing that they required the curative effects of secularization, Benedikt and Oppenheim—practicing in Vienna and Berlin respectively, cities where most Jews had already abandoned ritual—specifically targeted the Eastern, pious Jew. In their view, the Ostjude was the modern incarnation of what the German Jew had been before modernization—the bearer of ill health.

At the turn of the century, younger, dissenting voices among Jewish psychiatrists were beginning to be heard, and with them, the paradigm shift began to take root. In 1902, a Jewish physician in Vienna named Martin Engländer delivered a public lecture at the Zionist fraternal lodge, Zion. As a Zionist, Engländer drew a distinction between Eastern European and

Western European Jews that was very different from that drawn by Benedikt and Oppenheim. Despite what he deemed the physical inferiority of Eastern European Jews, brought on by their socioeconomic plight, their material poverty deprived them only of their physical, not their mental, well-being.[76] Conversely, the relative economic prosperity of Western European Jews had serious repercussions for the psychological state of this more assimilated group.

Capitalism itself came under fire by those who held it chiefly responsible for a variety of Jewish illnesses. Engländer's compatriot Richard von Krafft-Ebing pronounced that the Jew was an "overachiever in the arena of commerce or politics," spending his every waking moment "read[ing] reports, business correspondence, [and] stock market notations during meals. [For him] 'time is money.'"[77] To return to Karl Kraus, for whom "psychoanalysis is that mental illness for which it regards itself as therapy," the link between it and commerce was clear, the two of them being the principal "Jewish" diseases of the age. "The trading mentality," wrote Kraus, "is said to have evolved in the confines of the ghetto streets. In freedom they indulge in psychology.... What miracles a combination of trading mentality and psychology can produce, we see every day."[78]

Martin Engländer echoed the sentiments of those who identified modernity and especially commerce as the culprits in causing Jewish insanity: "Finally, I would like to mention that the degenerative process of the central nervous system—the main topic in the discussion about the condition of the Jews in the West—is also a consequence of over-striving and over-fatigue [*Überanstrengung und Übermudung*] of the brain. [This occurs] in the form of nervous disorders and mental disturbances, and is to be found considerably more frequently among Jews than among the non-Jewish population."[79]

In concurrence with Kraepelin and Krafft-Ebing, Engländer viewed Western European Jews as achieving a level of serious degeneration. But in contrast to their more organic or racially based view of Jewish mental illness, Engländer found the cause to be strictly environmental. The impetus for this manifest behavior of mental decline was release from the ghetto. It was at this point that the Jews had been cast onto the great battlefield of international competition and found themselves in the first line of combat. As Engländer observed: "This struggle, haste and drive, the hunt for happiness cannot but have left its trace on the nerves of the people."[80]

But this competition that Engländer so pejoratively described was an open one. Why, then, had Western European Jews been more severely affected than other Europeans? The answer lay squarely in Jewish history. While the recent struggle in the bourgeois marketplace had been a new experience for Christians, for Jews it was but a mere continuation of their ancient struggle for existence. This struggle, shared by all Jews throughout their history, came to have profound psychological consequences only for those Jews in the West. For when the time came for them to pursue their *embourgeoisement,* a necessary corollary of emancipation, they were an exhausted, spent people: "The struggle for a cozy existence is a struggle against the brain. The Jewish brain, however, has already fought a difficult fight for centuries. Up until emancipation it was just a naked struggle for the necessities of existence. The multifarious convulsions which the Jews have endured in their two thousand year Diaspora and life of suffering, cannot but have caused a reaction on their central nervous systems. By whatever measure, *the brain of the Jews was already, prior to their entrance into the above-described competitive struggle, less resistant, more vulnerable than the brains of non-Jews*" [emphasis added].[81]

Engländer's critique of Jewish life in the West constituted an attack on the Jews' preference for big cities, their participation in intellectual or business professions, their lack of physical exercise, their extreme susceptibility and emotion at the slightest instance, their timidity and helplessness. These were all taken as factors contributing to Jewish degeneration.[82] In a pointed criticism of Central European Jewish life, Engländer implored German Jews "not to be so unreasonable as to drag [your] children around to coffeehouses and restaurants. The youth need to sit inside less and move around and play more in the open."[83] Thus did the chord struck by Elcan Isaac Wolf during the Haskalah reverberate with clarity among Zionists well over a century later.

The specific features of modernity were not only seen by some as responsible for physical and mental breakdown, but were often specifically identified with Jews whose own symptoms were seen as presaging a universal fate for all humanity. The French historian Anatole Leroy-Beaulieu declared: "The Jew is the most nervous of men, perhaps, because he is the most cerebral, because he has lived most by his brain, [and is thus] the most nervous and, in so far, the most modern of men. He is by the nature of his diseases the forerunner, as it were, of his contemporaries, preceding them upon that perilous path upon which society is urged by the excesses of its intellectual and emotional life, and by the increasing spur of competition. The noisy army of psychopathics and neuropathics is gaining so many recruits among us that it will not take the Christians long to catch up with the

Jews in this respect." Thus could the Frenchman conclude on an unequivocally nonracist note: "Here, again, there are probably no ethnic forces in operation."[84]

It is worth noting that the differing environments in which Jewish physicians worked had profound consequences for their diagnoses of the Jewish condition. To take but one example, Maurice Fishberg in New York shared many of Hermann Oppenheim's attitudes toward Jews and Judaism and the relation of both to the host society. But despite identifying the Eastern European Jew as the principal victim of mental disorders, Fishberg's American setting precluded him from identifying class as a determinative factor in the profile of mental disease. His was a far more egalitarian and all-encompassing reading of the problem:

> The causes of this nervousness of the Jews are apparent to every one who knows the conditions under which they have laboured for the last two thousand years. In the first place, they have been town-dwellers for centuries, and only rarely engage in agricultural pursuits. Neurasthenia is known to be a disease of large urban centres, where the hurry and bustle of life is an appalling drain on nervous energy. These diseases are also most frequently seen among commercial people, speculators, and bankers; and considering the large number of Jews who depend on commerce for a living, and their ways of doing business often with a small capital, it is not surprising that many break down under the strain of speculation. It is, however, to be remembered that neurasthenia and hysteria are not only encountered among the richer classes of Jews. They are just as frequent among the poorer Jews, the artisans and labourers.[85]

In discussing the realignment of paradigms of Jewish mental illness taking place, mention must be made of those Jewish psychiatrists for whom Zionism was not a motivating factor. Rather, they advocated the development of a positive diaspora pride in order to alleviate insanity among Jews. In 1904, Fritz Wittels, a Viennese Jew, a disciple of Freud, and his earliest biographer, published his polemical work, *Der Taufjude* (The converted Jew). Wittels' fundamental assumption was that the Jewish convert was a psychologically tormented character, a prime example of the insane Jew. The convert is a congenital liar, not really aware that he is lying. His assimilation and conversion were not acts that were destined to "liberate" him from the persecutory environment of the Habsburg Empire. Because his conversion was not an act of faith, but one of opportunism, the Jew would, ironically, prolong the discrimination. Because the convert was unaware of this, his desire to advance socially was a grand act of self-delusion, the behavior of someone who is mentally deranged. The drive to convert was, for Wittels, as it had been for Herzl, a sign of moral bankruptcy. Jewish psychological solvency, on the other hand, could come about only as a result of a positive and forthright affirmation of Jewish identity.[86]

Otto Rank, who met Freud in 1906 and became a member of the inner circle soon thereafter, is one of the most important figures in the history of the psychoanalytic movement. His personal understanding of his own Jewish identity and the larger role he assigned Jews in the drama of the collective redemption of humanity mark his as an alternative Jewish contribution to the more parochial psychiatry of Zionist practitioners.

In his essay of 1905, *Das Wesen des Judentums* (The essence of Judaism), Rank made the bold claim that humanity had evolved from a state wherein initially, unbridled sexual gratification was the norm, but that had given way — as the human maturation process had developed — to repressed sexuality and neurosis. The Jews, however, had not followed this path of "backward" development. They remained in a more pristine sexual and thus less neurotic state. "They have yet to experience," wrote Rank, "the metamorphosis from a 'lower' organism to the state of isolated sexuality. . . . Generally, their religion, which they constructed thousands of years ago, appropriate to a stage in the repression process still prominent to this day, preserves the greatest part of the people in psychic balance."[87] Thus by not taking the Gentile path to *Kultur* (an advanced stage of the repression process) Jews resided in a state of psychological advantage vis-à-vis Christians. This placed them in a position of being able to cure non-Jews of their neuroses. Therefore, the role of the Jew is, through the therapeutic method, to lead the redemptive charge of all humanity. Hence their invention of psychoanalysis, "for the Jews thoroughly understand the *radical* cure of neurosis better than any other people, even better than the artistically and sublimely talented Greeks with their powerful tragedies. They brought matters to such a point that they could help others, since they have sought to preserve themselves from the illness."[88] Dennis Klein has perceptively remarked that this expression of Rank's "is an explicit example of the penetration of Jewish consciousness into the [psychoanalytic] movement's earliest phase of development."[89]

It is to be noted that Rank's according Jews the vanguard role in curing the world of its neuroses was predicated on a psychological diagnosis that differed from the analysis of Gentile, assimilated, and Zionist psychiatrists.

Rank's formulation was founded upon the belief in the psychological well-being of most Jews as a result of their conscious resistance to the advancement of Kultur, and the concomitant development of neuroses born of sexual repression. His arguing against the sexual promiscuity of Jews must also be seen as a direct refutation of stereotypical accusations of Jewish concupiscence, a standard claim in the antisemitism of his day.

While Wittels and Rank differed from the Zionist psychiatrists on the issue of where Jews should live as a collective entity, they shared their Zionist colleagues' basic anxiety about the diaspora. It was an environment full of risk for the Jew. Especially in Central Europe, it appeared that the danger lay in assimilation. This could take on its most radical form as in the case of Wittels' *Taufjude* or in the person of Rank's Jew, who, through mimicry, stood poised to adopt Christian sexual mores and, by extension, develop neurotic qualities, and possibly even express antisemitism.

The paradigm shift in Jewish psychiatry was, by the end of World War I, coming into sharper definition. The focus was no longer the maskilic image of the unhealthy yeshiva student, first elaborated in the eighteenth century, or the contemporary Eastern European Jew who is the psychopathic and sociopathic model. Rather, it was now the deracinated, culturally bankrupt Western European Jew who was the epitome of the neurasthenic, hysterical type. According to Zionist doctors, although emancipation, greater acculturation, prosperity, and embourgeoisement ensured that the physical condition of Westjudentum would be superior to that of Ostjudentum, their new lifestyles, the speed and way with which they integrated themselves into non-Jewish society, made them victim to myriad psychotic and neurotic disorders. By contrast, Jewish psychiatrists saw Eastern European Jews as physically unhealthy, victims of diseases brought on by poverty, but, because of their spiritual and cultural completeness, they were mentally sound in a way that Western European Jews, suffering above all from an identity crisis, were not.

This view was most fully elaborated by Rafael Becker (b. 1891), unquestionably the most prolific and influential of the Zionist psychiatrists. With this Russian Jew from Saratov, who took his medical degree at the University of Zurich in 1917, the paradigm shift can be said to have been completed. From the appearance of his first work on Jewish mental illness in 1918 to his final publications in the 1930s, he was the most widely quoted, oft referred to, and, indeed, controversial of all the Jewish psychiatrists discussed in this chapter. Aside from his high standing within the profession, what may account for his widespread contemporary recognition is that he published extensively in three languages, German, Yiddish, and Polish, and held various hospital appointments in Switzerland and finally in Poland, where he perished sometime during the Holocaust.

Following the completion of his medical studies, Becker took up an appointment as assistant to Eugen Bleuler at the famous Burghölzli clinic in Zurich, where Freudian psychoanalysis was being applied for the first time in a psychiatric hospital setting.[90] Becker's first research assignment was a comparative study of "Jewish and non-Jewish patients to determine whether the work done by earlier investigators could be validated with the new psychoanalytic approach."[91] Becker presented the findings of his research to a Zurich academic Zionist fraternity called Hechaver, on March 4, 1918.[92]

Becker's speech began dramatically. "All of humanity has become nervous," he declared. Not only did the war have terrible consequences for the people's nerves, but "the war itself was a product of the pathological spirit of man." It was in the context of this proposition that Becker sought to elucidate specifically the problem of the psychopathology of the Jews. While much work on this had already been done, Becker lamented, the results bore very little "goodwill." Typical of this genre was the view that mental illness had recently increased among the Jews and that many proclaimed them to be a "perishing and degenerate race" (3). It was exactly this view that Becker's study intended to test.

"Was there a specific Jewish mental illness or, in medical terms, a *Psychosis Judaica?*" Becker asked rhetorically. "There is no specific Jewish nervous disorder, just as there are no specific Jewish anthropological characteristics, the [supposed] existence of which are used to prove the inferiority of the Jewish race" (9). But Becker was forced to concede that on the basis of all modern research, Jews did indeed suffer from a higher frequency of mental illness than did non-Jews. Not only was the incidence of insanity among Jews higher than among Gentiles, but it was also on the increase. To substantiate his claim, Becker provided the following figures for Prussia and Bavaria, observing that they could be duplicated all over Europe. In 1871, per 100,000 of the population, 236 Protestants, 234 Catholics, and 423 Jews suffered from some form of mental illness. By 1895 those figures had increased to 291, 250, and 498, respectively.

Becker concurred with all other researchers that syphilis and alcoholism did not afflict Jews with great frequency. But they were, he lamented, on the rise in Western Europe. There, the crashing of the ghetto walls had led to the Jewish adoption of Christian morals, the subsequent increase in syphilis, paralysis, and feeblemindedness, as well as a newfound predilection for "Christian champagne"(10). According to other Zionist physicians, it was the very conditions of ghetto life in the East, such as the supposedly strict adherence to ancient customs, habits, and regulations that held luetic infection at bay. By way of contrast, one psychiatrist declared, "Thanks to his assimilation, his social position, his profession, and his prosperity, the emancipated Western European Jew [suffers] from a more frequent occurrence of [syphilitic] progressive paralysis."[93]

As Max Sichel argued in an article that appeared in the journal of the famous homosexual-rights leader and Berlin Jewish physician, Magnus Hirschfeld, the cause of the low incidence of syphilis among Eastern European Jews was the resistance they had built up as a result of living for centuries in a state of moral and ethical purity. By contrast, he argued, the Jew of Western Europe, by his very entry into the big city, had lost a good deal of his Jewishness and his religiosity. These were the surest protections against the inevitable consequence of wild and indiscriminate sexual intercourse — venereal disease. Sichel also pointed to the early marriage of Eastern European Jews as a custom of a biologically prophylactic nature, and a contributing factor to the infrequency of syphilis among those people.[94] In sum, Zionist psychiatrists, Becker foremost among them, concluded that insanity among German Jewry was a direct result of their assimilation.

In contrast to this, the ghetto, and the inbreeding that had taken place there for centuries, leading to the racial purity that the Eastern Jews currently enjoyed, was "the best security for the great psychical and physical productiveness of a people" (14–15). Central to the mental well-being of the Eastern Jews was the retention of religious faith. It is no wonder that Becker glorified medieval Jewish life, seeing its social and religious organization as the fountainhead of Jewish vitality and the source of Jewish perseverance. The Jewish Middle Ages were not a "period of suffering" (*Leidensepoche*), but, rather, a time characterized by Jewish spiritual integrity and, therefore, psychological contentment and well-being. To Becker, it was the contemporary period that witnessed the most Jewish suffering. According to him, the modern Western European Jew had abandoned his faith in his drive to assimilate. In this respect, Becker parted company with Freud, arguing instead for the psychological efficacy of religious observance.[95] Rather than regard religion as the collective analogue of individual neurosis, Becker held that it was profound piety and devotion to ceremony that had historically provided Jews with psychological stability and invincibility:

Yes ladies and gentlemen, in these modern times, Jews live in much greater torment than their forefathers did in the Middle Ages, and even the earlier times of persecutions, tortures, and autos-da-fé. At that time, the Jew went to his death without angst and fear, with firm faith in his religion . . . with proud readiness, with the *Shema Yisrael* on his lips. . . .

However, the earlier Jews were much more fortunate than we are now. They had the firm belief that God punished them for their sins and dispersed them to all the corners of the world, but that the time would come, that with their Messiah, the Jews would again be fortunate and be returned to their ancient homeland. This belief we do not have now.[96]

As a result of Becker's influence, the issue of religion and psychiatry became a celebrated theme in some of the Jewish periodical literature after World War I. Some reviewers of Becker's book *Die jüdische Nervosität* (Jewish nervousness) even questioned whether Becker had pursued the theme of religion and its prophylactic nature sufficiently. Felix Resek, writing in the leading periodical of German Orthodoxy, *Der Israelit,* found inadequate Becker's assessment that there were only two ways to cure the insanity of the Jews: assimilation and their ultimate extinction, or Zionism and their "strengthening" in Palestine. For him, only traditional religious observance would soothe soul and psyche. The simple modesty and piety of the patriarchs were the roots of the Jews' happiness, and the source of their capacity to resist all obstacles that had been placed before them. Accordingly, a readoption of these time-honored principles, plus a general return to the "village-soil and garden-city" (not necessarily in Palestine), would lead to the contemporary psychological and religious recovery of the Jews.[97]

The twin themes of mental health and religious observance also occupied Hermann Seckbach in his short feuilleton of 1919, "The Psychiatric Patient." In it the author told the story of a young Jewish woman who was committed to an asylum after receiving word that her husband had been officially declared missing during the war. Recounting her experience, the woman said:

It grips me with horror today when I have to say this word—[asylum]. . . . In addition, there was the agony of my soul when I realized I was in a non-Jewish institution. I wanted to die of shame when they removed the *Scheitel* [wig] from my head, and I almost went crazy, when out of hunger, I had to dig into the non-kosher food. How can I describe to you the unspeakable agony which I felt on Friday nights? . . . There were moments when only my trust in God could save me. It was like a dream to me. In the midst of a fog I saw Sabbath candles and I lost my poor mind. Who out of all these people who took care of me could guess what a Jewish woman feels if her religion is taken away from her?

Not only does the story end on a happy note, but it concludes with a resolution designed to benefit Jewish society as a whole. As luck had it, the woman's husband had not been killed, but only taken prisoner of war and had returned home. She concluded her story: "Then the first Friday evening we were together in unspeakable happiness, I decided to strive for, as much as it was in my power, the many Jewish welfare institutions. But for now the most important task was the establishment of Jewish mental asylums."[98]

One particular such institution deserves special mention because of its great cultural relevance to the theme of religion and mental health. It was established after World War I in Heidelberg by the Orthodox psychoanalyst Frieda Reichmann. The patients in her facility were treated with heavy doses of Torah study and Freudian psychotherapy. As Gershom Scholem relates in his memoirs, it was "a sanatorium which the wags called 'Torah-peutic.'" Such important figures as Ernst Simon, Erich Fromm, and Leo Löwenthal were regular outpatients there. This place, as memorable for its idiosyncratic approach to therapy as for its famous analysands, represents one possible type of institution the heroine in the above-mentioned feuilleton longed for. Established in recognition of the need for such a place, and with cognizance of the pre-war discourse about Jewish mental illness, the clinic sought to provide psychological and religious answers to troubled Jews. Just how successful Frieda Reichmann was in employing Judaism as therapy is debatable, for according to Scholem, all but one "had their orthodox Judaism analyzed away."[99]

While Rafael Becker extolled the faith of his ancestors, he did not remain at the simplistic level of lamenting a bygone age of Jewish piety and observance. He did not advocate the establishment of a theocratic Jewish state as the only salvation for his exiled, suffering people. Rather, what was needed, according to Becker, was a radical change in the political outlook of the Jews. For Becker, the Western Jews' loss of religious faith was symptomatic of their overall loss of faith; a loss characterized by those who believed neither in the Zionist dream nor in the Jews themselves: "And if some of us believe that our national rebirth, through our firm, great, will can come about, and that we can be freed from *Galut* [exile] and lead a new, normal, national life, then indeed another, and unfortunately a larger part of us, has lost its belief in this" (17).

Thus, it was the anti-Zionist, irrespective of his political or cultural persuasions, that Becker identified as the mentally ill Jew. For the path of assimilation had led many German Jews down the road of self-hatred. "The Jew," he declared, "whether he is a conscious assimilationist or even a nationalist, who sees how badly his national rebirth is going, begins to believe what the antisemites say—that his God is a wicked God, that his morals are base morals, that his entire race is not of high quality and is of no value. In a word, the Jew begins to feel himself inferior" (17).

Becker thus analyzed the social and psychological constitution of the Jews (primarily anti-Zionists), within the dissenting paradigm of neurosis developed by the one-time disciple of Freud, Alfred Adler (1870–1937), whose *Über den nervösen Charakter* (The neurotic constitution) (1912) Becker had read. For Becker, Adler's claim that "every neurosis can be understood as an attempt to free oneself from a feeling of inferiority in order to gain a feeling of superiority" was characteristic of a disturbed, Jewish mental condition.[100] It was typical of those Jews who refused to pursue the Zionist path to national rebirth. They were weak-willed, and further, they refused to do so because they suffered from a raging inferiority complex. And this complex was exacerbated, in part, because they had come to accept as fact the hostile evaluation of them by their enemies.

The hopelessness of Jewish life during the diaspora demanded the "most radical therapy"—a Jewish national homeland in Palestine. It could not be any other way. For as Becker assessed, the assimilationist Jew was still classified as a Jew by Gentiles, and the nationalist Jew was unable to garner any respect from his fellow Jews. Battered from without and within, the Jew was a helpless victim of his European environment.

Because the primary victims of these myriad mental disorders were the assimilated Western European Jews, then Zionism, in Becker's view, was the solution to the Western European Jewish problem. How far removed this is from Moritz Benedikt's and Hermann Oppenheim's analysis of the Jewish problem! According to Becker, the creation of a Jewish homeland in Palestine would cure the deracinated Westjude of his inferiority complex, the very source of his insanity.

In many ways, Becker's analysis is reminiscent of that of a fellow Zionist physician, Daniel Pasmanik (1869–1930). A peripatetic intellectual who was born in Ukraine, studied medicine in Switzerland and Bulgaria, and worked in Russia before finally settling in Paris, Pasmanik was one of the most important Zionist publicists and theoreticians of his day. In several works, including an essay on the history of assimilation since the eighteenth century, and a book on the psychology of Diaspora Jewry, Pasmanik described assimilation as "a sickness, [but] not a [sign] of the baseness of the Jewish people."[101]

In a rather sophisticated analysis, Pasmanik hypothesized that assimilation had two fundamental causes, the first economic, the second intellectual. In the first case, the economic interests of representatives of the haute bourgeoisie in Germany and France — military provisioners, financiers, bankers, industrialists, and physicians — forced them "to adapt to the dominant culture, and appropriate the language and customs of their Christian competitors." Rejecting a Marxist interpretation of history, Pasmanik refused to identify class and material interests as the sole reasons for Jewish assimilation. He suggested that by the end of the eighteenth century, cultural stagnation had set in among Western European Jewry. Devoid of poets, philosophers, and halakhists (legal scholars), Judaism was confined to the synagogue and the heder and was based upon fossilized traditions. Ignorant of their national language and history, and practicing a Judaism possessing only "form without content . . . the soul of the Jews had deadened."[102]

According to Pasmanik even though some of these deleterious developments were beginning to be detected among Russian Jews, "it was German Jews who developed and popularized the theory of assimilation" to its fullest extent. Similarly, like Wittels and Becker, Pasmanik accused the assimilationists of self-delusion, allowing themselves to believe in the "falsehood of assimilation," just as "the terminal patient deceives himself that with a morphine injection he has attained a state of apparent euphoria." For Pasmanik, "a cure can only come about through faith — faith in the possibility of attaining one's self-worth on one's own soil."[103]

Above all, Pasmanik was a diagnostician of the Jewish condition. Although he had been an instructor in the medical school at the University of Geneva, he never undertook clinical research on Jewish patients. So while his conclusions may have been similar to those of Rafael Becker, the Jewish medical paths of the two men did not show similar patterns of practical engagement. Pasmanik concentrated on political activity and medical-theoretical analysis, while Becker's work was concentrated in the areas of medical treatment and research of Jewish patients and the connection of such to the Zionist cause.

After the conclusion of his clinical research at Burghölzli, Becker took up a number of other hospital appointments in Switzerland, and published a monograph on mental illness among Swiss Jewry as well as a proposal for the establishment of Jewish mental institutions in Palestine and Poland.[104] Then sometime between 1920 and 1925 he left Central Europe for his native Poland, where he became director of the Jewish mental asylum Zofyowke in Otwosk, near Warsaw.

In Poland, working with a Jewish population of an entirely different character from that which he had treated in Switzerland, Becker was driven to ask new questions and challenge some of his older theories. He now confronted a traditional Jewish community, confident and proud of its heritage, speaking a Jewish language, Yiddish, possessed of a vibrant Jewish culture, and largely traditional. His paradigm of the "Jewish Complex," that feeling of Jewish inferiority that he used to explain the cause of insanity among Western European Jews, simply did not fit here.

To be sure, Becker was able to point to certain similarities between the clinical pictures of Eastern and Western European Jews. The infrequency of epilepsy, syphilis, and alcohol-related psychoses was also in evidence in Poland, but because of the tenacity of tradition, it seemed unlikely that an increase in such disorders, as was slowly occurring in the West, would take place here. However, important clinical differences between the two Jewries did exist. In the West, Jews suffered more from schizophrenia, manic-depressive insanity, progressive paralysis, senile dementia, and mental deficiency than did non-Jews. Cocaine and morphine addiction, on the rise among Jews in the West, was seldom found among their Polish co-religionists.[105]

In Poland, however, two forms of mental illness distinguished the Jewish population from both the Christian and the Western European Jewish communities. Schizophrenia and manic-depression struck Polish Jews at an even greater rate than it did Jews in Western Europe, and the incidence of both was significantly higher among Polish Jews in comparison to the Christian population. Schizophrenia and related psychoses affected 75 percent of all Jewish patients, while manic-depression was twice as frequent among Jews as Poles.[106] Despite the fact that these two disorders occurred most commonly among Central European Jewry, Becker was now convinced that there must be a psychogenetic or organic explanation for these diseases. He was not yet prepared to say that race played a factor in the spread of these disorders among Polish Jews, but he was stymied as to their etiology and called for more detailed research insisting on the need for genealogical, occupational, economic, and sociological studies.[107]

Even though Becker's large-scale studies of institutionalized Jewish mental patients enabled him to speak of the nosology of mental disorders among Polish Jews, he was unable to fit them into any etiological paradigm—other than adverse living conditions—that would explain the widespread existence of schizophrenia and manic-depression among them. As a consequence of this, when in Eastern Europe, he also proposed a eugenic solution to the problem, calling for the implementation of a program of negative eugenics, insisting on the need for Jewish society to self-regulate unhealthy marriages among the mentally and physically ill, or between cousins.[108] Encouraged by the success of such eugenics laws in the United States, England, Germany, and Czechoslovakia, Becker advocated a large-scale propaganda campaign among the Jewish masses.

In this discussion of the psychopathology of everyday Jewish life, a number of important themes have come to the fore and are worthy of reiteration and summation. It has been shown that the early twentieth century witnessed a paradigm shift in the way Jewish psychiatrists observed the mentally ill among the Jewish population. The Haskalah-inspired model of secular (German) Jewish sanity versus Orthodox (Eastern European) Jewish insanity was replaced with its mirror image.

Additionally, the work of the Jewish psychiatrists examined here is instructive in a broad sense in that it shows clearly the interaction of politics with science. We have seen how the political affinities of the psychiatrists, assimilationism versus Zionism, *Deutschtum* versus *Ostjudentum,* as well as cultural and class antipathies determined their medical diagnoses and prescriptions for cure. Even their places of residency had an enormous impact on their findings. This was as true for Hermann Oppenheim in Berlin, who looked down upon his Russian Jewish patients and co-religionists, as it was for Rafael Becker, who was forced to reconsider his understanding of the causes of insanity among Diaspora Jews once he returned home to Poland following his sojourn in the West.

We also see how all groups with medical-political agendas stereotyped each other. The physicians addressed here presented very little nuance in their description of Jews, painting them as monochromatically as possible: all German Jews are assimilated; Polish Jews are not; German Jews are drowning in a sea of craven materialism and reside at great remove from

Jewish tradition, while Polish Jews live lives of spiritual abundance and cultural authenticity. Neither assessment was accurate, of course.

By examining how Jewish psychiatrists constructed an image of the Jewish "other," an important event in modern Jewish history—namely, the encounter of the Western European and Eastern European Jew in the early part of the twentieth century—is broadened. With recourse to medical texts, we can see that the popular image of the German Jew holding Russian and Polish Jews in contempt was not a one-way street. Within the circumscribed, yet important field of psychiatry, Eastern European Jews were portrayed as models for a reinvigorated Jewish spirit and mentality, one that would serve Jews best in their quest for national liberation. By contrast, the thriving mental health of German Jews was presented as a thing of the past, for it was really they, and not their Eastern brethren, who bore the insecurities of the ghetto. In the view of Zionist psychiatrists, antisemitism and the concomitant craving for acceptance were the twin causes for one of the most tragic of all psychopathological conditions—Jewish self-hatred.

Above all, this exploration into the discourse about the mental state of the Jews provides some closure to the larger discussion about their bodies. After an examination of the sense of Jewish physicality at the fin-de-siècle, this chapter has explored the way Eastern and Western European Jews spoke about each other's respective psychologies. That such a discussion could take place at all required the emergence of a particular type of creature. He is—as made memorable from Freud's self-description—the "godless Jew." This does not necessarily mean "atheist." Rather, he is the person for whom "Jewishness," a psychological category, came to replace "Judaism," a religious designation. He is what Yosef Yerushalmi, borrowing from Philip Rieff, has called the "Psychological Jew."[109] He was a person whose emergence was possible only as a result of the breakdown of traditional Jewish society, whereupon he began his entrance into the world of the secularizing bourgeoisie during the course of the nineteenth and twentieth centuries.

The encounter between the religious and psychological Jewish archetypes—and it must be made clear that the modern religious Jew is also a Jew for whom "Jewishness" is a meaningful category and defining characteristic—and all the myriad variations and subclassifications stemming from each, go a long way toward contributing to the psychological profile modern Jews create for themselves, and the way they depict their fellow Jews. This deeply analytical, transferential process of self- and mutual awareness has become a characteristic mode of self-expression for the modern Jew. At the end of the nineteenth century, this undertaking, which can be said to have begun with the Marrano experience and continues unabated to this very day, saw Jewish psychiatrists contribute with professional expertise and personal passion to the ongoing discussion about the meaning and nature of modern Jewish identity, and the intimate relation of the Jewish body to that identity.

CHAPTER 6

# IN PRAISE OF JEWISH RITUAL
## MODERN MEDICINE AND THE DEFENSE OF ANCIENT TRADITIONS

To most Jews in modern Western Europe, science, and this includes medicine, did not pose a mortal danger to Judaism, notwithstanding the fear of rabbinical authorities in cases such as the burial controversy of 1772. Rather, science and Judaism have enjoyed a complementary relationship with each other. The Jewish scientist was not swayed by the nineteenth-century French philosopher Auguste Comte, who proclaimed that in the coming positivist order, scientists, rather than priests, would be canonized. Few Jewish scientists have ever suggested that a man in a lab coat would or should replace the rabbi in his long, black coat. On the contrary, among Central European Jews in the nineteenth century, there were many who sought to make use of science in order to help them bolster their links to Jewish tradition.

What this means is that for Jews in the modern period, science and religion have proven to be perfectly compatible. This raises a number of other questions. Are there ways in which they actually complement each other? Are there examples of ways in which Jews have sought to make use of science so as to affirm their Jewishness on a personal level, and are there ways in which science has been enlisted to defend the edifice of Judaism itself? The answer to all these questions is yes.

As the previous two chapters have demonstrated, medicine not only proved itself to be a weapon with which the Jews could be attacked, but it could also serve as a means of self-defense for modern Jews. With the Jewish body and mind under such close scrutiny, Jewish doctors responded forcefully to the dominant paradigms concerning the supposed predisposition of Jews to certain pathologies and mental illnesses. Those Jewish physicians who participated in the debates offered a variety of social explanations for disease etiology among Jews. And when the diseases affecting Jews were more apparent than real, Jewish physicians advanced historical and cultural reasons to prove that there was nothing inherently wrong with or biologically irredeemable about the Jewish body.

But at the intersection of the nineteenth and twentieth centuries, it was not only the Jewish body that was under investigation, but Judaism itself came under increasing and often hostile scrutiny. Observed by the fledgling disciplines of anthropology and theology, Jewish customs, rituals, and behaviors were examined with a view to unearthing the origins and meaning of the religion's rituals, and by extension, Judaism's relationship to Christianity.

This undertaking first appeared in earnest during the sixteenth and seventeenth centuries in the guise of travel or missionary literature and into the eighteenth century, when it was driven by the felt need of European intellectuals to distance and differentiate their own cultures from that of the aboriginal cultures with whom Europeans came in contact through imperialism.[1] For many, there lurked behind this undertaking an urgent need to justify European colonial ambitions and immoral behavior such as slavery, often by distinguishing between the "primitive" religions of the colonized and the "higher" religion of the colonizers.

The Jews became entangled in this debate because Judaism was the progenitor of Christianity and Jews were the principal non-Christian minority on the European continent; therefore, their religion, too, was subject to comparison with those of the Europeans.[2] Eighteenth-century critics of revealed religion often derided Judaism as primitive, or even savage, and contrasted it unfavorably with Enlightenment notions of a "Religion of Reason" or "Natural Religion."[3]

Later, Gentile critics of Judaism in Germany often operated under the influence of Immanuel Kant, who, in his *Religion Within the Limits of Reason Alone* (1793), denied that Judaism could even be regarded as a religion. For him, Judaism was "a collection of mere statutory laws upon which was established a political organization." The god of the Jews was a political autocrat who only demanded the outward observance of ritual, which was generally performed in an atmosphere of fear. This god made no moral and ethical demands on the individual and therefore, according to Kant, Christianity could not have sprung from Judaism. Rather, it was the product of a sudden religious revolution, and therefore all ties between Christianity and Judaism had to be severed.[4]

Such views were long-lived. The growth of Protestant New Testament scholarship in Germany after the 1860s, which was sometimes crudely antisemitic, saw liberal Christian theologians paint a negative picture of first-century Judaism in order to tear Jesus from his social and cultural milieu. Seeking to minimize Jesus' Jewishness by ignoring or denying the Jewish origin and content of his teachings, such scholars, according to Susannah Heschel, "elevate[ed] Jesus as a unique religious figure who stood in sharp opposition to his Jewish surroundings."[5] In response, Jewish scholars, such as the founder of Reform Judaism, Abraham Geiger, stressed the essential Jewishness of Jesus and his teachings, claiming that Christianity, a religion about Jesus, but not Jesus' own religion, was a distortion of those teachings.[6]

The Christian claims and Jewish counterclaims were made at that historical moment when intense nationalism and organized antisemitism were becoming palpable forces in Germany. The theological debates about Judaism and Christianity and Jesus' identity were immediately colored by the discourse on German national identity. Although many on the political right were forced to admit that Jesus had been born into the Jewish religion, they reclaimed him by asserting that he was, however, of Aryan and not Semitic *racial* ancestry. Others even launched an attack on Christianity itself, claiming that it was merely a modified version of Judaism and thus foreign and inappropriate to Germany. Later on, as part of the larger project to extirpate all that was Jewish from Germany, Nazi theologians would make much of the "Aryan" Christ.[7]

At stake here was whether Judaism and its detailed ritual code, or even a reformed version of it, could be accorded its due respect in Germany.[8] Were Judaism and Christianity so distinct in not only a theological but perhaps, even more important from a fin-de-siècle perspective, a racial sense that there was little hope for social harmony between adherents of the two religions? The debates were always about far more than abstract theology, going straight to the heart of contemporary social relations between Germans and Jews.

Although both Jewish and Gentile scholars were preoccupied with tracing the links and differences between the two religions, the outcome of their respective investigations could be very different. Jewish scholars tended to present Judaism and Jewish ritual as innovations that marked the historical advent of morality and ethics.[9] Entries in standard references of the era, such as Jewish encyclopedias, were apologetic in nature, seeking to inform and perhaps remind Jews and Christians who may have been unaware, or who had forgotten, that the roots of modern Europe's Christian culture were firmly planted in the soil of Jewish tradition.[10]

The Jewish response most often sought to challenge the more outrageous claims of the antisemites, whose central charge was that there existed an essential and insurmountable difference between Jews and Christians, at the core of which were mutually exclusive concepts of ethics espoused by the two groups. Jews refuted such claims by mounting arguments that affirmed the ethical and social compatibility of Jews and Christians. By contrast, German works that stressed the seeming pettiness or even savagery of Jewish rituals often intended to split asunder the cultural links between the two faiths.[11]

Into this religious and social debate stepped Jewish physicians. With their particular expertise, they attempted to counter the negative assessment that many Christians, and not a few increasingly assimilated Jews, had of Jewish rituals. While, for example, the era's basic textbooks on Judaism could still say of the dietary regulations that "holiness is . . . the only object of these laws," medicine could not be satisfied with such an explanation, as much as any individual Jewish physician may have believed it.[12] Rather, in this skeptical and often hostile cultural climate, medicine was employed by Jews as a rationalization and, indeed, a scientific justification for the continued practice of ancient rituals. Moreover, at this particular historical juncture, medicine was an important means of expressing and, if need be, shoring up flagging Jewish identity.

Pondering the relationship of science to Jewishness and Judaism, the German Jewish sexologist Max Marcuse declared in 1912: "What earlier differentiated the Jew from the non-Jew, as well as unified the Jews — was their religion and what evolved from their religious laws. This connection has been destroyed. The Jews no longer claim to be the 'chosen people,' no longer believe in the God of the Jews, and understand the laws of Moses to be only social and hygienic directives."[13]

Marcuse was not entirely correct. He was most likely speaking about his own person, or other religiously marginal Jews like himself. They may no longer have felt any attachment to ritual, but prior to World War I — and this is where Marcuse erred — the majority of German Jews would have subscribed to the notion that it was *precisely* religion, as opposed to nationality, that differentiated Jews from non-Jews. Where Marcuse is instructive, however, is in his drawing attention to the fact that Jews at this time do begin to see and tout the social and hygienic dimension of certain Jewish laws.

Still, Marcuse's extreme observation needs to be qualified, because he overstated the case. Jews did not *only* come to see the "laws of Moses as social and hygienic directives." Even those Jews who proclaimed the biosocial advantages to certain Jewish rituals never rejected the religious imperative behind their performance. Most were able to recognize their religious as well as medically prophylactic dimensions.

Nevertheless, the scientific efficacy of certain Jewish rituals was stressed as never before. Why? Partially, it had to do with the fact that the majority of Jews in Germany were now less dedicated to the fundamental religious ideas that lay behind these practices than were previous generations. Other rationalizations were sought to justify their continued performance, and here medicine played a useful role. But more decisive than this reason were the changed circumstances and context in which ritual practices were being performed by the minority. From the eighteenth century on, German Jewry, emerging out of the ghetto, and under sustained pressure to conform to the aesthetic and social demands of German middle-class life, felt pressured to justify those habits and behaviors that most clearly separated them from their non-Jewish neighbors.[14]

By the last third of the nineteenth century, Jews and an array of their religious practices came under renewed fire. According to Norbert Elias, Protestant interpretations of religious ritual and the impact of aesthetic changes that came in the wake of the breakdown of the feudal order helped drive criticisms of Jewish ritual.[15] In Central Europe, as the pressures born of increasing assimilation and a burgeoning antisemitic movement continued to mount, the ritual bath (*mikveh*), dietary laws (*kashrut*), ritual slaughter (*shehitah*), and ritual circumcision (*brit milah*) were challenged either as antiquated practices inappropriate to life in a modern, scientifically advanced land like Germany or simply as brutal and bloody practices that bespoke an indelible savagery at the core of the Jewish religion. The subtext of such criticisms was that their continued performance was obviously untenable in the heart of civilized Europe.

With its multitude of physicians and scientists, German Jewry mounted a spirited defense of Jewish rituals on the basis of science (as well as religion). Thus it was doctors who took responsibility for presenting and representing Judaism to a skeptical and often hostile public in order to explain the compatibility of the ancient religions' core customs with those of the modern nation-state.

## THE WRITING OF JEWISH MEDICAL HISTORY

The way Jews first elected to establish such a proposition was by undertaking studies of biblical and talmudic medicine. By writing the history of Israelite and rabbinic health care, Jewish scholars sought to demonstrate the farsightedness of ancient Jewish medicine, and by extension, drape in glory contemporary Jewish culture, which, they maintained, was still very much guided by the ancient medical precepts. While the late nineteenth century saw a proliferation of such studies, it is worthy of note that the first Jew to write such a history was Benjamin Wolff Gintzburger, the scion of a distinguished rabbinical family from Lithuania, and the first Jew to graduate with a medical degree from the University of Göttingen. On August 23, 1743, Gintzburger defended his doctoral dissertation, *Medicina Ex Talmudicis Illustrata*. For its day, this was a most unusual choice of topic for a graduating physician, especially a Jewish one, the majority of whom wrote dissertations that dealt with medical or scientific problems.[16] What added to Gintzburger's audaciousness was that his topic, medicine in the Talmud, attempted to capture the universal significance of the text's teachings on Jewish social hygiene.[17]

This study by a devout and learned Eastern European Jew—Gintzburger studied at various yeshivot and in 1735 even corresponded with Altona's rabbi, Jacob Emden, on whether it was permissible for him to participate in compulsory anatomical dissections[18]—is a remarkably proud assertion of his cultural heritage. At a time (as discussed in Chapter 3), when later physicians of the Haskalah were wont to encourage their fellow Jews to emulate Christian health care habits, Gintzburger was concerned with asserting the genius of Jewish medicine. Focusing on talmudic physiology, anatomy, animal pathology, surgery, internal medicine, dietetics, hygiene, prognosis, and preventative medicine, Gintzburger was at pains to show that Judaism's medical culture (and, by extension, the rest of its cultural edifice) was in no way inferior to that of the other ancients or, for that matter, the moderns. As he noted, "When I praise the masters of Hebrew medicine, to mention these here is necessarily only a beginning. They have enriched the art born of human endeavor and have furthered it by their ability and industry, [and, moreover] a small portion [of their writings] precedes the time of Galen while a large part is coeval. . . . No wonder then that much agrees with the Galenic tradition, and that some of it merits consideration for being special or familiar."[19] This perspective is a far cry from that of men such as Moishe Marcuze and Marcus Herz, who came to view the religious culture of the Jews as obscurantist and even life-threatening.

Gintzburger's research was that of a maverick. None of his contemporaries took up similar themes, and thus it was not until the nineteenth and early twentieth century that such scholarship blossomed among Jews. If Gintzburger sought to make a case for the Jews within the context of contemporary debates over Jewish emancipation, later scholars who took up the same theme did so in a thoroughly different social and intellectual climate. With the advance of scientific learning, the emergence of organized antisemitism, and the rise of Jewish nationalism, later Jewish presentations of ancient Israelite medical jurisprudence became more detailed, more scholarly, and more overtly political than Gintzburger's.

In 1865, Rueben Josef Wunderbar, a teacher and author from Riga, published a German-language study of biblical and talmudic medicine. Seeking to "do his bit to promote science in general and the national literature of the Hebrews in particular," Wunderbar produced a detailed, 165-page work of scholarship entitled *Biblisch-talmudische Medicin* (Biblical-talmudic medicine).[20] A work of considerable erudition, it included citations from classical Jewish texts that jostled for space on the page alongside references from Homer, the Koran, contemporary medicine, science, law, history, and archaeology.

Wunderbar tackled a wide array of subjects in order to demonstrate that the foundation of biblical and talmudic law was an overarching concern with the promotion of sound physical and mental health. For example, the biblical treatment of leprosy was designed to prevent contagion, while the laws concerning pederasty, sodomy, onanism, and menstruation stood, according to the author, in direct contrast to Egyptian and Canaanite licentiousness, and "were intended to promote the physical and moral well-being of the Israelites."[21] Wunderbar was medically graphic in his description of these acts, an innovation in itself in modern Jewish literature. In particular, he claimed that pederasty, sodomy, and onanism were responsible for a host of diseases, including syphilis, while abstinence from coitus during menstruation was not merely a matter of moral sensibility but a medical prescription in that Moses "assumed menstrual blood to have been infected." There were two other reasons for the prohibition against sexual activity for menstruating women and those who had just given birth. The first was that "a weakened uterus most likely needed to time to recover," and second, for the male it caused "inflammation of the penis with sores akin to syphilis."[22] As a measure of the scientific nature of Wunderbar's apologia and his desire to offer a nonpartisan appreciation of biblical medical law, he supported these claims with reference to contemporary European medical studies. Similarly, Wunderbar's remarkably frank and medicalized discussion of Judaism's laws concerning procreation and the age the Talmud deemed physiologically and psychologically appropriate for marriage and the onset of sexual activity was "confirmed by the most recent [medical] authors."[23]

Medicine, the law, and the needs of the state all came together for Wunderbar when he discussed the wide variety of baths mentioned in the Bible and Talmud. From the 1820s to the 1840s, Jewish ritual baths (*mik-

*vaot*) were the subject of intense debate in Germany. Both Jews and non-Jews criticized them on the basis of medical arguments that declared them unsanitary. When they did not call for their complete abolition, commentators demanded that state-appointed medical authorities police such institutions. The debate over the baths also demonstrates how medicalization and secularization were two elements of a larger process of social and cultural change for German Jews.[24]

Common to all cultures of the ancient Near East, but an especially rich tradition among Jews, ritual baths, thought Wunderbar, were praiseworthy institutions. He believed them to be particularly efficacious in warm climates, where regular usage was extremely helpful in warding off a host of skin diseases.[25] But times and location had changed, and Wunderbar railed against the state of contemporary European ritual baths. Like his predecessors, he claimed that they were in a "pitiable" state, often erected in dimly lit cellars, "rat infested," and filled with "stinking" and "muddy" water that was used by "hundreds of persons." Occasionally, he observed that in several mikvaot that were heated, no chimneys had been installed. Above all, the ritual baths now had the opposite effect of their original intent. They constituted a danger to one's health.[26] According to Wunderbar, sudden immersion in the cold and unclean water was painful and could cause a host of illnesses, including hysteria, rheumatism, gout, heart murmurs, body tremors, hemorrhaging, and the "gradual, organic destruction of the genitals."[27]

Wunderbar found it "puzzling that they could remain in the Jewish communities in such a state and be tolerated by the sanitation authorities." Naturally such conditions were worse in poorer rural communities than in the big cities, where he described their condition as "bearable, or good at best."[28] Especially shocking to him was that their existence was now religiously counterproductive in that because of their deterioration, ritual baths were being used by fewer and fewer women, and therefore the holy obligation to visit the mikveh was being undermined by the very institution as it currently existed. Although some communities were beginning to refurbish their ritual baths, not enough were, and Wunderbar was of the opinion that a far-reaching program of mikvah reform had to be instituted. To this end he offered three recommendations: the boring of holes into the sides of the bath so water could be drained off to allow for the cleaning out of the bath itself; the installation of a pump so that water could be regularly changed; and finally, the contrivance of a mechanism for the addition of warm water.

Given that Jewish society had become derelict in its duty to maintain such institutions — a far cry from biblical and talmudic times — the changes

Wunderbar proposed were best instituted by governmental decree. This had already taken place in Russian Kurland, where the imperial medical authorities, in conjunction with the locals, reformed the mikvaot. The most important point to note here is that Wunderbar did not suggest the abandonment of the ritual bath as an institution. In fact, the opposite was the case. Continuing to applaud the original religious and medical purpose of ritual bathing, Wunderbar wished to see mikvaot improved, modernized, and again made as prophylactically useful as they had been in antiquity, and the only way this could be done was through the rebirth of a national will to improve the health care of the nation. We can see clearly here how praising Jewish ritual could also entail a critique of contemporary practices and foster a demand for reform based upon modern science. With an eye to the future, Wunderbar — like Elcan Isaac Wolf when discussing the Jewish diet, or Marcus Herz when engaged by the burial controversy — looked backward, desiring a "return" to a medically imagined Jewish past where biblical figures lived sanitary lives in complete accord with Mosaic law.

Whereas Benjamin Wolff Gintzburger extended his praise to "the masters of Hebrew medicine" — that is, to individuals — this characteristic of Enlightenment thought was displaced by Wunderbar's emphasis on the achievements of the nation and the statist nature of medical jurisprudence and policing among the ancient Israelites. In this way, Wunderbar's study represents an entire cognitive shift, whereby ancient Israel's contribution to the welfare of humanity was now seen as an expression of collective genius and the product of superior national organization. From then on, nearly all Jews, especially physicians, who sought to defend the faith would couch their arguments in nationalist terms.

One of the most elaborate interpretations of Jewish law as a code of medical hygiene designed for the benefit of individual, family, and nation was constructed by the Zionist statistician Alfred Nossig.[29] In 1894, Nossig sought to contribute to the then raging European debate concerning public health policy by publishing a popular study of the legal codes of ancient China, India, Persia, Egypt, and Israel. For Nossig, these statutes were actually codes of social hygiene, the principal aim of which was "the preservation and advancement (*Erhaltung und Förderung*) of the physical welfare of the nations." According to Nossig, the civilizations he studied all displayed superior biological and moral traits as a result of their having developed advanced social hygiene codes and thus, perhaps, they could serve as models for contemporary European states.[30]

According to Nossig, historians of social hygiene had incorrectly dated its origins to Greek civilization, when in fact that honor belonged to the Jews. Precisely because among all the peoples who had originated in the Near East only modern Jews continued to adhere most closely to their ancient code of hygiene, Jewish civilization was extant, and the Jews as a group had developed and matured as a nation. This was because the Mosaic hygienic code, best epitomized in the ten commandments, recognized the "interlocking" (*Verflechtung*) of moral and physical health. Owing to the fact that "Moses stood on scientific grounds and that his elevated, penetrating intellect was not obscured by religious delusion" (*religiösem Wahn*), biblical law and later rabbinic legislation enabled the Jews to maintain their racial purity and to serve as a medical light unto the nations.[31] Endorsing such a view, the Scottish physician and devout Christian Alexander Rattray also noted that "the entire Jehovistic system of public hygiene, like His code of personal sanitation . . . was not merely public but of universal and worldwide application . . . many a nation nominally enlightened but sanitarily dark, even at the present day, would benefit materially by its adoption."[32]

Their farsightedness as a people permitted the Jews to anticipate all modern medical problems and to develop an effective social policy to best treat diseases that threatened both the individual and the nation. Thus, according to Nossig, long before modern nations, ancient Israel had created a working relationship between physicians and the state, the result of which was that ancient and modern Jews were healthier than their non-Jewish contemporaries.[33] The Jews had arrived at this point because their leaders — men such as Moses, Solomon and other kings, Ezra and Nehemiah, the rabbis of the Talmud, and the medieval sages, Rashi and Maimonides — were the nation's physicians and not merely its rabbis.[34] To make his case, Nossig engaged in an act of chronological and conceptual conflation in that despite his claim to write history, he recognized no distinction between contemporary and ancient Jewish ritual practice, or between modern, university-trained Jewish physicians and the medical-rabbinic luminaries of a bygone age. They were all part of a seamless whole — a scientifically grounded and hygienically vigilant civilization.

Nowhere was Nossig's disregard for history more evident than when he approvingly quoted the French scientist Guéneau de Mussy. Writing in the age of microbial discovery and germ-transmission research, de Mussy declared that "the idea of parasitical and infectious diseases, which occupies a predominant place in modern pathology, appears to have actively occupied Moses. One can say that it dominates all of his hygienic proscriptions." It is on this basis that Nossig evaluated the variety of "scientific" measures, including stringent quarantine rules adopted by the ancient Israelites to prevent the spread of infectious disease.[35] Citing several biblical examples such as public policy pertaining to the treatment and containment of leprosy (Lev. 13 and 14) and the disposal of human waste at military encampments (Deut. 23:12–13) as evidence of the scientific and medical basis of Jewish law, Nossig asserted that cleanliness, both physical and moral, was the core characteristic of the nation. Laws were designed to promote good health and, most important, given contemporary currents in medical practice and ideology, disease prevention.

In establishing a medically prophylactic purpose to Jewish law, Nossig was able to reinvent the meaning of Judaism by shearing it of religious significance and investing it with therapeutic relevance. Thus was he able to theoretically tailor Judaism to the intellectual demands of an overwhelmingly secular, political enterprise such as Zionism. By medicalizing and secularizing the religion, Nossig universalized Judaism and permitted a wider swath of the Jewish public to celebrate Jewish customs and rituals. He provided Jews, both Zionist and otherwise, with a reworked "mission" — to explain to the rest of the world that the secret of Jewish national longevity and good health lay in the strict performance of ritual that was based on a "medical," as opposed to a religious or political, constitution. In contrast to the enduring influence in Germany of both Kant and Hegel, Nossig maintained, Jewish law (*halakha*) was a rational compendium of rites and practices that promoted cleanliness, strength, and racial purity.

Nossig's subversive reading of Judaism served as a counterhistory to Christianity's interpretation of a Jewish fall from grace, one that was characterized by the Jews' physical deformity stemming from their moral inferiority. Just as he collapsed ancient and modern when discussing Jewish law and medicine, so too did Nossig see ancient and modern hostility toward the Jews as another seamless continuum. But whereas contemporary antisemitism saw in the Jews an effeminate, enervated, destructive, and degenerate cabal, Nossig's alternate reading of Jewish culture saw modern Jews as a masculine, vital, and creative force.[36] With their longer life spans, lower infant mortality rates, presumed immunity from a host of diseases, and sobriety, modern Jews became, in Nossig's hands, latter-day biblical superheroes.

Aside from the works of Gintzburger, Wunderbar, Nossig, and several others, the first and, to this day, most important study of ancient Jewish medicine is Julius Preuss's monumental *Biblisch-talmudische medizin* (Biblical-talmudic medicine) (1911).[37] In nineteen long and copiously noted chapters, Preuss, a physician and Semitic philologist from Berlin, was the first to undertake a thorough study of this type from the vantage point of doctor and classically educated Jew. The depth of Preuss's scholarship is both profound and incomparable, and it is certainly less polemical than that of his predecessors. In fact, he notes in the preface that "my previous works have been criticized as being 'cool all the way up to the heart.' I hope and pray that one can say the same about this book."[38] While it does appear "cool" compared to the more rambunctious texts of those who came before him, like theirs, Preuss's work must be placed in the larger context of contemporary German Jewish efforts at self-assertion, especially in the sphere of Jewish medical history. Herein lies his similarity to other Jewish scholars who worked on ancient Jewish medicine.

Significantly, however, Preuss was a superior historian to the others. This is most evident when, in contrast to Nossig's grander claims, Preuss stated that it would be as "foolish to criticize physicians in Talmudic times for not using ophthalmoscopes, as it is for us to use scholastic ingenuity to prove their acquaintance with bacteria, from incidental remarks concerning demonic influences (*mazzikin*)."[39] For Preuss, biblical figures were to remain just that. He was not prepared to turn them into modern physicians. Still, and here the resemblance to other scholars in the field does become manifest, it was impossible to put down Preuss's study and not come away convinced of the overarching concern that ancient Jewish culture displayed for healing and promoting good health. Although he stated that there is "no Jewish medicine in the sense that we speak of an Egyptian or a Greek medical science,"[40] he was the first to so completely document the myriad medical discourses in the Bible and Talmud that the effect was to establish the intimate relationship between medicine and the Jews and make clear the compassionate and healing qualities of Jewish culture. Concomitantly, while Preuss made no overt reference to the contemporary Jewish Question in Germany, *Biblical-Talmudic Medicine* must be read as a refutation of antisemitic accusations, which specifically charged the Jews with cruelty and inhumanity.

## KASHRUT

After about 1825 there was a noticeable decline in traditional religious observance among German Jews. While small and rural communities tended to maintain ritual practice longer than Jews in bigger cities, the overall movement was away from orthopraxy. What tended to be discarded first were those rituals that formed barriers between Christians and Jews and militated against full economic integration. Increased attendance of Jewish children at public schools only sped up the process of acculturation. By 1871 and the founding of the German Reich, large numbers of German Jews had already significantly reduced religious performance, confining observance to the home. After this date, which also saw them granted citizenship, the steady movement of Jews from small towns to large cities was accompanied by increasing and rapid secularization.[41] Foremost among rituals discarded in the wake of modernization and urbanization were Sabbath observance and dietary restrictions. Already by the middle of the nineteenth century there had been reports of Jews seen eating in taverns and restaurants, even at the same tables with Christians.[42] With time, this would, of course, prove to be true of Jews not only in Germany, but also in Western Europe as a whole.

However, German Jews, long faced with formidable antisemitism, were relentlessly called upon to defend practices that were regarded by the majority as incompatible with traditional German mores and values.[43] Moreover, these rituals were seen as being at odds with the practice of German citizenship — so recently gained and so long fought for. This was not only a Gentile view, but one shared by considerable numbers of Jews as well. In the early decades of the nineteenth century, Jewish critics had singled out the dietary laws (*kashrut*) as the ultimate expression of Jewish exclusiveness and self-segregation, seeing them as antiquated, nonsensical, and divisive at a time when hopes for social integration ran high.[44] But if Jews chose to avoid eating prohibited delicacies such as shellfish, or the omnipresent and infinite varieties of pork products available in Germany, that was their business. The debate over kashrut in the context of religious reform that took place in the 1840s was primarily a Jewish one. In fact, it was not even much discussed by the reformers themselves because they saw observance of the dietary laws as a private affair.

However, Christian complaints about kashrut could not be left unanswered. What ensued was a very heated debate about the dietary laws, with Jews this time mounting a vigorous defense of them. German Jewry had essentially adopted three principal positions regarding the dietary code. There were the radical abolitionists, the moderate reformers, and finally, the strict retentionists.[45] While it would appear that little could unite these disparate parties on this issue, confronted with Gentile criticism, they were able to find common ground by turning to and celebrating the supposed medical and physiological benefits of the Jewish dietary code. Even if the abolitionists and the reformers drew a distinction between biblical and rabbinic law, regarding the former as having been nullified with the destruction of ancient

Israel and the latter as nonbinding and the invention of mere rabbis, they often sought to salvage something from Judaism's dietary edifice by stressing the medical dimensions and farsightedness of kashrut. So seductive and appealing was this line of defense that even the Orthodox, inspired strictly by their faith, were wont to express to the outside world a scientific defense of the dietary laws. They were on safe ground when they did so, justifying themselves by explicitly drawing inspiration from no less a figure than Maimonides, the twelfth-century physician and rabbi who had himself explained the medical virtues of kashrut.[46]

Elcan Isaac Wolf in 1777 had already mentioned some of the advantages to health that were inherent in Judaism's dietary regulations. Such scientific defenses were made right throughout the nineteenth century and into the twentieth.[47] Bearing in mind that both Jewish and non-Jewish critics of Judaism stressed its irrational nature, the religion's defenders, especially when they were doctors, were at pains to point out its rational side, most often doing so by characterizing Jewish scientific genius.

In 1825, the same year that Prussia had introduced new procedures for medical examinations, thus contributing to the rising importance of university medical faculties and their stress on rationality and science, Ignaz Kahn, a Jewish physician from Augsburg, published a study wherein he sought to establish that Judaism had long been cognizant of and receptive to science. In this vigorous refutation of a contemporary claim that the Jews were ignorant of science, Kahn asserted that Jewish religious law itself was actually inspired by and based upon scientific understanding and medical wisdom. One of the primary examples he cited was the dietary code, which, he maintained, had evolved after centuries of accumulated medical knowledge among the Jewish people. According to Kahn, the Jews early on had recognized the link between food consumption and climate, and therefore had banned foods that spoiled easily in the heat of the Near East.[48] Specifically, Kahn noted that the prohibition against pork was a particularly wise and necessary innovation given that its consumption promoted skin diseases.[49] Finally, Kahn interpreted the strict prohibition against consuming blood not as an aversive Jewish response to pagan blood cults but simply as a response to the fact that the consumption of blood, especially when it was still warm, was deadly.[50]

Although the majority of religious reformers were in favor of dispensing with most if not all of the dietary regulations, their quest to highlight Judaism's rational side sometimes led them to even defend kashrut. An article that appeared in 1840 in the Reform periodical *The Israelite of the Nineteenth*

*Century* claimed that while kashrut had been designed to promote social segregation between Jews and others after the destruction of the Temple, the dietary laws nevertheless made sound scientific sense. Camel meat was considered to be heavy and indigestible, as were birds of prey, while pork from the Orient was a source of skin diseases, and shellfish such as mussels were said to promote colic. The author of the article was unable, however, to find any medical justification for the separation of meat and milk.[51]

Although they constituted the beginning of a new interpretive trend, such generalized and overly simplistic defenses of kashrut were themselves unsatisfying. Soon they too would give way to even more elaborate and complex scientific defenses of the dietary laws. In 1843, another proponent of religious reform penned an anonymous article entitled "Medical Discussion of the Mosaic Sanitary Laws." The Jewish dietary proscriptions, noted the author, were the product of indisputable scientific reasoning, based upon the close observation of nature. To make his case about the scientific and thus permanent validity of Jewish food laws, the author turned his attention to the prohibition against the consumption of carnivorous beasts and the restriction to ruminants. Like the previous author, this one claimed that the meat of carnivores was indigestible and that ruminants simply tasted better. But, he continued, "physiological chemistry" teaches that herbivores, animals whose diets are composed largely of carbohydrates, are more easily digested by humans, and thus constitute their principal source of protein. Carnivores, with a meat diet containing an excessive amount of nitrogen, are unable to provide humans with the chemical building blocks they require. The author's references to carbohydrates as *Vegetabilia* and protein as *Urstoff* (a primal substance) indicated that he was familiar with the latest scientific terminology and concepts — the term *protein* having been first used only five years earlier in 1838, and *carbohydrates* not long thereafter.[52] Finally, he was able to conclude with confidence that the rationality of Moses' legislation had been substantiated by the "most brilliant discoveries" of modern science.[53]

Other Reform Jews employed a two-pronged argument, appealing to the spiritual underpinnings of the dietary laws and the physical advantages to be enjoyed by observance of them. In a sermon given in German in 1881 by Rabbi Maurice Fluegel to the Benai Israel Temple in Kalamazoo, Michigan, we have the somewhat unusual situation of a Reform rabbi exhorting his congregation to observe kashrut for ethical, historical, and medical reasons. Decrying the fact that the modern world sees fit to dispense with all that is traditional, Fluegel chided the worshippers: "American Israelites! Haven't we, through giving up the discipline of the Mosaic dietary laws suffered a great loss, yet harvested spiritual torpor and physical invalidism? The statistician, the natural scientist, the philanthropist cannot avoid the disintegration, the decomposition, the physical and spiritual decadence of American Jewry in particular. This despite our Belgian carpets, mahogany furniture, our proud houses of business, and public schools. Is not the disintegration that we see before our eyes to do with every observance we abandon?"[54]

Fluegel went on to catalogue the illnesses to which Jews had now become prone as a result of having given up the Jewish dietary laws, suggesting reasons why it was essential for Reform Jews to be more observant. In so doing, he also opined about the fundamental nature of Reform Judaism itself and the ways it could further the cause of improving the health of the Jewish people: "But theory, just as pills, will not help. It has nothing to do with beliefs and opinions, but action. It has nothing to do with the Bible and the Shulkhan Arukh, nothing to do with sighting the Messiah or revelation, but how one can lead a rational life in order to win back [our] ancient vitality. It has to do with a healthy diet, and the sanitary and ethical rules of life. . . . But you say: 'We are Reformers and Reform has nothing to do with the kitchen.' Here is your error. Reform Judaism is the striving to harmonize religion and science."[55]

By the turn of the twentieth century an increasing number of studies had appeared in Germany that addressed the scientific dimensions of kashrut. Overall advances in medical science, especially in the field of nutrition, saw Jewish physicians attempt to interpret the dietary laws through the prism of the latest conceptual categories of medical analysis. In his *Manual of Nutrition* (1901), which bore the subtitle *With Special Consideration of the Jewish Dietary Laws,* a Nuremberg physician, Philipp Münz, noted that Jews seemed to suffer from a disproportionate number of stomach disorders. In fact, as a modern scientist under the influence of Lamarckian theories of inheritance, Münz contended that the full range of stomach disorders to which Jews had become predisposed had, in fact, become acquired and inheritable characteristics.[56]

Münz identified two principal reasons for this situation. The first is that having been restricted to trade from the Middle Ages on, Jews were subject to the uncertainty that comes from being dependent on the vagaries of the business cycle. Moreover, theirs was an intensive family life, characterized by excessive concern for materially providing for one's family, while finally, this overall "struggle for existence" was made even more precarious by the contemporary antisemitic movement. This constellation of factors led to nervous illnesses among Jews which, according to Münz, manifested themselves in a host of gastrointestinal disorders.[57]

Münz also suggested that the Jewish diet was itself a cause of stomach ailments among the Jewish population. Like his predecessor Elcan Isaac Wolf, Münz identified the way Jews ate as opposed to the dietary laws themselves as the root cause of the problems. As it was during the Haskalah, it remained an aesthetic problem. In their haste to modernize, the Jews had abandoned traditional Jewish customs, emulating their Christian neighbors. Modern Jews were in a rush. They took their meals in a disorderly fashion, "when and however they can, sometimes earlier, sometimes later, a little more, a little less, barely warm, nearly cold, rarely chewed properly. And as soon as the meal is ended, so do they begin their brisk activity again, which naturally impedes proper digestion." Finally, there was the problem born of excess. After a week of inadequate nourishment, the modern Jew would sit down to a sumptuous Sabbath or festival table and simply overdo it, consuming more than his stomach could bear. All this, declared Münz, was the result of an "irrational and unreasonable way of life."[58] And the irrational way of life was the life of the *assimilationist,* for it was he who had abandoned the rational and hygienic code that is kashrut.

Exacerbating the situation was the fact that many of the Jews who suffered from chronic stomach ailments attributed their condition solely to the consumption of kosher food, "holding it responsible for their suffering." Münz was especially galled by the fact that in most cases, despite their ignorance about the dietary laws, doctors advised their Jewish patients to abandon the regulations for the sake of their health. Münz adopted the opposite view. As both a medical practitioner and descendant of Orthodox rabbis, he asserted that the "dietary laws correspond not merely to the strictest requirements of hygiene (preventative medicine), but are especially salubrious and recommended for those with gastro-intestinal disorders."[59]

Münz was also unwilling to ignore the moral dimension that lay behind the dietary laws, claiming that "they promoted moderation and abstinence, a steeling and ennobling of the character, taking one above the level of a dull animal, elevating one to the status of a moral, ethical, and intelligent being." This was a crucial claim, for while it may appear that Münz was not saying anything that Jewish scholars had not already said before, the context—a modern medical textbook—is what makes it novel. Not only did Münz take aim as a Jew at the commonplace charges of Jewish immorality by highlighting the ethical impulse of the laws, he identified the ethical dimension of kashrut as being inseparable from the physiological, both operating together to produce a "hygienic, salutary effect."[60]

Münz's textbook, a primer on the most current findings of nutritional science, set out to demonstrate that behind the dietary laws lay a body of enlightened scientific knowledge. And despite the antiquity of Jewish food laws, their arrangement was commensurate with and verified by modern science. Münz first pointed to the basic foundation of the dietary code, Judaism's tripartite division of food groups into meat, dairy products, and those classified as neither, known as *parve* — the most important foods in this third category being fruit, vegetables, and fish. It was Münz's opinion that Judaism's orderly separation of foods into these categories served to ensure that "a mixed diet signifies the only rational, nutritional [regimen] for both healthy and sick individuals." What was particularly impressive about this arrangement for Münz was that Jewish law did not consider the groups separately, despite their formal division, but rather focused on how they were made to interact with one another. That is, considered from the vantage point of science, the law was concerned less with the provenance of each nutritional category than with its chemical composition, its corresponding fit with other nutritional categories, as well as the degree of various foods' digestibility and nourishment.[61]

For Münz, it was Judaism's holistic, scientific approach to food that enabled laws designed to aid digestion and promote good health. The bulk of the text was taken up with extremely detailed descriptions of the chemical properties of various foods, wherein he repeatedly stressed the extent to which the Jewish dietary laws conformed to common scientific and nutritional wisdom. Foremost among these were the highly detailed process of meat inspection in order to ensure the impeccable quality of the carcass, the process of making meat kosher by salting to extract all traces of blood, the strict separation of milk and meat products, the stipulation to wait six hours before eating dairy products after having consumed meat and half an hour when the order is reversed, and periodic fasting.[62]

Although the wholesale adoption of Jewish dietary laws for the general population was an impossibility, Münz did endorse the notion, derived from kashrut, that all people, whether sick or healthy, require a strict dietary regimen. To that end, he recommended a diet characterized by the moderate intake of alcohol, tea, coffee, and spicy foods, even indicating the specific temperatures at which a host of beverages and foodstuffs should be consumed. Münz also made specific recommendations concerning the kitchen, which, he asserted, should be free of food odors and heated to no more than a chilly 15°C.[63] Further, as part of his all-encompassing approach to good nutrition, Münz insisted upon a program of regular exercise and offered a host of other directives concerning personal welfare, all of which he claimed worked to the benefit of those with stomach disorders.[64]

Because for Münz the entire Jewish dietary code was scientifically grounded, it was of universal applicability. Perhaps not in all its details, but certainly in its practical intent — the "harmonization of ethics and hygiene" — in his view the laws were not time-bound but, rather, for the ages. For as presented by Münz, they were rational, humane, moral, and thoroughly modern, in keeping with the demands of contemporary life. Therefore Christians who confronted similar, if not identical, pressures stemming from modern life had much to learn from ancient Jewish legislation. In all, Münz identified the dietary laws as the most important sign of an ethical and scientifically intuitive civilization.

Whereas Münz examined Jewish dietary laws and their advantages in treating stomach disorders, Wilhelm Sternberg, a Jewish physician from Berlin, studied the possible links between the supposed prevalence of diabetes among Jews and kashrut in his 1903 treatise, *Is Diabetes a Consequence of the Ritual Kitchen and Orthodox Lifestyle of the Jews?* Like Münz, Sternberg compared the three kosher food groups with the three scientific classifications of food — proteins, carbohydrates, and fats — in order to show that the Jews had discovered the scientific existence and meaning of these nutritional categories long before modern science. The predisposition of Jews to diabetes was not the result of kashrut, according to Sternberg. He believed (as discussed in Chapter 4) that racial factors, the laws of inheritance, and nervous disposition explained the high incidence of diabetes among Jews. This organic explanation enabled Sternberg to defend Jewish culture and the scientific affinity it displayed. Rather than causing the dreaded disease, the balanced diet that resulted from following kashrut was protective. In fact, a comparison of modern medicine's teachings on diabetes with those of the Jewish dietary laws showed that the "dictates and prohibitions of science with regard to diabetics conforms to those of Jewish ritual, and are thus closely followed by Orthodox Jews."[65] Therefore, neither kashrut nor an Orthodox lifestyle were to blame for the high proportion of Jewish diabetics.

Sternberg concluded that because diabetes occurred to a greater extent among Jews than non-Jews, and because the majority of Jews did not lead strictly kosher lives, then a kosher diet was *not* the cause of the disease among them.[66] In fact, given that the majority in the West did not keep kosher,

Sternberg suggested that the food Jews ate should be seen as a "national" rather than a "religious" cuisine. And although that national cuisine was characterized by its sweetness, a preference Sternberg described as so "extraordinarily conservative" that it was in evidence even among converts who had "given up the religion of their fathers, but not the cooking of their mothers," high sugar consumption had not been proven scientifically to cause diabetes. Indeed, to the modern medical community the onset of diabetes appeared to be independent of dietary factors.[67]

If the food Jews consumed did not have a negative impact on their health, it may nevertheless have had one on their political culture. In a thoroughly bizarre supposition, Sternberg asked his readers to consider whether there was a connection between the Jews' predilection for sweets and the state of their political development. Children, according to Sternberg, almost exclusively favor the taste of sweet food. This preference changes with age when one sees a "manliness" of the palate develop that manifests itself in the consumption of more savory foodstuffs. Now, given that the Jews, especially the males, have tenaciously preserved their collective sweet tooth, Sternberg asked, "Should one seek an explanation for the predilection among male Israelites for sweets in the fact that they have retained a kind of childishness, reflected in an unmanly and effeminate indulgence of sweets? This is due to the absence of political freedom which the Zionist visionaries and utopians will certainly seek to change."[68] Food, politics, gender, and the health of the Jews all come together here in a classic example of fin-de-siècle medical discourse. For physicians such as Sternberg, progress, both political and pathological, could be made, but it did not have to be so at the expense of ritual and Orthodoxy. In fact, there may even have been an unintended physiological advantage that stemmed from Jewish cookery. Sternberg suggested that the Jews' predilection for sweets and fats may have given them an aversion to the taste of alcohol, and thus did they enjoy the benefits of sobriety.[69]

What this all meant for Wilhelm Sternberg, and all the other Jewish medical commentators before him, was that the culinary culture of Central European Jewry was not inherently inferior to that of their Gentile neighbors, and that any pathological defects that Jews displayed were not due to kashrut. Whether that food was declared medically prophylactic or was nostalgically celebrated, as the poet Heinrich Heine had done in his ode to the sweet pudding known as *Schalet* in the poem "Princess Sabbath," the message that Jewish doctors were sending out was that for the sake of their health, Jews did not have to sacrifice kosher food on the altar of assimilation.[70]

## IN PRAISE OF JEWISH RITUAL

### SHEHITAH

Above all, Jews defended the dietary code in the larger context of debates about the pros and cons of ritual animal slaughter — what the Germans called the *Schächtenfrage,* or "slaughter question." Seen by opponents as inhumane, the Jewish method of slaughter, known as *shehitah,* came under attack from the middle of the nineteenth century in both Europe and the United States. While in all countries where the debate raged Jewish communal authorities and rabbis responded defensively, it was principally in German-speaking Europe that we see, in addition to the traditional spokesmen, Jewish physicians and specialists in animal physiology enter into the fray.

Leading the crusade against Jewish animal slaughter were animal protection societies who charged that the way Jews killed their animals was cruel and torturous.[71] The method of slaughter they protested has essentially remained unchanged since antiquity. It entails cutting the throat of the animal above the larynx almost completely across, severing windpipe, gullet, and all veins and arteries. By this means, the blood is permitted to flow freely and rapidly from the carcass until it is completely drained. What sustained the charge of excessive cruelty was based on the cursory observation of opponents that following the cutting of the throat, there takes place a torrential discharge of blood, followed immediately by several convulsive shudders by the beast — all of which are a reflex, and not indicative that what is being experienced is either consciousness or pain.[72] Indeed, according to some animal physiologists who supported the Jewish method of slaughter, loss of consciousness was coterminous with the rapid drop in blood pressure experienced by an animal whose throat is cut.[73]

By contrast, the most common mode of slaughtering four-legged animals among Christians in the nineteenth century was through the deliverance of a stunning blow to the head, usually with a mallet or poleax. An incision in the neck was then made and the blood drained. The opponents of shehitah were unshakable in their belief that the non-Jewish method of slaughter was of superior moral and humanitarian worth to the Jewish one.[74] Jewish participants in the debate ridiculed this notion. The British rabbi Philip Benny, from Sheffield, spoke for many Jews when he noted, "When we now bear in mind that in the ordinary [non-Jewish] mode of slaughtering, the butchers are not in any way restricted, but may knock, hack and cut, when, where, and how they please, without any fear as to the consequences, without pecuniary loss, and remember that the carcase, though suffering while alive from the most disgusting and loathsome diseases, may freely be sold so long as the flesh *appear* healthy, all must acknowledge that the Jewish mode of

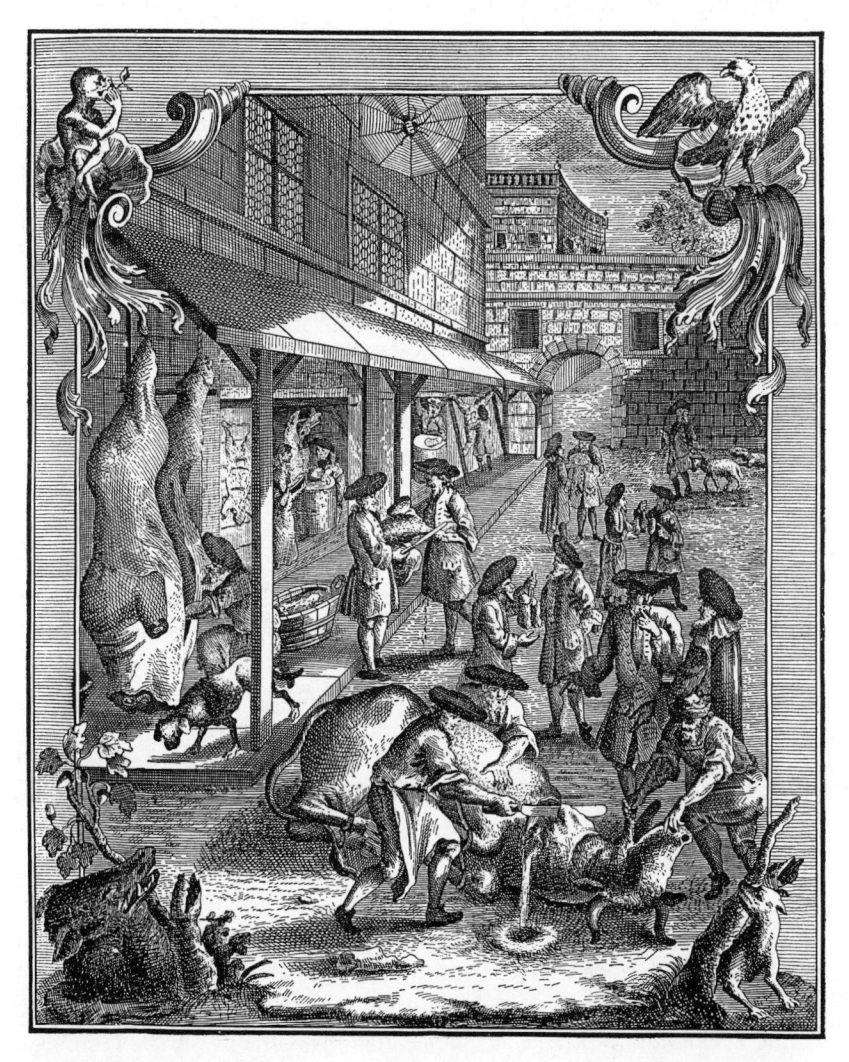

FIGURE 7. This depiction of an eighteenth-century German Jewish slaughter yard is an engraving from Johann Christoph Georg Bodenschatz's *Kirchliche Verfassung der heutigen Juden, sonderlich derer in Deutschland* (Strassburg, 1748). Note the gushing blood of the slaughtered cow in the foreground and the fact that the Jews in the background continue their transactions unperturbed by the violence of the scene. The representation of Jewish ritual practice as Oriental and thoroughly un-German was commonplace into the twentieth century. Source: *The Jewish Encyclopedia* (New York, 1905).

slaughtering can *per se* claim these advantages."[75] In Germany, one commentator even saw shehitah as the reason for Jewish nonviolence, noting that "given the care and humanity with which Jews carry out rites of death with animals whose flesh they intend to eat, an act which is clothed in solemnity, surely it [shehitah] is not without influence on the infrequency of violent crimes and cruelty against people and animals by Jews."[76]

Switzerland was the first European country to adopt an anti-shehitah law. Beginning in the 1850s, a grass-roots campaign opposing shehitah began to emerge in the canton of Aargau. The agitation spread to the canton of St. Gallen in the following decade, where articles decrying shehitah as counter to humanitarian ideals appeared in local newspapers. Although the articles professed outrage and claimed the moral high ground, they were written, according to the rabbi of St. Gallen, Hermann Engelbert, for purely venal and malicious reasons, having been orchestrated by Swiss butchers as a means of winning public support for their narrow economic and professional interests. The rabbi also declared the butchers to have been driven by outright antisemitism—a point that lies at the heart of the entire shehitah debate.[77]

The published articles were effective, for they launched the campaign that saw both cantons outlaw Jewish slaughtering in 1867, St. Gallen characterizing it as practice that "disturbed public order and caused unnecessary pain [to the animals]."[78] The Jews of Switzerland launched a vigorous campaign to defend their practices. While they mounted arguments based on traditional expressions of Jewish ethics and humanitarianism, they included something new in their arsenal. Rabbis and communal leaders turned to renowned scientists, asking them to render expert opinion as to whether shehitah was cruel and painful and what its merits were relative to other forms of animal slaughter.[79]

This was a major innovation in the form of Jewish apologetics—Orthodox Jews seeking to defend Jewish ritual through the solicitation of support from Gentile scientists. The rabbis' faith in science was justified, for in rendering its opinion the scientific establishment was unanimous in its support of shehitah. The director of the Veterinary College of Zurich, Dr. Zangger, stated that death from the Jewish method comes "within seconds, not even a whole minute. In this period of time the suffering cannot be said to be cruel." Both the Jewish and non-Jewish methods, he concluded, were equally good. Similarly, the principal of London's Albert Veterinary College, John Gamgee, certified that he "consider[ed] the Jewish system of slaughtering at least as good as any other in practise in this or other countries." Professor Roloff in Halle commented unequivocally that "the Jewish method of slaughter is an entirely suitable and humane procedure." Admitting that observing any form of animal slaughter is not for the fainthearted, the city of Augsburg's police veterinarian, Theodor Adam, testified that "according to the proof I have furnished, Jewish slaughtering can in no way be regarded as cruel," while Professor Gerlach, director of the Royal Veterinary College in Hannover, declared without hesitation that "Jewish slaughtering, as I have observed it, is not cruel, but, rather, the opposite, it being the most humane method of animal slaughter, and it would serve to introduce it into general usage."[80] The protests and the summoning of expert veterinary testimony had the desired effect, for the municipal council of St. Gallen revoked its ban against shehitah in March 1867, after it had been in effect for only some nine months.

There the matter lay until suddenly, in 1874, St. Gallen again banned shehitah, this time employing the underhanded means of permitting the slaughter of animals only according to the newly introduced Bruneau method, one that was said to "not only stun, but kill animals immediately." After a predetermined examination of shehitah, the municipal report stated that "according to the modern conception of cruelty to animals . . . [Jewish] slaughtering is not compatible with our present requirements, and must therefore be banned as constituting animal cruelty." Canton authorities again passed into law the prohibition against shehitah, effective as of January 1, 1875.[81]

Approximately coincident with these local developments, the 1874 revision of the Swiss Constitution took place, by means of which Jews were granted freedom of residence as well as civic and legal equality.[82] Most important, in the context of the anti-shehitah campaign, religious liberty was ensured in Article 50:1 of the Constitution, which guaranteed religious freedom for all citizens. A resolution issued from Bern specifically affirmed the right of Jews to practice shehitah.[83]

Despite this concession, the spirit of religious freedom enshrined in the Constitution remained under attack as animal protection societies and prominent antisemites escalated their campaign against shehitah. In 1891, Aargau, indefatigable in its opposition to the practice, passed a resolution that "*shehitah* is not a religious rite, and therefore may not enjoy the protection of Article 50:1 of the Federal Law." This conclusion was arrived at by making tendentious use of the comments of a small but vocal chorus of German Jewish opponents of shehitah. In particular, the Swiss quoted liberally from the writings and speeches of two Reform rabbis, Leopold Stein of Frankfurt and Jacob Stern of Stuttgart. Both these men and their supporters made the argument that the method of Jewish ritual slaughter of animals was not of biblical origin and was merely an innovation of the rabbis. It was therefore not divinely inspired but the human product of another time and place, one that was no longer binding on modern Jews.[84] Yielding to pressure from a host of interest groups, the Swiss Confederation resolved that while any restriction on shehitah might contravene the religious liberty enshrined in the Constitution, individual cantons were free to adopt laws that prevented cruelty to animals. The government of Aargau wasted no time in mobilizing the anti-shehitah forces again, this time voting to hold a popular referendum on the adoption of an anti-shehitah law, the proponents of which won the day.[85]

Heady from their victory, the Aargauers pushed for the extension of such legislation to the national level. The passage of such a law required that a national plebiscite be held.[86] August 20, 1893, was the date set by the National Council in Bern for the plebiscite aimed at determining whether shehitah be permitted or outlawed, nationwide. In an act reminiscent of the ancient Jewish response to impending catastrophe, August 10 was declared a fast-day for the Jews of Switzerland. But neither the depredations nor the support from such quarters as Swiss professors of veterinary science, the Swiss Consul in the United States, and the National Council in Bern—which in addition to running the plebiscite voted 61 to 49 to recommend the people vote against the anti-shehitah measure—were able to sway the voters.[87] The abolitionists triumphed by a vote of 188,668 to 116,592. Thus was Switzerland's Federal Constitution amended, and to this day, Article 25 reads: "It is expressly forbidden to bleed animals being slaughtered without stunning them beforehand. This applies to all methods of slaughtering and all types of animals."[88]

The successful campaign in Switzerland buoyed the hopes of anti-shehitah forces everywhere, and nowhere more so than in Germany, where agitation was most keen. It is worth mentioning that contemporary observers of the national plebiscite noted that it was German-speaking Switzerland that was in the forefront of the assault. The newspaper *American Hebrew* reported: "It is stated that this majority was obtained chiefly in the German cantons and among the Lutheran population, where anti-Jewish feeling runs the highest."[89] A report prepared by the Anglo-Jewish Association observed: "To the credit of the Roman Catholics it should be stated that their votes were solidly cast against the new clause, their priests having made it known that the movement was a religious attack on the Jews."[90] Shared culture, language, and, often, religious sensibilities meant that the Swiss discourse and the contours of the debate over Jewish ritual slaughter would translate easily over the border.

The German associations for the prevention of cruelty to animals were scarcely far behind their Swiss brethren. Already at their first conference in Gotha in 1879, they decided that shehitah had to be stopped by legislative means. For several years thereafter, the associations mounted an energetic propaganda campaign among the general public. Deeply fearful, Jews appealed directly to Otto von Bismarck. On a visit to the town of Kissingen in 1886, the chancellor personally assured a local rabbi, Moses Löb Bamberger, that the German government would never agree to a ban on shehitah.[91] Undeterred by Bismarck's comments, the opponents of shehitah petitioned the Reichstag, which eventually met to discuss the subject in plenary session in May 1887.[92] Mobilizing quickly, the orthodox rabbis Hirsch Hildesheimer and Samson Raphael Hirsch assembled 2,300 petitions from Germany's Jewish communities against the animal protectionists. This aggressive approach, together with the artful parliamentary skills and the principled stand of the Catholic Center Party head, Ludwig Windthorst, was enough to win the day. The antisemites' petition never made it out of committee.[93] Despite their defeat, the animal protection societies sought to achieve their goal by having restrictive legislation passed at the state as opposed to national level. It will be recalled that this, too, had initially occurred in Switzerland.

Despite the 1890 report of a special veterinary commission called by the Prussian government that demonstrated the widespread, scientific approval of the Jewish method of slaughter, as well the reassurances of the chancellor, Berlin refused to pass an imperial law that would have prevented the passage of municipal laws banning shehitah. Thus, with this guarantee of states' rights and independence of action, the anti-shehitah advocates pursued their goals with some confidence of success. In Saxony in 1892, the reactionary forces secured an order from the Minister of the Interior declaring shehitah illegal. The state's Jews petitioned the minister for an exemption against the order, to which he replied: "It is apparent that any ritual custom, of however long standing, and having its origin in variable human decrees, does not deserve any consideration if it is calculated to give moral offense. . . . The Ministry of the Interior cannot decide to allow the petitioner exceptional treatment of Jewish slaughtering, especially since it would be considered by the great majority of the people as an unjustified favor to an isolated minority."[94] And that comment twenty-two years after the Jews of Germany had been granted citizenship!

Emboldened, the forces aligned against shehitah kept up the pressure to have the ban extended. According to Hirsch Hildesheimer, with "their impudence only exceeded by their ignorance," the opponents had the temerity to declare that not even the Orthodox were scrupulous in all the laws concerning slaughter and thus they had no grounds to continue to resist the adoption of stunning prior to killing.[95] In response, the non-Jewish Committee for the Defense Against Antisemitic Attacks published an extensive report in 1894 detailing the antisemitic character of the anti-shehitah campaign, and appended to it the expert opinions of 254 men of science who had affirmed that the Jews' method of slaughter was bound up with their concern for the welfare of the animal.[96]

This distinguished panel of experts from all over Europe found, like previous commissions, that the Jewish method was equal if not superior to all other forms of animal slaughter. The list of internationally recognized scientists that offered expert testimony bespeaks the importance of the issue. Nothing, thought the enemies of shehitah, so starkly separated Jews from Germans as this fundamental question of how each group treated animals. To the chagrin of the "abolitionists," scientific opinion again came out on the side of shehitah. Among them was the distinguished pathologist and Progressive Party politician, Rudolf Virchow, who responded to critics by praising Jewish religious custom, ethical enlightenment, and scientific cognition. The renowned scientist stated that "the form of [Jewish slaughtering] is based upon religious proscriptions that are intended to avoid unnecessary cruelty to the animal and to make for the complete removal of blood from the meat so that it is better for human consumption. . . . When the procedure is followed completely, as ordained, the aim is achieved with greater surety than with any other killing method."[97] Perhaps of greatest comfort for Jews who sought to make their case by turning to the Gentile medical and veterinary establishment was the declaration of Swiss professors Alfred Guillebeau and Ernst Hess. Commenting on the unanimity of responsible opinion, they observed that this "state of affairs says that *science has rendered its judgment in favor of shehitah*" [emphasis added].[98]

So vociferous was the agitation in Germany that it occasioned the single most important and exhaustive scientific defense of shehitah undertaken up until that point. In 1894, Russian Jewish physician Isaac Dembo published his German-language study, *The Jewish Method of Slaughter Compared with Other Methods from the Humanitarian, Hygienic, and Economic Point of View*. In 1891, Dembo had been invited by the steering committee of the Russian Societies for the Prevention of Cruelty to Animals to prepare a report on the different methods of slaughtering, to be read before a congress of the various chapters of the society in St. Petersburg in 1891. This Dembo did, but according to his own testimony, the heated discourse surrounding the practice of shehitah, especially in Germany and Switzerland, was such that it prompted him to spend a further four years studying the methods of slaughter throughout Europe.

Dembo's studies were undertaken according to the most exacting standards of modern scientific investigation. Characterized by close observation of the methods employed in European abattoirs, the use of control groups, and his own participation in slaughtering a variety of animals according to the numerous methods then used, Dembo's work remains the standard by which all comparative studies of slaughtering techniques must be measured.

It is significant that in the tripartite division of his investigation, Dembo commences by comparing shehitah with the other current methods of animal slaughter in order to test the relative "humanitarianism" of the various approaches. It must be borne in mind that for the shehitah abolitionists, it was the alleged absence of a humanitarian ethos that distinguished "cruel" Judaism from a "loving" Christianity, something for them that was most apparent in the area of animal slaughter.

By the late nineteenth century, a vast array of methods and devices had been employed by Christians to slaughter cattle. With the introduction of each new method there came claims that the latest technique was more humane that the one it was said to replace. These included: the use of a mallet to stun the animal; a poleax to render it unconscious; Bruneau's mask, which allowed for a bolt to be driven through the skull; Sigmund's mask, which had a revolver attached to it; the neck-stab; electrocution; and the introduction of narcotics to render the animal unconscious. That Judaism, by contrast, had never altered its technique was construed as a further indication of its stagnant character and primitive value system.

Having observed literally thousands of slayings, Dembo described all the new methods employed in European slaughterhouses in gruesome detail.[99] His huge scientific sample permitted him to answer the most pressing questions that animated the debate over shehitah. How long did it take animals to die by the respective methods? How much did they suffer? Which means were least cruel? What happened to each animal physiologically with each method of slaughter? Did the various methods have a decided impact on the quality of the meat?

Now, although Dembo was Jewish, and his defense of shehitah was cast on behalf of his co-religionists, he shied away from employing biblical ref-

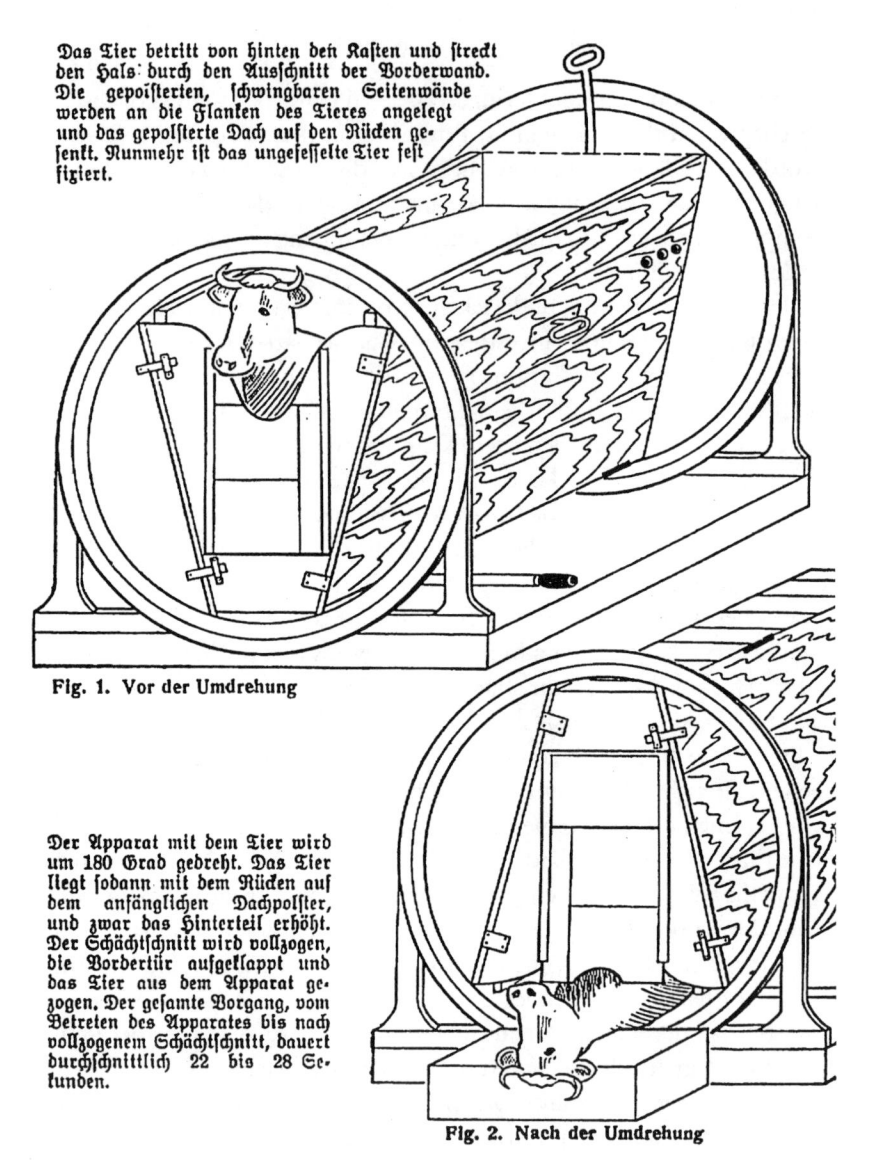

Das Tier betritt von hinten den Kasten und streckt den Hals durch den Ausschnitt der Vorderwand. Die gepolsterten, schwingbaren Seitenwände werden an die Flanken des Tieres angelegt und das gepolsterte Dach auf den Rücken gesenkt. Nunmehr ist das ungefesselte Tier fest fixiert.

**Fig. 1. Vor der Umdrehung**

Der Apparat mit dem Tier wird um 180 Grad gedreht. Das Tier liegt sodann mit dem Rücken auf dem anfänglichen Dachpolster, und zwar das Hinterteil erhöht. Der Schächtschnitt wird vollzogen, die Vordertür aufgeklappt und das Tier aus dem Apparat gezogen. Der gesamte Vorgang, vom Betreten des Apparates bis nach vollzogenem Schächtschnitt, dauert durchschnittlich 22 bis 28 Sekunden.

**Fig. 2. Nach der Umdrehung**

FIGURE 8. In response to accusations by animal rights groups that the Jewish method of slaughtering animals was cruel and should be outlawed, or at least modified to include stunning prior to death, German Jews mounted vigorous scientific defenses of the traditional practice. They also invented the contraption pictured here to minimize the animal's distress, whereby it was led calmly inside this half-barrel, spun around 180 degrees onto its back, and then slaughtered. The entire process, from the entrance of the animal into the apparatus until its slaughter, averaged a mere 22 to 28 seconds. Defenders of *shehitah* claimed repeatedly that the Jewish method was quicker and thus less cruel than Christian slaughtering. Source: Isak Unna, *Das Schächten vom Standpunkt der Religion und des Tierschutzes* (Berlin, 1931).

erences, citations from rabbinic literature, or religious arguments to rationalize Jewish slaughtering techniques. Rather, this is a highly technical, although passionate, work written in scientific language. It is a mark of the new apologetic possibilities offered by science and the particular demands made on Jews at the end of the nineteenth century that allowed for the production of such a text as this.

Dembo established that it took an animal killed by the Jewish method a mere three to five seconds to lose consciousness (8). With regard to non-Jewish slaughter techniques, this occurred at different times according to the chosen method, but it always exceeded five seconds. The question of the extent of the pain felt by the animal was central to the attack on shehitah. In a very matter-of-fact way and using the most technical of medical language, Dembo made his case for the relative painlessness of Jewish slaughtering:

> Moreover, the anatomical fact that in the Jewish method of slaughtering the pneumogastric nerve (n. vagus) is divided below the point where its sensory branches to the larynx are given off, that thus the sensory branches need not be divided at all, is a circumstance which of course goes far to lessen the pain of the animal. The student of the Jewish ritual law, when carefully reading the directions on this point, will find that the incision is allowed to be made lower but never higher than the level of the lower edge of the larynx. It is difficult to decide whether this rule has been laid down lest the knife be damaged by the cartilage of the larynx, or because the teachers of the religion already had a knowledge of the above-mentioned pneumogastric nerve. At any rate, it is a fact that those very sensitive nervous filaments are not severed by the knife in the Jewish method of slaughtering. (12)

In terms of the common Christian method of animal slaughter and one that was most vigorously pushed by animal protection societies, namely stunning, Dembo opined that "it is quite impossible to fell an ox in every case with a single blow" (17). Rather, from statistics he compiled based on observations at Swiss and German slaughterhouses, he calculated that "on average five to six blows are required to stun an ox completely. If we assume that the lifting of the hammer, the blow and the interval between one blow and the other, each occupy but one second, the animal's suffering must not last less than twelve seconds before it ceases to feel" (23).

As for the method known as Bruneau's mask, the whole procedure took up to forty seconds, and sometimes longer to complete (27). Dembo examined all the other methods and found that they prolonged and even intensified the animals' suffering. The charge of the callous disregard by Jews for the "feelings" of animals did not hold up under the light of medical scrutiny. As Dembo concluded, "On analysing all these symptoms with critical and experienced eyes, and on taking into account all the facts of physiology, surgery, and medicine relating to the subject, one is driven to the conclusion that, from the humanitarian standpoint, *the method of slaughtering with previous stunning cannot bear comparison with the Jewish method of slaughtering*" (24).

The second category of analysis employed by Dembo was that of "hygiene," concerned as he was to measure the relative quality of the meat garnered from the various killing processes. Considerable medical opinion held that kosher meat was rarely infected with tuberculosis, an explanation offered by physicians for why the disease seemed to strike Jews less frequently than it did non-Jews. Thus it was of paramount importance to Dembo to ascertain whether the hygienic quality of kosher meat was indeed superior to that of nonkosher.

According to Dembo, "It is obvious that the more blood there is left in the meat, the sooner the meat will become spoiled—this connection between the quantity of the blood and the preservation of the meat being an incontestable scientific axiom.... The Jewish method is the one which leaves the least blood in the body, since during the whole time of bleeding the nerve-centres regulating the flow of the blood in the vessels are not interfered with" (56). This was the exact opposite of most of the other methods then in vogue, almost all of which entailed causing an injury to the brain of the animal. Such violence led to paralysis of the vasomotor centers, which in turn prevented bleeding to the greatest extent possible.

In addition to scientific evidence, Dembo relied upon the expert lay opinion of Christian butchers, many of whom wrote to Dembo in support of his scientific enterprise. Their evidence provides surprising testimony to the influence of shehitah in certain German abattoir circles. Recognizing the link between the extent of bleeding at the time of slaughter and the potential for putrefaction, Carl Friedrich Hoffmann, a wholesale butcher at Berlin's central cattle market, testified, "I am myself not a Jew, but, as is well-known in Berlin, I have for the last fifteen years had just the same instrument used for killing as the Jewish '*shochet*' or slayer.... The flesh of cut animals keeps much longer than that of stunned." In 1893, another Berlin butcher, Hermann Kersten, responded to Dembo that for about fifteen years he had oxen killed for "non-Jewish consumption" according to the Jewish method because "1. An ox slaughtered by this method loses more blood, and the meat has a better appearance; [and] 2. The meat keeps in summer at least a day longer than that of oxen killed by stunning and afterwards bled." Similarly, in Cologne, a group of butchers co-signed a letter to Dembo in which they claimed that "the flesh of animals slaughtered according to Jewish ritual keeps from one to two days longer in summer than that of animals killed by any other method, in consequence of the more thorough draining-off of the blood."[100] Sixteen Christian butchers from Karlsruhe even used the word *shehitah* to describe the method of slaughter they personally employed (50–53)!

It is noteworthy that in his scientific and cultural quest, Dembo undertook unusual experiments to prove the scientific efficacy of shehitah, experiments that could only have been undertaken by a modern Jewish physician seeking to make the case for the defense of ancient ritual. Dembo slaughtered three rabbits (animals that are nonkosher), one according to the Jewish method of slaughter, a second via stunning, and a third with a combination of stunning and shehitah. The first rabbit lost 72 percent of its blood, while the latter two lost 29 percent and 46 percent, respectively (75). Dembo's aim was to establish the exsanguineous efficacy of shehitah and its attendant advantages. Only in the name of science and modern Jewish apologetics could we see the rationale for killing an inherently nonkosher animal according to ancient Jewish practice.

Dembo's final category of analysis was an economic one. The Jewish method of slaughter required less time and fewer slaughtermen. Moreover, Dembo demonstrated that the earlier onset of rigidity of kosher meat made it fit for consumption sooner than meat slaughtered by other means, the delay in decomposition of such meat being up to two or three days longer in summer. Finally, the lower content of blood and water in the meat of cut animals was of decided economic advantage to the buyer. Dembo calculated that a government that supplied an army of half a million men with the meat of animals that had been stunned prior to slaughter "would be cheated by its contractors to the extent of half a million marks per year (£25,000)." Again, Dembo's economic argument was predicated upon scientific experiment (96–99).

Ultimately, what must be borne in mind here is that Dembo's *The Jewish Method of Slaughter* is a Jewish text. On first glance, his presentation of seemingly dry scientific data and the detailed description of his experiments bear no relation to Jewish literature of the past. Its point of reference is modern science, and not the traditional, Jewish canon. Nevertheless, Dembo and other modern Jewish physicians were in the midst of creating a new kind of Jewish literature — a secular and scientific Jewish apologia.

## IN PRAISE OF JEWISH RITUAL

Isaac Dembo, a distinguished physician, is a classic example of the modern Jewish doctor who used medicine in order to defend Jewish ritual. To read Dembo's text is to go on an excursion across the terrain of contemporary medical disciplines such as animal and human physiology, pathology, biology, and bacteriology. The latest findings pertaining to brain and central nervous system research also assumed a prominent place in Dembo's study. It was, of course, only his medical training that provided him with the discursive and methodological arsenal to refute his opponents on their own terms. As for what prompted his study, Dembo made clear the role of antisemitism in the debate over shehitah. Perhaps somewhat naively, he noted that those who expressed their opposition to the Jewish method of slaughter in the 1850s and 1860s were sincere in their belief that shehitah was tantamount to animal torture. But when they were presented with scientific evidence to the contrary, they desisted and accepted that "the Jewish method was absolutely no more cruel than any other. However, during the last ten years, which have witnessed the growth of Antisemitism in Germany, those attacks have been of a quite different character." Dembo observed that "agitation against the Jewish method flashed up like lightning the very instant that any new apparatus for slaughtering loomed on the horizon, without the least trouble having been taken to test its effectiveness" (104).

Blind faith in technology, combined with implacable opposition to Jews, caused the animal protection societies to seek to impose modern, "scientific" methods on what were considered antiquated and barbaric Jewish rituals.[101] Seeking to root out Jewish "primitiveness," the antisemites stopped at nothing to make their case against Jews, even totally misrepresenting distinguished scientists such as Emil Du Bois-Reymond. In 1893, through its official organ, the Berlin Society for the Protection of Animals declared that "the profound scientific researches of the eminent physiologist, Professor Du Bois-Reymond, have thoroughly established the extremely important fact that the fear and suffering endured by an animal killed in the Jewish manner before and during the slaughtering has such a deteriorating effect on its flesh as to make it unfit for human consumption." Dembo, who was familiar with Du Bois-Reymond, was so shocked that he wrote to the German physiologist for clarification and received the following reply: "In accordance with your request, I hereby declare . . . that the above statements, in so far as they concern me, have not the slightest foundation in truth. I have never undertaken such researches as are above ascribed to me, and I further regard them as absurd, and their so-called result as false" (107–108).

Dembo was quite certain that the outrageous tactics of the opponents of shehitah would backfire. In fact, he was convinced by the evidence he saw in European slaughterhouses that the Jewish method had already been widely adopted and might even spread further thanks to government legislation. And this because shehitah, "instead of being rejected and suppressed shall have incontestably established before the tribunal of science its full, its exclusive, right to existence" (111).

It is an irony that the defense of shehitah was taken up by all streams among German Jews, despite the fact that perhaps the majority no longer kept kosher. Why did they, for whom kashrut was something only their parents or grandparents adhered to, become so actively involved in the debate? There are three principal reasons. First, the timing of the attack and the content of the oppositional discourse indicates that the anti-shehitah campaign was not merely about animal slaughter, but was part of the larger antisemitic movement that had snowballed in the late nineteenth century.[102] The leader of the anti-shehitah forces, royal court veterinarian Sondermann, pronounced in 1879, "And now to put a quick and certain end to shehitah, we wish to propose that no Christian be permitted to consume the meat of animals that have been killed by means of shehitah and that no Christian butcher be permitted to slaughter in this way, [for] *shehitah* is an evil custom from antiquity."[103] The Swiss newspaper from Bern, the *Bund,* was brutally honest about its anti-Jewish stance when in 1884 it wrote:

> Our paper is antisemitic. . . . Whether shehitah is really a bit more or a bit less cruel to animals than other methods of slaughter is immaterial to us. For us the crucial point of the whole question is whether or not a special place should be cleared away for the Jews [in the state] because of their religion. . . . It is a fundamental principle of every civilized state that within its borders religious freedom be permitted to religious communities only in so far as the latter, through the centuries, has made advances for the good of civilization. . . . Should a religious minority whose ceremonies conflict with the ethics of the vast majority be permitted? There exists in this civilized land a race from the desert who still practices ancient and barbaric customs. It must either give them up or be expelled.[104]

In 1911, the debate over shehitah was brought directly to the attention of the medical profession when W. Back, editor of the *Medical Bulletin,* the official organ of the Union for the Protection of the Economic Interests of German Physicians, an organization with approximately 24,000 members, published an article entitled "*Shehitah* or Stunning?" Explaining why such an article would find its way into this particular medical journal, the author declared that "German physicians were honor-bound to take a stand in the slaughtering-question . . . and not only leave it as a matter for our veterinarian colleagues." According to Back's sternest critic, the physician and rabbi Eduard Biberfeld, the decision to publish an anti-shehitah article in a magazine for physicians was intended to influence public opinion, something that could best be achieved through disseminating such propaganda in a widely circulated, prestigious journal. Moreover, recent changes in German insurance law and the findings of a parliamentary commission to root out medical quackery meant that German medicine "had nothing to lose and everything to gain" by attacking the Jews and possibly making political capital out of such a campaign. As Back himself admitted, German doctors had a unique role to play in the struggle against Jewish influence in German society.[105]

Above all, it was economic competition that drove the animus of Back's organization. Its members stood first and foremost to accrue personal and group advantage by being at the forefront of the antisemitic assault on German Jewry. Taking a decisive stance would put them in league with powerful political and social forces who would presumably return the favor by parliamentary lobbying for legislation that in some way or another would redound to the advantage of German physicians. A further point has to do with the central social and cultural role played by physicians in Germany. Their prestige and authority meant that the appearance of an antisemitic diatribe in one of their major medical publications, the *Medical Bulletin,* carried great weight and was indicative of the depth of antisemitism among important sections of the German medical establishment.

As was the case in the Middle Ages, toward the end of the nineteenth century Jews across Central and Eastern Europe were once again being accused of murdering Christian children in order to use their blood ritually. Antisemites linked this alleged ritual to the discourse about the practice and mode of Jewish animal slaughter, identifying shehitah as yet another bloodthirsty Jewish practice, in keeping with the Jews' inherently cruel tendencies. The charge went: if they could kill innocent children then certainly the Jews would have little compassion for animals.[106] According to Rabbi Eduard Biberfeld, "Tales of ritual murder and the struggle against shehitah are worthy sisters, adorning the main plank of the antisemites' program."[107]

In summer 1891 the body of a five-year-old Christian boy, Johann Hegmann, who had had his throat slit was discovered in the largely Catholic town of Xanten. The antisemitic uproar that followed led to the arrest of the local Jewish butcher, Adolf Buschhoff.[108] Although he was later released for lack of evidence, the fact that antisemitic forces focused their attention on the Jewish butcher illustrates the intimate connection in the public mind between Jewish animal slaughter and imagined Jewish cruelty and even murderousness.[109]

In fact, one of the Jewish opponents of shehitah, Rabbi Jakob Stern, made this a theme of his abolitionist campaign. In his misguided interpretation of the causes of the 1883 Tisza-Eszlàr affair in Hungary, wherein a Jew was charged with having ritually murdered a Christian boy, Stern suggested that the whole situation "would never have taken place had the Jews long ago abolished *shehitah*."[110] Years later, this explanation still proved attractive for other Jewish opponents of shehitah. While at a May 1908 meeting of Baden-Baden's Society for the Protection of Animals, the son of a rabbi, Edgar Loewi, represented the position of radical Reform Jews when he told the gathering that "for me it is an established fact that the foolish old wives' tale of ritual murder that refuses to die has, for centuries, filled the heads of the uneducated, brutal, and persecutory masses. Peaceable, industrious, and upright people have been killed by the thousands, *and the reason for it is to be found in shehitah*" [emphasis added].[111]

Of course, the group most directly affected by the anti-shehitah campaign was Orthodox Jewry. In response to general developments, several Orthodox rabbis even joined animal protection societies to both agitate from within for moderation and, above all, to show that Judaism was completely at one with the ethical stance these organizations took. In addition, they also organized petitions and called upon zoologists, physiologists, and veterinarians, to attest to their claim that shehitah was the most humane way of killing an animal.[112]

In their defensive strategy, Orthodox and Reform Jews differed in the degree to which they placed their faith in science as evidence for the case they were making. The Orthodox were skeptical of too great a reliance on science for proof of the efficaciousness of shehitah. In their opinion, even if science were now on their side, future scientific findings might run counter to previous claims and be used to undermine the validity of shehitah. It is for this reason that while they were prepared to employ the findings of science and make use of science's celebrated figures, such as Rudolf Virchow, the Orthodox were most content to turn to explanations that had to do with faith, for the Law of Moses was eternal and not subject to paradigm shifts.[113] So in traditional Jewish fashion, science and faith were compatible and could even be jointly used to fight the good fight, but faith and God's law counted for more among the Orthodox than did scientific observation.

Haunted by renewed, medieval accusations and fearful of the growing antisemitic movement, the entire German Jewish community, sensing it was under siege, banded together as Reform Jews lined up alongside the Orthodox in a pact of mutual self-defense.[114] But the campaign had still wider ramifications, ones that went beyond the immediate and obvious interests of the Jewish community. The hundreds of Gentile scientists who provided expert testimony on behalf of shehitah were also fighting a larger political battle, for most of them were either apolitical or maintained liberal political sentiments. This pitted them against the antisemitic and fundamentally anti-democratic political parties of the far Right, for it was they who joined up with the animal protection societies in the campaign to abolish shehitah. Thus, much was at stake for Jew and non-Jew alike, because the Jewish Question in Germany was always a barometer of more general, political winds.

In Germany, expert testimony in favor of Jewish ritual slaughter was gathered on at least five separate occasions, in 1885, 1894, 1902, 1908, and 1927–1929.[115] The 1908 report, one of the most comprehensive ever undertaken, was composed of 457 testimonials from university scientists, directors of veterinary colleges, government and slaughterhouse veterinarians, butchers, and meat inspectors. A Dr. Rosenthal, professor at the University of Erlangen, wrote for the majority when he stated that "the so-called [Jewish] cut (*Schächtschnitt*) is one of the best means of killing an animal, sparing it needless cruelty, and bringing about its loss of consciousness as quickly as possible. *My testimony has nothing to do with the question of religion or ritual. It is supported only by physiology*" [emphasis added].[116] This is precisely the grounds upon which German Jewry sought to make its case. An appeal to science rather than to goodwill and tolerance seemed to make the most sense in this environment.

## BRIT MILAH

As was the case with the dietary laws and shehitah, ritual circumcision was the subject of a wide-ranging debate in nineteenth-century Germany.[117] Circumcision had been long regarded as the most distinctive and separatist of all Jewish rituals, and the discourse surrounding it went to the heart of the "willingness" of the Jews to fully participate in the "act" of being German. The ritual was interpreted as a signal of the Jews' refusal to rid themselves of their differences, imprinting on their own male bodies, as an aboriginal would his tribal markings, an ineradicable expression of national identity. For some, it was circumcision itself that made the Jew. In the seventeenth century, the Jewish philosopher Baruch Spinoza declared that "the sign of circumcision is, as I think, so important, that I could persuade myself that it alone would preserve the nation forever."[118] For figures of the German Enlightenment such as Wilhelm and Alexander von Humboldt, circumcision was one of those Jewish practices that "unnecessarily" separated Jews from the rest of society. The brothers were of the opinion that circumcision should be either significantly reformed or abandoned altogether. Expressed at the time of the debates over Jewish emancipation in the eighteenth century, the von Humboldts' suggestion was designed to help foster the assimilation of the Jews, and thus promote the cause of their emancipation.[119] In 1831, Heinrich Paulus, professor of Oriental languages and theology at the University of Heidelberg, declared that for Jews to merge fully with Christians they had to abrogate circumcision, for unlike the universal act of baptism, it served only to ensure their isolation and distinct national identity.[120] At the fin-de-siècle, the opinion that circumcision was the key to Jewish separatism and national identity was highlighted in one of the most important anthropological surveys of the Jewish people to appear in the nineteenth century, Richard Andree's *Ethnography of the Jews*. According to the author, "Circumcision was the pride of the Hebrews and a sign of their covenant and their separateness from other, non-circumcised peoples, and that upon which their nationality was conditioned."[121] Further, Andree remarked that the consequence of circumcision is that it breeds in the circumcised an "arrogant and haughty" attitude toward the uncircumcised.

Given that circumcision among German Gentiles was (and still is) extremely rare, Andree's remark went beyond the mere historical or anthropological to constitute a negative commentary on what he imagined were the hostile Jewish perceptions of Germans. In response to such claims, Jewish physicians downplayed the religious and nationalistic aspect of the ceremony and instead emphasized its medically beneficial and thus universalistic qualities, for there was nothing particularistic about the desire for good health. By stressing the hygienic advantages of circumcision, German Jews could offer Germans the benefit of millennial medical wisdom.[122]

The offer to share with large numbers of Germans the alleged pathological advantages of circumcision (and other Jewish rituals) first took place in 1911, at the International Hygiene Exhibition in Dresden. Attracting well over a quarter million visitors, the exhibit, and all those that followed until the rise of the Nazis, was akin to a modern world's fair, but specifically focused on those positive health and social habits that served to promote good health among the world's different nations and races. The Jews manned their own pavilion, and in explaining their customs and life cycle events, the exhibitors considered their expository performance an act of generosity rather than a display of haughtiness.[123]

In addition to having been the subject of historical, anthropological, and theological speculation, circumcision came under legal scrutiny, as it became highly regulated over the course of the nineteenth century. While this was reflective of the general trend of the German state to enforce ever more control over public health, the desire to assert authority over the Jewish body had, as we saw with the burial controversy, an established precedent. Various state governments and local authorities, often in conjunction with interested Jewish parties such as physicians and advocates of religious reform, passed legislation and decrees in their attempts to control Jews, seeking to sanitize in both surgical and aesthetic terms the procedure and make it conform as best as possible to German sensibilities. For example, in 1799, the Prussian Oberkollegium sponsored the preparation of an expert report on the dangers of circumcision and how they could be avoided. The result was that in 1819, Prussia promoted the practice of having a physician attend all circumcisions. This was expanded upon in 1824 when it was decreed that the *mohel* had to pass an examination to prove his medical proficiency in treating the wound. By 1830, the Jews of the Rhineland had reached an agreement with the state's health officers that only their officially recognized mohelim would be allowed to practice. Nevertheless, a physician still had to be in attendance, and by 1843, noncompliance resulted in a monetary fine of between 5 and 20 taler for the boy's father, and from 10 to 50 taler for the mohel. In 1852, the Jewish community of Hamburg decreed officially sanctioned rules and instructions for mohelim, which were later supplemented at a general session of the mohelim commission of 1900. In 1885 the government of the district of Wiesbaden offered instruction for mohelim, and finally, by 1887 in Vienna, only physicians were permitted to perform circumcisions.[124]

During the 1840s, when Reform Jews held conferences to discuss issues of religious modification, debates about the nature and practice of circumcision also emerged.[125] For a minority, circumcision was a bloody ritual, more fitting for what were deemed savage tribes than for middle-class German Jews. Still others questioned whether circumcision was itself an absolute requirement as a sign and marker of Jewish identity. In 1843, the radical reformer Samuel Holdheim maintained that the ritual was no longer binding on Jews and that the sign of the covenant was to be symbolic rather than real. This view was soundly rejected by the overwhelming majority of German Jews. But all these were theological, not scientific arguments, and the majority of Jews were simply not prepared to argue over the religious nature of brit milah. As a Jewish ceremony it was a sanctified rite of initiation to be practiced in perpetuity.

Still, brit milah was under assault and needed defending. To this end, Jewish communities early on acted in consultation with state authorities and Jewish physicians to transform and modernize circumcision by focusing on the medical aspects of the ceremony. As early as the decree of 1819, wherein the Jews agreed to permit a physician to attend every brit milah, a creeping concession to modernity was countenanced. The ceremony became more of a public performance and was conducted under the "impartial" and "scientific" eye of the modern physician. To satisfy the demands of German society, Jews sought to accommodate the ancient ceremony to the rigors of modern science. They set out to prove that the operation, without abandoning its basic elements, still met the surgical standards set by modern medicine.

In 1844, a Jewish physician and staunch advocate of ritual circumcision from Berlin, Joseph Bergson, responded to the circumcision abolitionists by promoting medical reforms to make the procedure safer. For Bergson, circumcision served a religious, symbolic, medical, political, mythological, and, even quite possibly, a military purpose.[126] In his view, the sheer antiquity of brit milah, plus its centrality in the cultural life of the nation, justified its eternal practice. But to defend brit milah from attack, Bergson proposed the introduction of modifications into the ceremony.

Because in matters of public health it was "the duty of the state to protect all its subjects, irrespective of religion and class," Bergson recommended that circumcision come under tighter regulation. Precisely because of its "bloody character," he wanted to see it more closely observed by both physicians and state medical authorities. Concerned about the possible abuses that could come from state intervention in religious affairs, Bergson suggested that the state tread lightly, embarking with the "greatest possible forbearance" on a "suitable" program of education and "enlightenment" in order to promote the "physical well-being" of the child—an advantage to be later accrued by the state itself.[127]

Among the technical changes Bergson advocated were the abolition of *periah* by the traditional method, that is, the peeling back of the entire foreskin and splitting it with a razor sharp fingernail in order to expose the glans, and *metsitsah,* the sucking of the wound by the mohel to draw out the blood. Claiming that neither had biblical sanction, Bergson noted that the former procedure had long been rejected by "rational and . . . modern

2

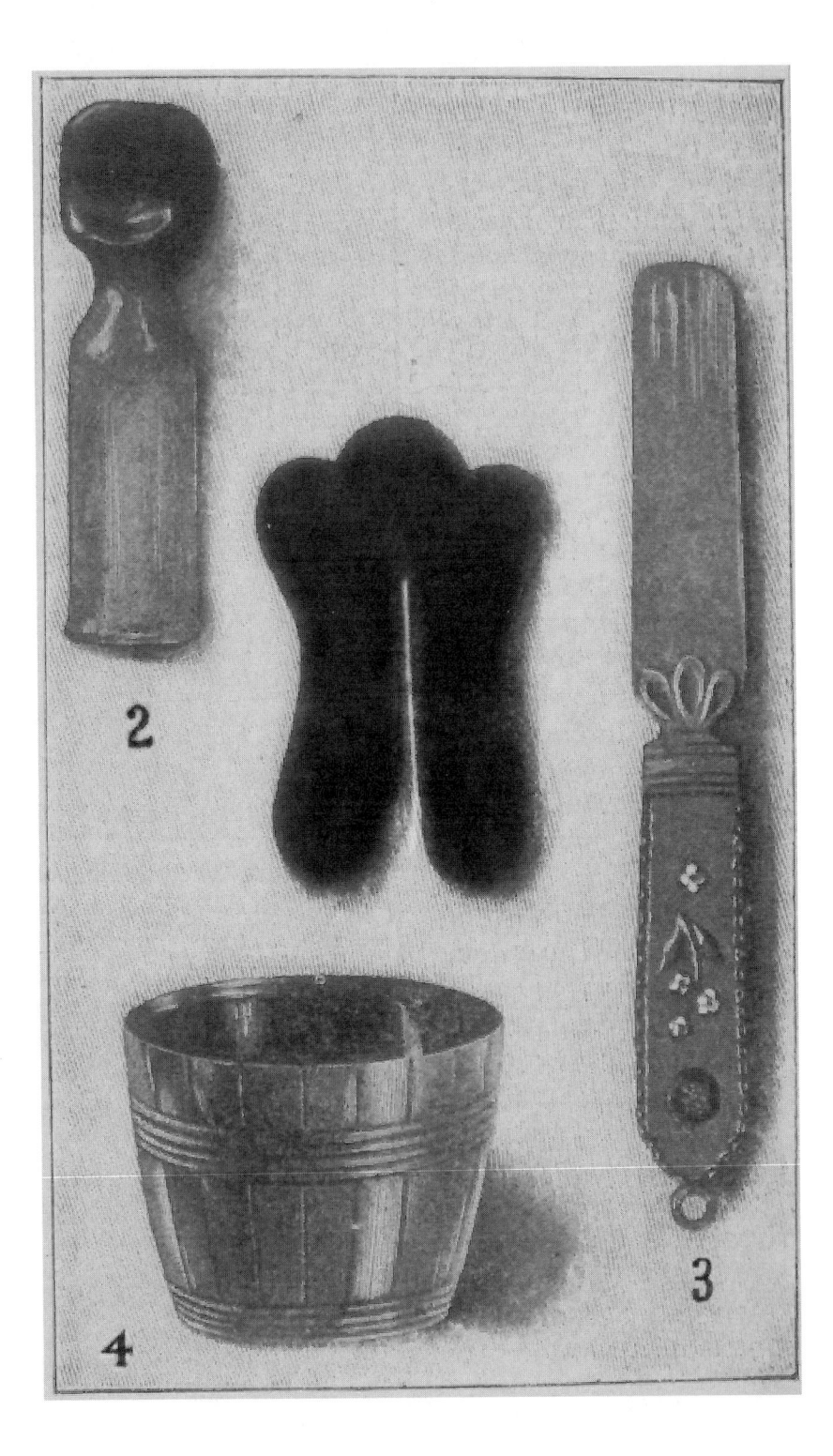

3

4

surgery, a barbaric remnant from medieval field-surgery." In its stead, he recommended the use of recently invented scissors and other surgical implements, specifically designed for the task, and the application of the latest salves, balms, and elasticized bandages.[128] Another Jewish physician who likewise sought to reform brit milah, D. Salomon, also recommended a postoperative surgical procedure that involved stitching the wound, a procedure that was never accepted in the Jewish world but was nevertheless endorsed by Bergson.[129] According to Bergson, metsitsah played no prophylactic role whatsoever, and only increased the chances of transmitting a host of infectious diseases, including syphilis. It had to go entirely.[130]

In addition to changes in surgical procedure, Bergson wanted mohelim to receive fundamental instruction in anatomy and surgery, claiming that it was "little wonder that in recent times the opinion had been expressed that the operation should be taken out of the hands of mohelim and entrusted to qualified doctors." He lamented the fact that in antiquity, circumcision among Israelites had been performed by physicians, whereas it was now performed by the unqualified![131] This is reminiscent of the call by *maskilic* physicians in the eighteenth century to remove the control over what Jews did with their own bodies and hand it over to duly certified professionals. It also recalls a common *Haskalah* refrain, echoed by nineteenth-century Jewish social critics, that idealized and glorified the health care culture of biblical Israel while at the same time emphasizing the extent to which modern Jews seemed to have deviated from that ideal.

With advances in medical knowledge, criticism and advocacy of circumcision took on a more scientific tone by the late nineteenth century. The medical profession at this time expressed two diametrically opposed views of circumcision: one for, and one against. As for the negative assessment, Jews had been long accused of hypersexuality and of being chronic practitioners of what a liberal French cleric, the Abbé Grégoire, called, the *libertinage solitaire*.[132] Similarly, Jews had long been linked to the spread of syphilis. Indeed as early as the fifteenth century, the Genovese ambassador

---

FIGURE 9. Circumcision implements from the early twentieth century. The item in the center of the frame is the shield; to its right is the knife. The cup is for the performance of metsitsah, the sucking of the wound. This act came in for considerable criticism at the end of the nineteenth century as being unhygienic and morally dubious. In response, physicians invented a special glass tube (labeled here as number 2) for metsitsah that was widely used in Germany. Source: *The Jewish Encyclopedia* (New York, 1903).

to Charles VIII called it the "Peste of the Marranos." At the close of the nineteenth century, because of their association with skin diseases, antisemitic claims of their immorality, and the fact that Jews predominated in the nascent medical specialty of dermatology, Jews played a prominent role in the medical literature on venereal disease, and medical opponents of circumcision rarely failed to draw a causative link between alleged Jewish concupiscence and sexually transmitted diseases and the rite of circumcision. One German opponent of circumcision, a physician from Halle, even claimed that the majority of patients he treated for gonorrhea were Jewish.[133]

The opposite medical assessment was that Jews were to a large extent protected from a variety of diseases precisely because they were circumcised.[134] Stressing the prophylactic quality of circumcision, physician-advocates of the procedure regarded it as a mode of prevention against sexual malfunction and deviance, sexually transmitted diseases, and what some physicians even called "sexual neurasthenia."[135] Proponents also saw it as a means to prevent childhood bed-wetting, and prolapse of the rectum, hernia, and hydrocele, caused by overexertion of the abdominal muscles in order to overcome impediments to urination caused by inflammation of the prepuce.[136] One Zionist physician, Felix Theilhaber, held circumcision responsible for the lower incidence of uterine cancer among Jewish women.[137]

Much like people today who display a seemingly insatiable appetite for medical news, the Jewish public at the turn of the century likewise sought out the latest information about medical breakthroughs, especially when they pertained to Jewish pathologies. In a lecture to a Breslau synagogue in 1902, Jewish physician Carl Alexander told his audience that there were several diseases that could be prevented by circumcision, for example, phimosis, a constriction of the penis opening, which was congenital in 12 percent of boys, and elephantiasis, a chronic enlargement of cutaneous and subcutaneous tissue, especially of the legs and scrotum. Alexander also believed circumcision helped stem the tide of diabetes.[138] He and other Jewish advocates also stressed the humanitarian aspect of performing circumcision on newborn males because at that tender age, there would be no memory of either the event or the discomfort.[139]

Another physician noted that just as the dietary laws had a "hygienic basis" in addition to a religious one, circumcision was to be interpreted similarly. Circumcision and the attendant admonition of God to "be fruitful and multiply," he argued, was a holy prescription that for the Jewish people "led to a curative function." Fulfilling both requirements was "a sure protection against the inclination to onanism."[140] Many Jewish physicians concurred that circumcision lessened if not eliminated entirely the instinct to masturbate—an act, they suggested, that was the end result of a buildup of irritating secretions under the foreskin.[141] The subtext of this observation was that because they were uncircumcised, it was Christians rather than Jews who challenged nineteenth-century bourgeois morality, which condemned masturbation as a vice that in addition to constituting a complete "loss of control" was "opposed to all that was manly and virile."[142] Here could Jewish doctors turn the tables on those who had long accused Jews of unbridled passion and predatory, deviant sexual behavior.

Critics of ritual circumcision were particularly hostile to the act of metsitsah, sucking the wound. For many Jews, primarily those who had joined the German middle class and had come to share the culture and aesthetic sensibilities of that group, metsitsah appeared to be an atavistic, sexually deviant act.[143] Part of the traditional circumcision ceremony, the practice of metsitsah was widely condemned throughout the nineteenth century by medical and lay authorities, Jews and Gentiles alike. Charging that the practice promoted the spread of a host of sexual and infectious diseases, the arguments made against the practice were not confined to Western Europe but made their way east as well. A commission established in St. Petersburg in 1891 composed of physicians and "specialists in Jewish ritual" recommended that in the name of hygiene, metsitsah and the "tearing off of the *lamina interna* by hand" (periah) be abolished.[144] A German Jewish physician named Bamberger also shared some of the more common misgivings about the procedure, such as the fear that syphilis or tuberculosis could be spread from child to mohel or vice versa. In a comprehensive study of brit milah Bamberger published in 1912, he advocated the use of a glass apparatus to suck the wound, citing in particular the device designed by a Professor Pettenkofer of Munich at the urging of Rabbi Michael Cahn of Fulda.[145] What Bamberger sought to impress upon his readers was that science and religion were not only compatible in theoretical terms, but that religion could be the mother to science's invention. Working together, they were capable of tackling the problems confronting the modern Jew, arriving at creative solutions that permitted ancient tradition to be adhered to.

Technical innovation was not only used to modify tradition and reconstruct ancient rites in order to harmonize them with modernity; scientific evidence could even be employed creatively to defend all aspects of brit milah, including the most derided. In 1913, Emanuel Rosenbaum, a German Jewish physician practicing in Paris, published a thorough scientific defense of metsitsah. Drawing copiously upon classical Jewish sources, he supplemented these with evidence from contemporary medical science to endorse the prophylactic nature of the act.

In defending metsitsah Rosenbaum made two principal points. The first was the hypocrisy inherent in the campaign against the practice, in that double standards of hygiene were employed to make unrealistic demands upon Jews. The goal in the "rational treatment" of a wound, according to Rosenbaum, is to stave off infection by creating an "aseptic" environment. But even in a hospital setting, the attainment of asepsis "in the surgical sense of the word is an absolute impossibility."[146] Why, he demanded to know, were Jews required to observe standards of hygiene in domestic environments that were unattainable even in a hospital? Rosenbaum's other method of supporting metsitsah was to use expert testimony on the treatment of snakebites. International authorities were quoted, all of whom testified that standard medical procedure in the case of such an injury entailed sucking poison from the wound. From this, Rosenbaum extrapolated that metsitsah was not only harmless, but efficacious.[147]

Rosenbaum directly tackled the issue of the transmissibility of syphilis and tuberculosis through metsitsah, claiming that not one case had been reported in the medical literature of contagion having been spread in this way. At any rate, the mohel's use of alcohol — "one of the most outstanding disinfectants" — prior to performing metsitsah ensured an antiseptic oral environment. And again highlighting double standards, Rosenbaum asked rhetorically why restaurateurs and hoteliers were not compelled to disinfect cutlery, crockery, and glassware in carbolic acid or Lysol after use by their customers if the threat of orally transmitted infection were so great and so roundly acknowledged.[148] The fact that they were not required to do so only confirmed his sense that the attack on metsitsah was biased.

Not only did the ceremony of brit milah require defending, but the mohel had long been an object of scorn. The mohel, who had no medical training, was clearly seen as inappropriate. Berlin Jewry had required a physician to attend each brit milah since the early part of the nineteenth century, and various reforms had been instituted throughout the course of the century in order to "medicalize" the procedure.[149] Although Bamberger defended the mohel, who was attacked most often because of his inadequate surgical training and because of the perception that his personal hygiene constituted a threat to the infant, he did note that rabbis were concerned about the surgical qualification and dexterity of the mohel, disqualifying from service anyone who suffered from "shortsightedness, nervous disorders, shaking of the hands, and internal diseases." Indicating that a sea change had taken place in the sensibilities of German Jews, Bamberger observed that "today, here and there, the religious character [of circumcision] has been stripped away and it is regarded as a medical operation."[150] To this end, and in response to various accusations concerning the hygiene of the mohel himself, Bamberger offered the following inventory:

> Before the [*mohel*] performs the act, he must thoroughly disinfect his hands. Today's *mohelim* wash their hands and in this same warm water they soap themselves up with carbolic acid or Lysol and use a brush, especially around the nails. The same happens to the instruments which are boiled just before their use. These are: 1. a double-bladed knife, 8–10 cm long; 2. a metal clamp and forceps; 3. a common pair of tweezers to fasten the area around the wound; 4. 2–3 bolted tweezers to squeeze the bleeding; 5. different bandages, plasters, and swabs — all sterilized; 6. a scissors and a surgical sewing needle; 7. a glass tube for the metsitsah. In Hamburg the doctors have put together a 'sterile first-aid kit for circumcision.' Also the instruments, which are afixed inside a utensil for boiling, are sterilized at the scene of every circumcision.[151]

Here there is no God, no Abraham, no Covenant. This stark and clinical description of the mohel's instruments was designed to construct a clean counterimage of the Jews. Here, in Judaism's most elemental rite of passage, one long derided for its supposed savagery and uncleanliness, Bamberger sought to demonstrate the antiseptic nature of brit milah as it was performed in contemporary Germany. Although the mohel was not a physician, let alone a trained surgeon, every precaution had been taken to ensure that he upheld the most stringent rules of modern medical hygiene. As much as it could be, the ceremony had thus been "de-orientalized," indeed Germanized, tailored to conform to German, not traditional Jewish notions of cleanliness.[152]

One of the most important claims made about circumcision by its opponents in the medical world was that it was an unnecessary procedure, one that "deformed" a perfect organ, a view expressed, for example, by Paul Ascherson, professor of medicine at the University of Berlin.[153] In stark contrast, a Jewish physician, S. N. Kutna, declared circumcision to be an act of bringing about "bodily perfection," the foreskin being, "in a biblical sense, a defect."[154] Jewish countercharges notwithstanding, the accusation of their bodily deformity goes to the issue of how Jews fit into the aesthetic of human physicality in Wilhelmine Germany. Antisemites interpreted cir-

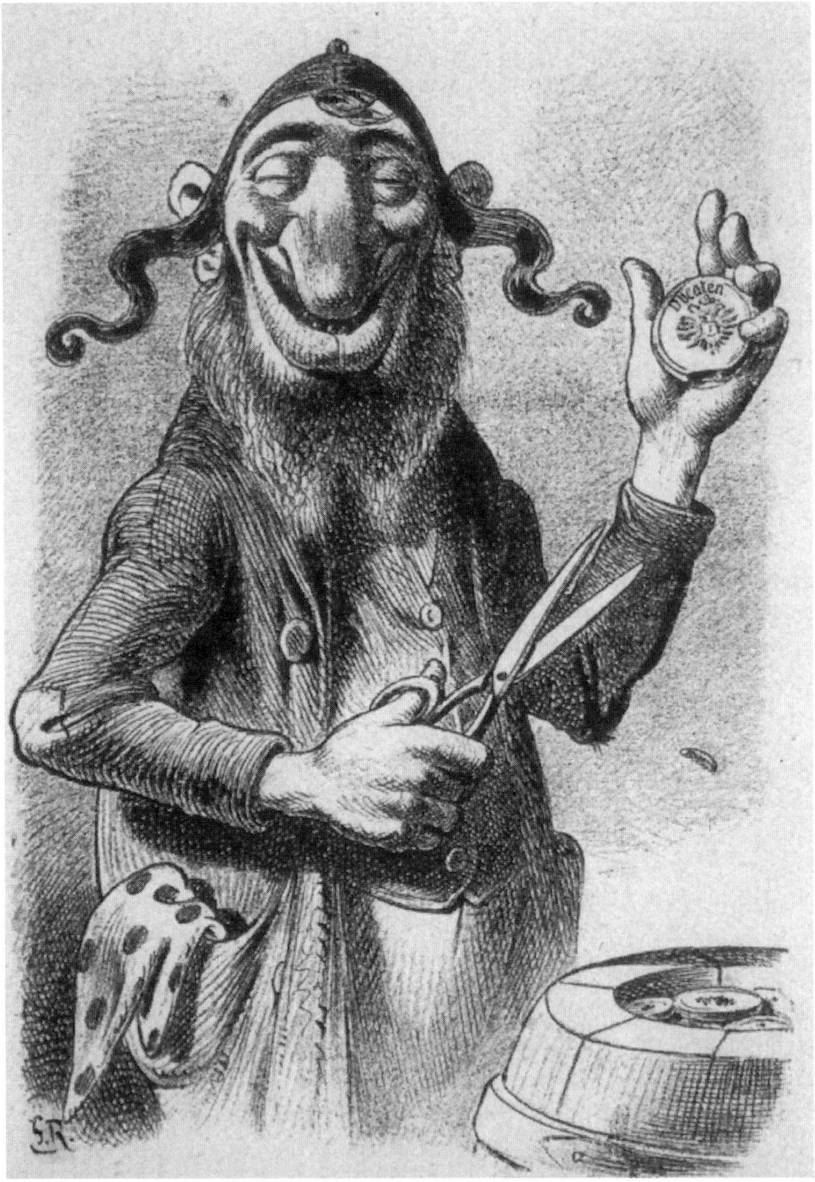

FIGURE 10. Entitled "The Circumcision," this antisemitic caricature appeared in the Viennese magazine *Kikeriki* in 1912. The *mohel* is represented as dirty, Orthodox, and avaricious as he proudly holds up a ducat that he has just clipped. The caption (not shown) reads: "Circumcision leads to profit — that's why it is in common use among the Jews." The word used for *profit* is *Vortheil*, which can also mean "advantage." The play on this word can also be a reference to the pathological advantages that Jewish physicians at the time claimed for those who had been circumcised. Source: Eduard Fuchs, *Die Juden in der Karikatur: Ein Beitrag zur Kulturgeschichte* (Munich, 1921).

cumcision in political and nationalistic terms. For them, a deliberately misshapen body, such as one that had been circumcised, was an imperfect body, and an imperfect body was, by definition, inadmissible into the body politic of the nation. For example, the 1894 statutes of the fiercely antisemitic organization, the Deutschbund, claimed that "the Jew cannot belong to the Deutschbund, nor become eligible by baptism, because his circumcision harbours his nature."[155] In this radical assessment, circumcision constituted a permanent taint that prevented the integration of Jews into German society.

For many, the separatist rite of brit milah distinguished Jews from Germans in the most tangible way, permanently impressing upon Jews a mark of national otherness. Thus circumcision was akin to the notion of race, in that for antisemites it too was indelible. The Jew, because he was circumcised, would forever remain "physically" Jewish, even if he had converted to Christianity.

It was not only brit milah but the entire array of Jewish customs and ritualistic behavior that contributed to a sense that the Jews were essentially different from the Germans. Even those Germans who were well disposed to the integration of Jews into German society were quite convinced that the social product of the performance of Judaism's most important rites was Jewish separatism.

In response, Jewish physicians in modern Germany enlisted the help of medicine to answer crises in and challenges to Judaism and Jewish culture itself. Sometimes, for example, in the case of the methods of animal slaughter, the challenge was driven by blatant antisemitism. On other occasions, such as with the discussions of the ritual bath or the dietary laws, the agitation for reform could come from within as well as from without. Whatever the case, the challenges were generally the product of the Jewish encounter with the modern, secular world. And, in what is a wonderfully intricate paradox, German Jews were able to use one of the defining characteristics of the modern age — science — to reinforce their Jewish identities, justify their ancient traditions, and help them navigate their way through the turbulent waters of modernity.

CHAPTER 7

# BEFORE THE STORM
## JEWISH DOCTORS IN THE KAISERREICH AND WEIMAR REPUBLIC

At the close of the nineteenth century, coterminous with the antisemitic claims and counterclaims about the Jews' body and the influences of Jewish ritual on it, attacks and polemics against the Jewish doctor were revived in Germany. Resuscitating many of the identical claims to those of the early modern period, the new ones added novel, modern twists but retained a pre-modern quality that is striking. One of the elements that distinguish the older campaign from the modern one is that in the sixteenth and seventeenth centuries, the Jewish doctor was vilified as a medical outsider. He was denounced for his charlatanism and his reliance on practical experimentation. In other words, he was accused of not being grounded in theory because he lacked a university education.

By the end of the nineteenth century, that situation had changed completely. University trained, and no longer professional outsiders, Jewish physicians were targeted precisely because of their increasing and formal presence within German medicine.[1] And that presence was indeed palpable. At the end of the eighteenth and turn of the nineteenth century, Jews constituted approximately 2 percent of Germany's doctors.[2] But by the turn of the twentieth century, Jews, who composed just over 1 percent of the total population, now made up 16 percent of all physicians in Germany. So fundamental had medicine become to the social structure and thus self-perception of German Jewry that nearly one half of all Jews attending universities in 1900 were there to study medicine.[3]

More specifically, these figures represent only native-born German Jews. Because of quotas restricting the entrance of Jews into Russian universities, there was, after the turn of the century, a large influx of Eastern European Jews into German institutions of higher education.[4] At the end of the nineteenth century, over 600 Russian Jews were studying in Germany, and the most popular area of study among them was medicine. To take but one example, by 1911, foreign Jews outnumbered German Jews in the medical school at the University of Königsberg. Overall, while foreign Jews were a mere 7 percent of all Jewish university students in 1891–1892, that figure had skyrocketed to 56 percent by 1911–1912.[5]

Furthermore, Jews, both native and foreign-born showed a definite preference for the type of universities they chose to attend. These tended to be the larger universities in bigger cities. Some were located in the eastern regions of Germany, making trips home to Eastern Europe somewhat easier.[6] Other reasons Jews tended to eschew attending smaller schools ranged from the Christian character of many of them to the desire of Jews to live in more cosmopolitan urban centers. There they could draw on the resources and largesse of local Jewish communities, and for Eastern European Jews the presence of Russian Jewish immigrants in big cities ensured familiarity born of cultural and linguistic affinity. Consequently, the preferred schools of both German and foreign Jews were the universities of Berlin, Frankfurt, Breslau, Heidelberg, and Baden. Although the latter two were located in small towns, they were in the liberal state of Baden, where the universities had since the early nineteenth century displayed a more welcoming attitude toward Jewish students.[7]

The situation that existed in Germany was basically replicated in Austria, but with even more pronounced characteristics. By 1910, approximately 90 percent of all Austrian Jews lived in Vienna. The imperial capital was home to 175,318 Jews, who constituted 8.6 percent of the total city population. By contrast, Berlin's 144,043 Jews were 4.3 percent of the Reich's capital.[8] Generally less affluent than their German co-religionists, and with a greater proportion of workers and Eastern European Jews among them, Austrian Jews elected to study medicine in similar numbers to German Jews. At the turn of the century, about 50 percent of Vienna's doctors and 63 percent of its dentists were Jewish. Most of these graduated from the University of Vienna.[9]

The picture that we are left with for both Germany and Austria is that Jews were highly concentrated in only a handful of institutions, and within those, the medical (and law) schools accounted for the lion's share of Jewish students. Figures for the 1887–1888 academic year indicate that among Prussian medical students, 59 percent were Jews. More specifically, a third of all medical students at Berlin and Breslau were Jewish, and one-fifth at Königsberg were Jewish.[10]

Just prior to the outbreak of World War I, German and Austrian institutions of higher learning began admitting women. Jewish women chose to attend the same handful of institutions as Jewish men. Moreover, medicine proved to be a highly popular area of study for them as well.[11] In Prussia in 1914, among all women medical students, 30 percent were Jewish, and at the University of Vienna, 43 percent of all women students were Jewish. In 1932, on the eve of the Nazi takeover, 40 percent of Berlin's 722 women physicians were Jewish, while the percentage in Vienna was even higher.[12]

There are several reasons for the identifiable presence of Jews in German medicine. Primary is the disproportionate engagement of Jews in all levels of education. In 1906–1907, although only 8 percent of Prussian children received an elementary education, the figure for Jewish children was 59 percent. The respective percentages for those attending secondary school are almost identical. The situation was similar in Austria, where in Vienna in 1912, Jews, who were just under 9 percent of the population, accounted for 47 percent of all high school pupils.[13] In both Germany and Austria, this phenomenon found its analogue at the university level. To take the academic year 1911–1912 as an example, we see that for every 10,000 males attending Prussian universities, 13.19 percent were Protestant, 9.19 were Catholic, and 66.22 were Jewish. In all, Jews claimed 5.4 percent of the Prussian student population and 17 percent at the University of Berlin. Similarly, in 1904, while Jews accounted for 18 percent of all Austrian university students, fully 25 percent of the student body at the University of Vienna was Jewish.[14]

In a social and cultural sense, it was this unquenchable desire for secular education that characterized German-speaking Jews, and paved the way for their entrance into the educated middle classes and their overrepresentation in the liberal professions. Notably, these were goals that were shared by all classes of German Jews. Whereas university education for Christians was traditionally the preserve of elites, even lower-class Jews strove to provide this for their sons. Rural Jews such as cattle dealers and hawkers of second-hand goods, as well as those from the urban petty merchant class, all made it a priority to send their children to *Gymnasien,* and then on to university. In fact, in the last quarter of the nineteenth century, Jewish students in Prussian universities came principally from the heavily agricultural eastern provinces of Posen and Silesia.[15]

For those already entrenched in the rising middle class, seeking to enter occupations commensurate with their elevated economic status, German Jews found that the two most prestigious occupations in Germany — upper-level positions in the military and civil service — were all but closed to them. Here medicine proved to be an attractive alternative. For the doors of opportunity were open to aspiring Jewish doctors. Not only were there no restrictions on medical school entrance for Jews, but medicine as a professional undertaking was a means to financial security and, just as important in the Victorian age, elevated social status.

This latter point is crucial, for status could now be derived from a source that was noncommercial, and commercial pursuits were looked upon with derision in Central European culture. As the historian Peter Pulzer put it, "We may spurn the millionaire for having once been a ragpicker, even while we drink his martinis. No one spurns the surgeon for having been the son of a ragpicker."[16] In 1907, 61 percent of all employed German Jews were in business.[17] Thus the majority of Jews who took up medicine had fathers who were in one branch of commerce or another. Among Jewish scientists (there are no figures specifically for those in the field of medicine), 51 percent had fathers who were businessmen, while only 33 percent came from academic, artistic, or journalistic backgrounds. Medicine, of all the sciences, was by far the most popular for Jews because it offered the most security. And here, the commercial environments in which they were raised were of benefit to Jewish physicians. A majority of the 61 percent of employed Jews who were in business were self-employed. And although the sons may have sought careers outside of commerce or manufacture, they inherited the ethos of self-employment from their fathers. In Berlin, where approximately 50 percent of the city's doctors were Jews, three quarters of them were in private practice.[18] Again, the situation was similar in Vienna.

Contemporary Jewish claims about the shared culture of Germans and Jews notwithstanding, widely divergent value systems, class background, national origins, religious affiliation, and faculty preference all conspired together to clearly distinguish Jews from their Christian neighbors and fellow students. The differences manifested themselves in the development of specific social aspirations among Jews and, very often, in expressions of envy and outright antisemitism by non-Jews.

With the production of so many Jewish doctors in Germany and Austria, the expectations of the young physicians and, indeed, their parents began to change. Whereas at one time becoming a doctor was a mark of success, Jewish aspirations had intensified, and simply becoming a doctor was insufficient for many. Now, becoming a professor of medicine became the ultimate goal. In his memoirs, Jewish physician Hermann Zondek, who began his medical practice in 1912, recounted how the social distinction between the "physician" and "professor" was freighted with enormous worth in the contemporary "Jewish value system" (*jüdischen Glaubenskatechismus*). "Simply put," he wrote, "the physician was valued and respected. However, one looked upon the professor with unshakeable trust. And the Jewish

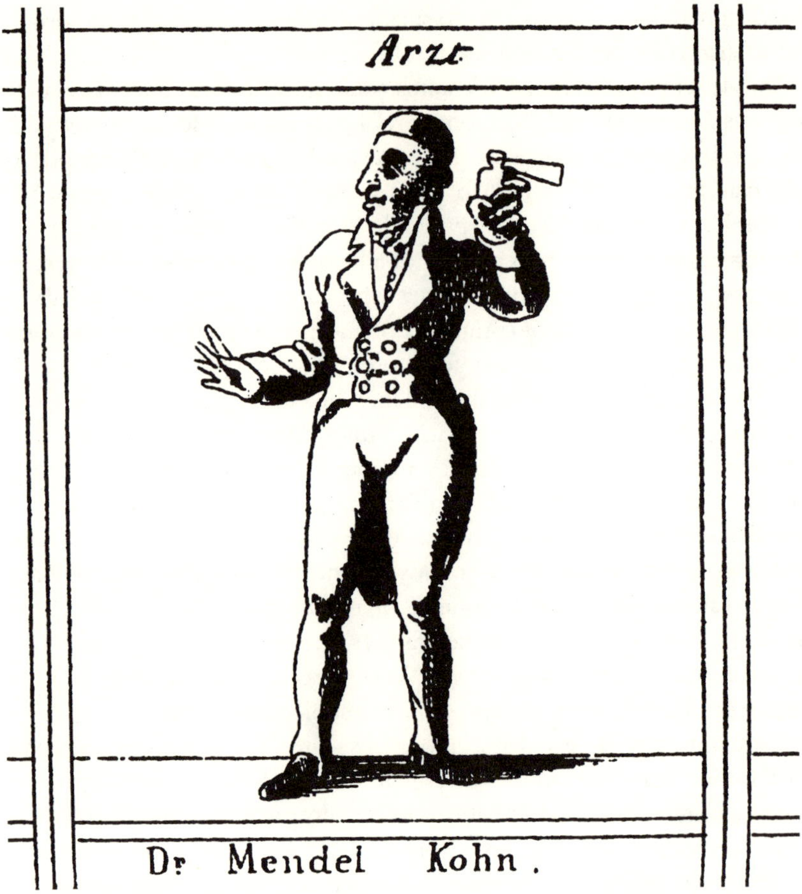

FIGURE 11. A caricature of Dr. Mendel Kohn, a Jewish physician in modern dress, from c. 1825. This was published in an antisemitic illustrated magazine, the *Nürnberger Bilderbogen*. Source: Eduard Fuchs, *Die Juden in der Karikatur: Ein Beitrag zur Kulturgeschichte* (Munich, 1921).

mother was especially covetous that her marriageable daughter would form a golden union with a Privatdozent or titled professor."[19]

But this would remain an unfulfilled aspiration of many a German Jewish parent. One of the reasons private practice proved so attractive and indeed so necessary an option for Jewish physicians was antisemitism. While many Jews wished to join the academy and enjoy the elevated status that was the privilege of members of the professoriate, teaching at the universities, which was, in effect, a civil service position, was essentially off limits to Jews. Although constitutionally guaranteed access to academic appointments, Jews were in actuality barred from taking up such posts.[20] Hence, when they did, they largely remained unsalaried lecturers (*Privatdozenten*), generally relying on family support. And those relatively few lucky Jews who had been promoted from Privatdozent to salaried professor had to wait inordinate periods of time for the honor to be bestowed upon them — for Freud it was seventeen years, while the average for non-Jews was four years.[21] For many, promotion never came. The world-renowned neurologist, Hermann Oppenheim in Berlin, remained a Privatdozent for seventeen years. Giving up any hope of promotion, he voluntarily vacated his position. Similarly, the distinguished Jewish cardiac and pulmonary specialist at the University of Berlin, Albert Fränkel, languished for twenty-seven years in the rank of Privatdozent before relinquishing his post, certain that he would never be promoted. In both cases, it was the Prussian ministry of education that refused to confer the promotion, even though the medical faculties had recommended them.[22]

In the above cases, the Jewish physicians triumphed, carving out stellar careers in spite of the obstacles. But the hostility they experienced and the hurdles placed before them on the path to professional advancement were typical of the lot of all aspiring Jewish academic physicians. We cannot write the history of the humiliation of Jewish physicians, some of them men of international stature, most of them not, and what they must have felt when denied their due. But painful it must certainly have been. For some, the rejection was too much. In 1905 a young Jewish doctor in Berlin, Friedrich Borchert, a recent graduate who had already been recognized as destined for greatness in the world of science, was denied even the lowly position of Privatdozent. According to a contemporary account, Borchert had been denied an appointment because he was Jewish. With dashed hopes of making it even to the first rung of the academic ladder, Borchert took his own life.[23]

A non-Jewish periodical that tracked antisemitism in Germany ran a story on the discrimination against Jews in the medical school at the University of Berlin in 1908. It found that of 19 full professors at that university, there were no Jews. Of the 11 associate professors, 3 were Jewish, while there were 9 Jews among the 43 assistant professors. Of the faculty's 113 unsalaried lecturers, or Privatdozenten, 44 were Jewish. "Is it really true," the periodical asked rhetorically, "that among so many Jewish unsalaried lecturers there is not one who could fill a regular academic position? In contrast to their Christian colleagues, do these men lose their skills through such lengthy periods of activity in the ranks of *Privatdozenten?*"[24]

Nothing illustrated the problem so starkly as the case of the hematologist, immunologist, and father of chemotherapy, Paul Ehrlich.[25] One of the most important medical scientists of the twentieth century, Ehrlich sought to discover chemical compounds that could destroy bacteria without killing their host cells. In 1909, in the course of his experimentation, Ehrlich, together with his Japanese assistant, Sahachiro Hata, discovered Salvarsan. In its day, this compound was the most important therapeutic breakthrough in the fight against syphilis up to the discovery of penicillin. Despite his impeccable scientific credentials, Ehrlich, who also happened to be an active member of the Jewish community, held the modest rank of assistant professor when he won the Nobel Prize for his work on immunology in 1908 at the age of fifty-four.[26] He did not become a full professor at the University of Frankfurt until 1914. For the overwhelming majority of German Jewish doctors until 1918, the prerequisite for climbing the academic ladder was not so much talent as it was religion. One had to be Christian, and most Jews who had professorships, and this was mostly in the natural sciences, had been baptized.

Exclusion from teaching appointments was only one manifestation of a pervasive antisemitism. In 1880, nearly 40 percent of all medical students at the University of Vienna were Jewish. For quite some time before this, the atmosphere was hostile, and the first to feel its effects were the Eastern European Jews, who found themselves discriminated against by the German nationalist student fraternities. Because admission to the medical school was intensely competitive, provincial Jews from the Empire's hinterland, especially those from Galicia or parts of Hungary, were met with considerable vehemence. The hostility was not lost on one particular Jewish medical student from the provinces. Sigmund Freud, who entered the university in 1873, recalled that "I experienced some appreciable disappointments. Above all, I found that I was expected to feel myself inferior and an alien because I was a Jew."[27] For a short while he may well have. However, this would change with the Billroth affair.

In 1875, antisemitism in the Vienna medical school became a public matter with the publication of a study of medical education at German universities by the distinguished professor and surgeon Theodor Billroth. The report argued vigorously against the open admissions policy for citizens of the state. He claimed that Eastern Jews came unprepared to receive a medical education, "lacking the talent for the natural sciences, and [were] absolutely unsuitable to become physicians." For Billroth, these disadvantages were not temporary. Coming to Vienna poverty-stricken and culturally at sea, the Jewish immigrant would be constantly scrambling to exist, and thus valuable study time would be lost. Most important, these Jews threatened to compromise the high standards of the Vienna medical school. According to Billroth, "Backward, ignorant, starving students could only become backward, ignorant, starving physicians."[28]

To reduce competition and maintain "high academic standards" in the medical school, Billroth recommended the imposition of a *numerus clausus* against the Eastern Jews. Although Billroth sought to distance himself from the rabble-rousing antisemitism of his day, which targeted all Jews indiscriminately, noting that "the important men among the Jews are for the most part visionaries, idealists, and humanists," he contrasted them with those Jews who strove for professional success but lacked the talent. This was a different matter altogether, and their ambition was to be neither applauded nor encouraged. "To begin a medical career," he noted, "with insufficient means and with unfounded optimism as well as unrealistic confidence in luck and raw energy is a specifically Jewish characteristic." Billroth's belief in an essential difference between Jews and Germans lay at the core of his attempt to limit Jews from the study of medicine at the University of Vienna:

> It is often forgotten that the Jews are a well-defined nation and that a Jew—just as little as a Persian, Frenchman, New Zealander or African—can never become a German. Whatever is meant by Jewish German, it is only coincidental that they are speaking German, only coincidental that they are educated in Germany. . . . They lose their [Jewish] national tradition just as little as the Germans lose their German manner no matter where they live. . . . It is thus neither expected nor desirable that the Jews ever become German-nationalists or participate in the national struggles like the Germans themselves. Above all, they cannot possibly be sensitive to the accumulated influence of medieval romanticism, upon which our German sensibilities—more than we want to admit—are based; for, the Jews, have no occasion to ponder with special delight the German middle ages. . . . It is certainly clear to me that, in spite of all reflection and individual sympathy, I deeply feel the cleavage between pure German and pure Jewish blood.[29]

Billroth had clearly moved beyond merely singling out Eastern Jews. Now it was a question of all Jews and the stark, mystical, and irreconcilable differences between them and Germans. Despite their penchant for mimicry, their celebration of German culture, and their striving to be accepted as Germans, the Jews remained apart. But in particular, for Billroth, it was the "foreign forty-percent" at the Vienna medical school. Their peculiar sensibilities engendered a "cleavage" that had been brought on by "blood." In Billroth's view, this meant that Jews could never make competent, responsible physicians in the German mold. So where it was once Judaism that made Jewish physicians a threat to Christian patients, now it was race. Biological determinism characterized modern antisemitism, but the sentiment, as applied to Jewish physicians, remained essentially the same as it was during the early modern period. Jewish doctors were still held to be dangerous charlatans, poised to inflict harm upon unsuspecting, Christian patients.

Just days after the appearance of Billroth's book in December 1875, antisemitism at the Vienna medical school turned violent. The air was thick with hate as German nationalist students quoted liberally and publicly from Billroth. The cries of "Juden hinaus!" (Jews get out!) could be heard throughout the medical faculty. On December 10, a clash between German and Jewish students broke out in Billroth's own classroom. The Jews were beaten back and expelled from the lecture hall. For the next week, German nationalist students continued with their disruptions, while Jewish medical students staged counterdemonstrations. In the end the Jews were evicted from the classes of other professors and the affair moved beyond the confines of the medical school and became a cause célèbre in the press.[30]

For a short time after the affair, many assimilated Jewish students joined German students in protesting the high proportion of Eastern Jews at the university, and also voiced disapproval of the self-assertive Jewish response to Billroth. For Freud, who had expressed German nationalist sentiments as well as a disdain for the Eastern Jews, the virulent antisemitism in the medical school was also the beginning of the end of his flirtation with German nationalism, and marked the start of his positive assertions of his Jewish identity. As he later said of this period, "My language is German. My culture, my attainments are German. I considered myself a German intellectually, until I noticed the growth of anti-Semitic prejudice in Germany and in German Austria. Since that time, I consider myself no longer a German. I prefer to call myself a Jew."[31]

Although Billroth later regretted his stance and became a champion in the fight against antisemitism, he succeeded in unleashing the floodgates of Austrian Jew hatred. From the early 1880s, Viennese antisemitism both in the university and without continued to grow. There were demonstrations, riots, boycotts, and open vilification. In response, Jews either resigned from or were thrown out of German national organizations or nationalist student fraternities, a trend that had actually begun in the 1870s.[32] In 1883, one of the University of Vienna's most famous Jewish alumni, Theodor Herzl, quit his fraternity, Albia, in a storm of indignation after it became openly antisemitic.[33]

Other Jews became even more openly assertive. Freud, for example, recounted an ugly incident on a train in 1883, when he opened a window and was told to shut it, to the accompaniment of racial slurs that included "dirty Jew." He wrote to his wife, Martha, "Even a year ago I would have been speechless with agitation; but now I am different; I was not in the least frightened of that mob, asked the one to keep to himself his empty phrase which inspired no respect in me, and the other to step up and take what was coming to him."[34]

At this time, the medical profession outside the university became increasingly hostile to Jews. The Vienna General Hospital, with a large number of Jewish physicians, proved itself an increasingly inhospitable environment for them. In 1884, a Jewish friend and colleague of Freud's at the hospital, Carl Koller, got into an argument with a surgeon who then called him a "Jewish swine" (*Saujud*). Again reporting on the event to his wife, with obvious satisfaction, Freud wrote that "we would have reacted just as Koller did, by hitting the man in the face. . . . We are all delighted; a proud day for us. We are going to give Koller a present as a lasting reminder of his victory."[35]

The tension between Austrian and Jewish doctors was palpable and growing. Eventually, radical propositions were floated, such as the demand made in 1911 by one antisemitic medical fraternity that Jews and Freemasons, "enemies of God and his Holy Church," be excluded from becoming physicians. Strikingly identical to charges made hundreds of years before, it was claimed that "these godless, conceited doctors comport themselves with such haughtiness that they [assume] that the entire Catholic population is just there so that they can be treated [for the purpose of acquiring] ill-gotten gain." The agitators went on to assert that with the population of Austria being 96 percent Catholic, the people needed to be treated by Catholic doctors, and to that end a Catholic university needed to be founded in Salzburg in order to train them.[36]

Art soon came to imitate life. Medical antisemitism in Austria had an impact that was felt by more than just the immediate parties involved in this or that incident. It was a theme that resonated with the public at large, and as such, Jewish artists at the fin-de-siècle represented it in their work. Arthur

Schnitzler, the preeminent Austrian dramatist of his day, was also a doctor, as was his father before him. In 1912, Schnitzler wrote *Professor Bernhardi,* a play set in Vienna in 1900 about the fate of a Jewish physician and the injustice meted out to him. It was Schnitzler's attempt to render dramatically the Jewish Question as it pertained to medicine in Central Europe.[37]

The drama begins toward the end of the first act when the twenty-five-year-old Oskar Bernhardi prevents a priest from entering the room of his dying patient, a young woman suffering from blood poisoning after a botched abortion. Partly because she has lapsed into a state of euphoria and is under the illusion that her recovery is imminent, Bernhardi aims to make the patient's last hours as comfortable as possible and not cause her any undue stress. Although a nurse had sent for a priest, Bernhardi determined that the receipt of last rites would certainly have made the patient aware of her fate, and acting from purely humanitarian motives, feared that "it might hasten the end, perhaps only by minutes, but still — ."[38] The patient, however, dies before the priest can perform his religious duties, and then the recriminations begin.

The plot turns as Bernhardi's behavior is interpreted as an expression of his anti-Catholic sentiment. His enemies read the entire situation as indicative of the Jews' power, especially their disproportionate participation in Austrian medicine. Now, in Catholic Austria, a Jew is suddenly in a position to prevent a man of the cloth from carrying out his sacred responsibilities. The situation becomes intolerable. Reporting what has happened to the authorities, the priest and his supporters turn the incident into a scandal that is eagerly taken up by unscrupulous politicians and the press. Bernhardi is the victim of false testimony given by the nurse on duty at the time of the incident, and betrayal, as his deputy, Dr. Ebenwald, colludes with a government minister and feeds lies and trumped-up charges to the antisemitic press. Because an action of sacrilege is to be brought against Bernhardi, and because his institute has been the recipient of partial government funding, the matter makes its way onto the floor of the parliament. There, to the accompanying cries of "Jews are overrunning the Universities," the rancorous debate sees members split along party lines.[39] The whole scandal has the makings of an Austrian Dreyfus Affair as Bernhardi is eventually imprisoned for two months after having had his license revoked. Even after it becomes evident that his incarceration was due to the manufacture of false testimony, Bernhardi chooses not to fight for a retrial to clear his name. Rather, he goes silently, electing to finish out his professional career in private practice.[40]

As had happened with the Billroth affair, not all the Jewish doctors in Bernhardi's clinic side with him. Some side with the nationalists, while others are scared into a timid and confused silence; this is especially the case among the converted. Bernhardi is denied an adequate defense because he retains the services of Goldenthal, a converted Jewish lawyer who fears that if he puts up too rigorous a defense his conversion will be cast into doubt. On the other hand, the Zionists marshal demonstrations in support of Bernhardi, but he is embarrassed by their aggressiveness.

Thus did Schnitzler, through this incident involving a Jewish doctor who occupies an elevated yet precarious position in this fiercely antagonistic society, succeed in highlighting the severe fault lines that characterized the topography of Viennese Jewish life at the turn of the century. As such, it is more than the story of one wronged individual. To be sure, the protagonist represents beleaguered Jews, but in particular, Bernhardi stands for all the overrepresented Jewish professionals in Germany and Austria. Among the "liberal" professions of medicine, dentistry, law, and journalism, the naked visibility of Jews became a central platform in the campaign of German antisemites.

But Schnitzler's choice to make Bernhardi a physician was not an arbitrary one. The ubiquitous presence of the Jewish doctor in the social reality of the Habsburg capital allowed Schnitzler to tackle the issue of Austrian antisemitism and the Jewish response to it in a thoroughly believable and easily recognizable way.[41] In the end, the failure of even Bernhardi to rise in righteous indignation at the miscarriage of justice perpetrated upon him reflects some of the "weariness and skepticism" and "disillusionment" that characterized the Jewish encounter with Austrian antisemitism. It was omnipresent and psychologically devastating. And in *Professor Bernhardi,* the resignation to its ugly reality among the Jewish characters is illustrative of Schnitzler's own sentiments born of personal experience.[42]

According to one historian, "The multi-ethnic Habsburg Empire was the cradle of the most successful modern political movement based on anti-Semitism to emerge anywhere in nineteenth-century Europe."[43] And as Schnitzler well knew, the charges leveled in the universities, on the floor of the Parliament, and in the press made clear that the Jewish physician was a lightning rod for antisemites. This was so because according to their enemies, Jewish physicians did not so much cure the ill in society as they did bring about society's ills. A clear example of this occurred in October 1892, when Emperor Franz Joseph condemned the rising tide of antisemitism, specifically referring to charges raised in the Lower Austrian Diet by antisemitic deputies that Jewish doctors had sought to kill off Christian patients by admitting them to cholera hospitals.[44] The charge was distinctly medieval.

Beginning in the 1890s, according to one contemporary Jewish observer, the steady decline in the number of Jews entering the field of medicine "was in no small measure due to the antisemitic disturbances that many Jewish students in Vienna have suffered in their stay there."[45] In this climate, antisemitism and the metaphor of medicine were also linked to each other. After he had recanted his earlier views, Hermann Bahr, the former fraternal brother of Herzl who had given the antisemitic speech that led to the latter's resignation from the lodge, declared that antisemitism was "a new madness," designed to restore to modern man his "wilted nerves." According to Bahr, "The rich resort to morphine and hashish. Those who cannot afford drugs become antisemites."[46]

The antisemitism that grew like an uncontrollable weed in the narrower confines of the University of Vienna and in the medical profession found its parallel in the rise of antisemitic political parties and organizations.[47] In 1897, Vienna became the first European capital to elect an antisemite, Karl Lueger, to be its mayor. Peter Gay has written that Lueger's advent "sealed the bankruptcy of Austrian liberalism with irrevocable finality."[48] No one summed up the prevailing mood better than Theodor Herzl. In September 1895, he wrote an entry in his diary about the raucous Viennese mayoral elections to which he was a witness: "Towards evening I went to the Landstrasse district. A silent tense crowd before the polling station. Suddenly Dr. Lueger appeared in the square. Wild cheering; women waving white kerchiefs from the windows. The police held the people back. A man next to me said with tender warmth but in a quiet voice: 'That is our Führer.' Actually, these words showed me more than all declamation and abuse how deeply antisemitism is rooted in the hearts of these people."[49]

In Germany, meanwhile, the antisemitic movement also continued to grow, and the specific backlash against Jews in medicine proceeded apace. While less virulent and violent at German universities, antisemitism in that environment manifested itself largely in the exclusion of Jews from medical student fraternities and the refusal of German dueling fraternities to accept challenges from slighted Jews, whom they deemed to be unworthy of fighting.[50]

The antisemitism of the students was matched by that of many of the professors, and that which had been learned at the universities was carried into the public realm by the graduates. It was in the larger public domain that antisemitism against Jewish doctors struck a resonant chord. One of Germany's most extreme racial antisemites and successful agitators in the Kaiserreich was Theodor Fritsch. In 1887 he founded an antisemitic publishing house, The Hammer, whose first product was Fritsch's own work, *The Antisemites' Catechism,* later called the *Handbook on the Jewish Question.* By 1933, the year Fritsch died and Hitler became chancellor, the *Handbook* had gone through forty editions.[51] In 1944, the *Handbook* was in its forty-ninth edition; Fritsch was therefore one of Germany's most widely read authors, with perhaps millions of readers.

Theodor Fritsch constituted something new in the dark world of German antisemitic politics at the end of the nineteenth century. Unlike his predecessors who grafted antisemitism onto their larger political agendas, Fritsch made the struggle against the Jews the raison d'être of his political worldview. It was a program he pursued with intense zeal and singular focus. Sure that an antisemitic party could never capture the reins of power in Germany, Fritsch believed passionately that if fed a steady diet of anti-Jewish propaganda, Germany could become an even more antisemitic country than it already was. He maintained that through the implementation of a slow but constant regimen of indoctrination, especially in the schools, all political parties, social groups, and religious organizations would eventually absorb the gospel of hate.[52]

In his *Handbook*—he also put out an antisemitic newspaper called the *Antisemitic Correspondence*—Fritsch catalogued the supposed misdeeds of the Jews, compiling a list of charges that he excerpted from all writers dating from the classical period to his own day. Unusual even among his coterie, Fritsch called for violence against Jews and their eradication from German lands. More typical, however, was his railing against the overrepresentation of Jews in a variety of occupations, and the damage done to German culture as a result of that disproportionate presence. Among those he targeted were Jewish doctors. So great was the number of Jews practicing medicine that Fritsch envisioned a "time when the German doctor, at least in the big cities, will be an exception."[53]

In Fritsch's view, the large numbers of Jews choosing to study medicine could not be accounted for merely by their "acquisitiveness." This was because the overproduction of physicians in Germany had severely hampered the earning potential of all doctors, a situation that only threatened to get worse. On the other hand, those who were successful and enjoyed wide public acclaim stood to "build up their reputations as well as their bank accounts." In the 1919 edition of his *Handbook,* Fritsch claimed that famous

Berlin doctors earned between 200,000 and 300,000 marks per annum. How could this be, given that regulations existed to protect patients by strictly limiting the fees doctors could charge? The answer was that fee restrictions did not apply to medical specialists. Naturally, according to Fritsch, the Jews chose to become specialists in order to enrich themselves, and at the same time impoverish Christian patients.[54]

In fact, there was a kernel of truth in what Fritsch had to say. Where once a medical degree was a guarantee of a handsome income, after the 1880s too many graduating physicians made the economic outlook for doctors ever more bleak. A study of the earnings of Berlin physicians in 1891 showed that 59 percent failed to earn 3,000 marks per annum, not enough to live on. By way of comparison, 80 percent of lawyers in Berlin earned what the top 10 percent of physicians brought in. And, of course, the expenses to study medicine were greater than in any other field. In 1893 the average cost of a medical education was 1,479 marks per year. By comparison, the study of philology, law, and theology cost 580, 466, and 432 marks, respectively. Paying back such tuition costs was extremely difficult for young doctors just leaving the universities. As a consequence, many physicians' organizations began to officially discourage the study of medicine.[55] No other liberal profession had experienced similar pressures, and this is one of the critical reasons that between 1886 and 1905 the percentage of Jews studying law in Prussia rose from 17 to 41 percent, while in medical schools the percentage actually fell, from 57 to 24.5 percent.[56]

Partially in response to the economic situation, Jews, as Fritsch said, did indeed flock into medical specialization. In fact, they were twice as likely to be specialists than their Gentile colleagues. Before 1933, roughly 52 percent of all Jewish doctors were specialists, while the corresponding figure for non-Jewish physicians was 26.1 percent.[57] Fritsch, of course, did not explain what was really behind this development. Jews became specialists for a number of reasons. The first, as he hinted at, was the overproduction of doctors and the imposition of fee restrictions, which made earning a comfortable living as a general practitioner increasingly difficult. The unfulfilled promise of financial reward was a reality that few doctors, irrespective of religious background, would readily tolerate. Therefore, in order to either attain or maintain a comfortable, bourgeois lifestyle, German Jews came to realize, medical specialization made good financial sense and fit in well with their socioeconomic aspirations.

Antisemitism also played a decisive role in the professional choices graduating Jewish medical students made, leading a majority to enter a specialty field. In addition to the very limited potential for unbaptized Jews to become professors of medicine, other areas of employment, such as the armed services, were closed to Jews. They were prevented from becoming military medical officers—another civil service appointment—in the midst of a widely recognized shortage of expert army medical personnel.

The prohibition against Jews entering the military as physicians, while contrary to the spirit and letter of the constitution, was the result of endemic antisemitism in practice. As the editor of a conservative Silesian newspaper put it, "And Jewish officers in the army? No. Our army is too dear to us to wish for [the inclusion] of the Jewish element on a large scale into the officer corps."[58] It would appear from this statement that for the author of these lines, even one Jewish officer constituted "large scale" infiltration.

When reasons were offered for barring Jews from becoming medical army officers, they were spurious and insulting. According to one newspaper, "The Jewish physician has no heart for [treating] soldiers. Rather, he sees in him a subject on which to perform medical experiments, and later, with his adroitness, a means by which he can earn money. Woe to the soldier who falls into the hands of the Jewish surgeon."[59] Commenting on the 1898 debate in parliament that Jews be admitted as medical officers to the armed forces, a nationalist, antisemitic newspaper moved beyond the specific matter at hand to address the role of Jews in medicine in general. It challenged the widely held assumption that Jews had a "particular aptitude" for medicine, stating that "the particular aptitude they have lies less in the way they practice [medicine] than in the way they commercialize the profession."[60] In that same Reichstag debate another antisemitic member denied that either the military or the state was to blame for the absence of Jewish army doctors. Bluntly, he declared, "If the pay for military doctors was better, then more Jewish physicians would apply for the military."[61]

That Germany was both perpetrator of discrimination and victim of its own bigotry was recognized at the time in liberal German circles. In a letter to a Berlin newspaper, one physician suggested that a "rational balance" be implemented that would allow Jewish doctors to serve not just in civilian life but in military life as well. Implementation of this policy, he said, would relieve the pressure on the medical profession as a whole brought about from the overproduction of doctors.[62]

From the late nineteenth century, antisemites tirelessly repeated the claim that the Jews had introduced the culture of commerce into medical practice. Echoing the sentiments of those who railed against Jewish doctors in the Middle Ages, polemicists charged that Jewish doctors substituted business principles for the basic humanitarianism of medicine, thereby undermining and perverting the whole profession. "The Jew," went a common charge, "does not see the healing of the sick as his profession. Rather, it is the earning of money."[63] The majority of antisemitic claims concerning Jewish doctors and the military involved reiteration of well-worn charges about Jewish cowardice and unmanliness. When these were combined with the equally ancient accusation of Jewish greed, an airtight explanation for why Jews avoided the armed forces and chose to practice medical specialties in big cities was in place.[64]

Finally, the Jewish preference for specialization could be explained by the fact that older, more established medical specialties such as surgery sorely restricted the number of Jews they would accept into their ranks.[65] Consequently, Jews were almost forced to move into newer medical specialties such as internal medicine, gynecology, psychiatry, dermatology, and aesthetic surgery.[66] Specialization in medicine was in its infancy at the turn of the twentieth century, just at that moment when Jews had graduated from medical schools in large numbers, but found that were they to have remained general practitioners, their opportunities for advancement would have been severely curtailed. Ironically, discrimination may have resulted in Jewish medical and natural scientists excelling in the marginal clinics and institutions that would employ them, places where both time and freedom to pursue cutting-edge research were more readily available. As historian Fritz Ringer observed, "Anti-Semitism produced outsiders among Jewish intellectuals, and the status of the outsider, no matter how it is attained, often makes for radicalism as well as for creativity."[67] The excitement of essentially creating new fields of medical research proved especially alluring to Jews. In a country with a distinguished reputation as a world leader in science and medicine, young Jews anticipated reaping the rewards of scientific discovery. For ambitious and marginalized Jewish doctors the greatest reward would be the winning of respect.

The advent of specialization heralded a new age in the history of medicine.[68] Up to the eighteenth century in universities, specialization meant concentration on a particular organ or disease. However, the specialist was more of a scholar than a practicing physician, shying away from treatment, confining himself to the theoretical explication of illness and disease. In contradistinction, there were a host of medical providers such as barber-surgeons, midwives, dentists, broken-bone setters, and bathhouse attendants who provided "hands-on" care. Principally motivated by the desire to alleviate pain, these caregivers were little concerned with the origin and cause of disease.[69]

By the nineteenth century, the self-understanding of doctors had undergone a change. Specialists saw themselves not as university-based theoreticians but rather as a professional class of men who "did not shy away from laying on hands." Thus the new specialist was a sort of composite of the two previous types of medical specialist. He combined the theoretical knowledge of his university-based predecessor with the direct approach to healing that had previously been the preserve of medicine's less prestigious workers. Diagnosis, once the central element of the specialist's craft, was replaced with therapy.[70]

Not only did this shift mark a change in medical practice, but it also fundamentally altered patient-doctor relations, for it resulted in the emergence of a new, educated, and more demanding kind of patient. Once content to entrust their medical needs to whomever was available and seemingly qualified to treat them, patients now elected to secure the services of trained specialists. No longer willing to be passive participants in the doctor-client relationship, patients were becoming sophisticated medical consumers. "Medicalized," just as doctors were becoming professionalized, patients now sought to place themselves under the care of "experts."[71] In a majority of cases these "experts" were Jewish.

One of the major consequences of the restructuring of German medicine that came about with the rise of the specialist was the increasingly hostile split between specialists and general medical practitioners. General practitioners experienced a decline in business and a commensurate drop in status. According to this formulation, it was the Jews who orchestrated the process that would eventually lead to the redundancy of the general practitioner. With their preference for medical specialization, Jews were seen as the cause of the major problems that beset German medicine at the turn of the century.

The fact of medical specialization is of critical importance in understanding the virulent antisemitism within the medical profession and the eventual fate of Jewish doctors under the National Socialists. More than merely causing pecuniary and social disadvantage, however, the drive of Jewish doctors to become specialists was seen by antisemites as indicative of something larger and of greater and more damaging consequence to German culture as a whole.

To be sure, specialization was an inevitable development facilitated by the burgeoning growth of scientific knowledge. But to its opponents, especially those who were stridently anti-modernist, medical specialization was representative of the disintegrative, fractured nature of modern life. Most specialists were to be found in big cities. Rarely, if ever, did they make house calls and thus get to know the extended family, and they had next to no relationship with the patient outside of a professional one. Whereas the general practitioner, especially in the countryside and in small towns, shared the values and culture of his patients, big city specialists treated people from lower social orders, people with whom they had very little in common. Socially detached from their patients, they "tended to view their activity from the standpoint of medicine as an exact natural science, supported by experimental data."[72]

New and without roots in medical tradition, specialization was seen as a uniquely Jewish invention. It had emerged from an urban setting, and the clear hierarchical arrangement of the doctor-patient relationship — one that had been based on and maintained by social and cultural boundaries — was a direct challenge to volkish, nationalist notions of an organic community of healers and healed. Above all, specialization was seen as the peculiar product of the Jewish intellect. To the antisemites, the tendency to divide, to split hairs, to avoid conceptualizing holistically was typical of Jewish thinking. Here we can see how older antisemitic canards of Jews as casuistic, materialistic, and devoid of spirit were modernized and introduced into the attacks on Jewish doctors, whose penchant for medical specialization was thus held to be illustrative of the very foreignness of Jewish thought patterns.[73]

According to Theodor Fritsch, specialization threatened the integrity and nature of German medicine, jeopardizing its "comprehensive science of healing."[74] In contrast to the Germans, "the sick body is," for the Jews, "a machine-like composite, and not a living unity, to be treated accordingly." Above all, Jews possess "cold sobriety and mechanistic ways of thinking and [with it] have brought about an immense disintegration of medical-care."[75]

In this age of mass movements, parliamentary politics, organized labor, and political antisemitism, disgruntled elements in German society suggested that distinctly modern tactics be employed to deal with what they regarded as the recent "Jewification" (*Verjudung*) of German medicine. Advocating Christian solidarity and collective mobilization as a means of combating the presence of Jews in medicine, as well as the deteriorating material circumstances of the medical profession, polemicists offered instruction to German doctors on what to do about Jewish competition:

> As a result of the overgrowth of the Jewish element, the reputation of doctors has sunk deeply. So long as Aryan doctors do not arrive at the complete conviction that there can be no alliance with Jewish powers,

that because of his collegiality, the Christian doctor will always be the victim; in short, so long as Aryan doctors do not form a tight bond with one another in opposition to Jewish machinations and Jewish hypocrisy, and so long as there are Jews in medicine, the poverty of the medical class will not disappear. Aryan doctors must unanimously rise up and expose the machinations of Jewish doctors to the public. They should then persuade the Volk to only use Aryan doctors.[76]

At the turn of the century, it was a common yet untrue charge that Jews held the leading positions at most clinics and hospitals. According to Julius Kleeberg, a German Jewish immigrant physician to Palestine, "Talented and ambitious Jewish assistants" were denied positions in "clinics and scientific institutes for fear that a non-Aryan would 'contaminate' the Germanic alma mater."[77] And yet, as one alarmist line in an antisemitic newspaper asked in 1898, "Are there still Germanic doctors in Berlin?"[78] In response to such perceptions, and as a practical measure to curb the employment of Jewish doctors, it therefore became a common tactic at that time for advertisements announcing hospital and clinic openings to specifically call for Christian doctors only. Essentially promoting the boycotting of Jewish physicians, such advertisements requested that the applicants supply proof of baptism. But increasingly, the advertisements took on a decidedly racist quality when they insisted that job applicants be "Aryan" or "Christian by descent." In a foretaste of German racism, Jewish converts to Christianity were regarded as no more Christian than their Jewish colleagues.[79]

In 1905, the German Medical Association met at Strasbourg for its annual convention, and the wording of the above-mentioned job announcements came up for discussion. Obviously, the association, whose mandate it was to protect the rights of all German physicians, irrespective of religion, could not countenance open discrimination. However, in deference to and out of sympathy with the prevailing sentiment, it suggested a compromise to antisemitic members, recommending that in job listings, the words "where possible" follow directly after the stipulation that the applicant be Christian or Aryan.[80]

Discrimination was also meted out to Jewish nurses, who were finding it increasingly difficult to find employment in non-Jewish hospitals. The first Association for Jewish Nurses was established in 1893, but because of a hostile atmosphere and limited professional prospects the Jewish Nurses' Training School did not open its doors until 1895. Affiliated with the Berlin Jewish Hospital, the school undertook to train and then place Jewish nurses in Jewish institutions. In addition, because of the rise of Jewish nationalist sentiment, Zionist voices in both Germany and Austria had begun calling for Jewish women to take up nursing. Aside from providing honorable work for middle-class Jewish women, the call was part of a larger philosophy of Zionist-inspired Jewish self-help. Jewish doctors and nurses, it was believed, should provide care for the army of Jewish sick and poor.[81]

Unlike the discrimination against Jewish nurses, which was real and painful but was not accompanied by a fully developed set of beliefs, the attacks on Jewish physicians were expressed in an elaborate liturgy of denunciations. In 1899, a Jewish physician named Joseph Lewy drew attention to the issue of antisemitism in the German medical profession in a lengthy article he published in one of Germany's major Jewish periodicals. Lewy acknowledged that German medicine was in crisis, and he identified three factors in particular that were responsible for the difficulties faced by German doctors at the fin-de-siècle: intense competition among private practitioners for patients, many of whom had been denied access to private physicians because of recent changes in health insurance laws; an overproduction of doctors; and the fact that "quackery was in full bloom and increasing due to the absence of strict regulations [against it]."[82]

According to Lewy, these three developments not only caused the financial difficulties that beset German medicine but also brought about the worsening image of physicians in the eyes of patients. German doctors were indeed caught in the vice of economic competition and social vulnerability. But the thrust of Lewy's thesis was that the frustrations of many German doctors were being vented in the form of antisemitism. Although Jewish doctors were also precariously positioned, the fear of the majority Christian medical community manifested itself in a backlash against their Jewish colleagues. And if German physicians did not take up cudgels against Jewish physicians themselves, the stridently antisemitic press waged the battle on their behalf.

The causative factors that Lewy identified as responsible for the worsening condition of the German physician were indeed of great import. The most important social issue in German medicine in the late nineteenth century concerned "insurance doctors."[83] After the passage of health insurance legislation in 1883, the number of insured Germans increased dramatically — from 10 percent of the population initially, to about 50 percent in 1914. This meant that the treatment of insured patients now became the principal source of physicians' incomes, whereas previously, private patients had been the mainstays of a doctor's practice. Assured of a roster of regular patients, insurance company doctors were, therefore, protective of their positions, while physicians shut out of the system sought ways to enter it. In 1890, the German Medical Association first suggested that patients be given free choice of doctors. In effect this meant that insurance companies would no longer employ physicians. Instead, insured members could freely choose to be treated by any doctor practicing in a particular locale. It was a move the insurance companies and their physicians strenuously resisted. The result was that the system promoted tension and rivalry among German doctors.

In addition, even those physicians employed by insurance companies had cause for grievance. They did not enjoy job security, for they could be dismissed for a host of reasons ranging, from the purely commercial interests of the company to issues involving treatment and therapy. In the latter instance, physicians often found their professional autonomy curtailed through the cost-cutting measures of the insurers. It was they who had the ultimate say in patient treatment, determining which medical services would be covered by insurance plans. With this challenge to their freedom to practice medicine as they saw fit, many in the system, while guaranteed steady, albeit low incomes, found themselves beholden to higher, nonmedical powers. This was an encroachment of a humiliating kind.

As Lewy observed, the overproduction of doctors in the late nineteenth century had serious repercussions. Between 1889 and 1898, the number of doctors in Germany had grown by 56 percent, while the population increased by only 11.5 percent.[84] This resulted in tremendous competition among doctors. In this situation, good business sense may well have given an advantage to those physicians who possessed it. Coming from commercial backgrounds, many of the Jewish medical practitioners may well have been able to weather the storm better than most. And as is so often the case with antisemitism, envy of the perceived financial acumen of Jews played a significant role in fanning the flames of hostility toward Jewish doctors.

Another consequence of competition was that fee undercutting became commonplace, as did the paying of bribes by physicians to the directors of insurance firms in order to get on their employee rosters.[85] Thus, in addition to forcing doctors to hone their business skills, the system inadvertently promoted corruption, which in turn created an impression that the medical profession had become riddled with moral corrosion. It was easy to make the causative link that the turpitude coincided with and resulted from the great influx of Jews into the field of medicine, and the prominent role Jews played as directors of health insurance firms.

Finally, in the period 1869 to 1871 medical practice was liberated from bureaucratic supervision and accorded the status of a "free trade."[86] This promoted a sense of self-confident elitism among doctors, whereby they assumed as a group the social and cultural characteristics of society's upper orders. As a professional group, physicians, practicing a new and highly scientized profession, desperately sought to win and maintain respect and social standing. Thus, according to Michael Kater, "German full professors of medicine, who were then universally recognized as the leading experts in their fields, exuded an atmosphere of regality and papal infallibility."[87] Often mistreating and, indeed, abusing their students, professors inculcated in their young charges, "the importance of rank and subordination, of command and discipline which medical students were meant to adhere to as a way of life after graduation."[88] An important venue for the indoctrination of such values was the system of dueling fraternities, so favored by medical students. There, where violence in the name of honor was a dominant cultural code, they made important social connections with wealthy potential benefactors, or even members of the aristocracy. In the fraternities, members underwent an intense program of "social militarization" where, seeking to emulate the aristocracy, they learned to display that most Prussian of behaviors, *Obrigkeitsdenken,* a deference to authority and hierarchy. And because of their exclusivist and nationalist nature, the German fraternities and the culture they spawned were closed to Jews.

Bestowing upon medicine the title of a "free trade" had another effect. It granted, as Joseph Lewy said, almost free rein to a host of quacks and charlatans. The unintended impact of creating an elite caste of healers trained in the universities was the simultaneous creation of a counter-cohort of untrained, nonscientific medical care providers. With their emergence, which led to the establishment of the German Medical Association in 1873, doctors redoubled their efforts against all "out-groups" that they imagined compromised their status. And in this environment it was Jews, outsiders in every sense, who were targeted for attack.

In sum, these developments resulted in a closing of the circle of accusations and recriminations around Jewish physicians. Insurance laws that provided medical coverage to workers were seen by opponents to be part of a larger Socialist plot, at the forefront of which were Jews. On the other hand, the capitalist culture that had developed in tandem with the insurance legislation was also seen as the nefarious contribution of the Jewish "trading mentality." And specialization, so preferred by Jewish physicians, was, to many, quackery and a betrayal of the humble code of medical practice that the idealized German doctor supposedly embodied.

It was in this context that ancient charges against Jews and Jewish doctors were resuscitated. For example, the cholera epidemics that struck Hamburg in 1892 and again in 1902 were blamed on Russian Jewish immigrants.[89] Although Gentiles were among those arriving from the East, the antisemites focused only on the Jews, and conservative agitators sought to have Germany's borders closed to them. As one newspaper put it: "Russia may wish to keep its infected Jews to itself, just as it may its infected pigs."[90] However, Jews were accused not only of causing the epidemics but also of profiting from them. Not coincidentally, it was claimed, did business activity increase for Jewish-owned pharmaceutical concerns that produced cholera vaccinations.[91] Thus could a neat conspiratorial web be spun that charged Jewish carriers of disease with working in league with Jewish entrepreneurs to infect Christians, who then sought treatment from Jewish doctors, the latter two groups reaping the rewards that came from curing the afflicted.

Vienna was the site of exceptionally resilient and vitriolic accusations that Jewish physicians were engaged in research designed to kill Christians. Here, at the dawn of the twentieth century, the medieval charges against Jews were revivified and clothed in modern guise. Jewish doctors were accused of deliberately inoculating Christians and healthy animals with doses of plague and other diseases, performing vivisection, and promoting the passage of the Vaccination Act of 1874, which required compulsory inoculation against smallpox for every child in the German empire.[92] Antisemites believed that Jewish deputies, as part of a Jewish plot, had pushed the vaccination legislation through the Reichstag in order to infect the German race. According to one such politician, "To inject someone with cow-pox vaccine is an un-German way of thinking."[93] Obviously the accuser was unaware that Edward Jenner had not been Jewish.

Typically, accusations of Jewish criminality are allied to the pornographic depictions of Jews, which are an iconographic staple of modern antisemitism. They also occupied an important place in the campaign against Jewish physicians. One of the more popular areas of specialization among Jewish doctors was gynecology. Certain that Jewish gynecologists would commit sex crimes against their unsuspecting and vulnerable patients, perhaps even using the widely maligned practice of hypnosis and suggestion, antisemites warned German women not to use them. Moreover, they insisted that more German women gynecologists be trained in order to reduce the possibility of placing German women at risk.[94]

Racist literature of the period likewise expressed such themes. In 1893, Oskar Panizza, a German physician, published a short and ghastly porno-

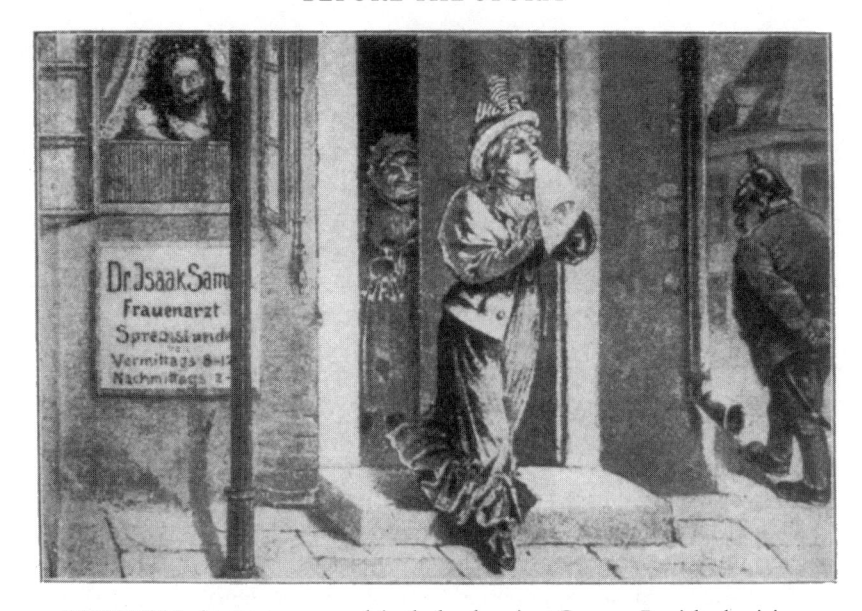

FIGURE 12. A common complaint lodged against German Jewish physicians from the late nineteenth century onward was that too many of them were gynecologists. Antisemites constantly raised the specter of Jewish doctors taking advantage of innocent German women. In this turn-of-the-century illustration from the *Dresdener Bilderbogen,* a tearful young German woman leaves the practice of a Jewish gynecologist under the watchful and hateful eye of the doctor's assistant, an old Jewish woman. In the window, one can see the Jewish doctor, his eyes ablaze with lust as he is about to ravish yet another young German. A policeman walks by the scene, his head bowed, offering no assistance. He is powerless, while the Jews are in complete control. The caption (not shown here) reads, "The devil in Germany." Source: Eduard Fuchs, *Die Juden in der Karikatur: Ein Beitrag zur Kulturgeschichte* (Munich, 1921).

graphic tale entitled *The Operated Jew.* The story recounts the efforts of Faitel Stern, a rich, Jewish medical student who, desperate to "become German," submits to, among other things, a series of excruciating orthopedic operations, painful cosmetic procedures, blood transfusions from "seven strong women from the Black Forest," and elocution lessons to achieve his desired goal. The final act in the attempted metamorphosis is his wedding to a Protestant woman. But there, at the reception, Jekyll and Hyde–like, Stern suddenly begins to return to his previous physical self. Horrified, the guests are transfixed by the "bloodthirsty, swelling, crimson visage [which] spewed saliva from flabby drooping lips." Stern then began "clicking his tongue, gurgling, and tottering back and forth while making disgusting, lascivious and bestial canine movements with his rear end."⁹⁵ Here we can see the threat posed to German patients by the Jewish doctor. Possessing all the traits that were part of the antisemitic arsenal of accusations, Stern was a cruel charlatan, a revolting beast, and a frenzied sex maniac. Despite his best efforts, Stern's Jewish racial character could not be denied—his Aryanization a much desired, but impossible to attain, chimera.

In Austria, the field of medicine and Jewish involvement in it became a lightning rod for those with grievances about the nature of modern society, modern science, and liberal politics. An outbreak of bubonic plague in Bombay in 1897 saw teams of European scientists descend on the Indian city to bear witness to the disease and retrieve bacteria samples to take back to Europe for investigation. Toward the end of 1898, at the Bacteriological Institute of the Vienna General Hospital, a tragic accident occurred when a young laboratory assistant named Barisch was infected with the plague. While escorting him for treatment to the clinic of the famed Hermann Nothnagel, a physician by the name of Müller and a female attendant also became infected. All three died.⁹⁶

While most of the press treated the matter in a sober fashion, the antisemitic press had a field day. According to them, an epidemic was on hand and it had been spread deliberately. In fact, the connection of Jews to the incident had been tangential at best. Apparently, one of the young scientists at the Bacteriological Institute named Mayer, was Jewish. He, it was claimed, had participated in plague research in order to make a name for himself. Nevertheless, the antisemites highlighted the fact that Nothnagel—a Christian whose only connection to the case had been that Barisch had been brought to his clinic—was in the forefront of liberal politics and was especially energetic in defending Jewish doctors against attack.

Further accusations stemming from this episode serve as an accurate barometer of antisemitic opinion concerning modern society. One newspaper said that the affair "threw a glaring spotlight on modern medical research" and demanded that the state regulate closely all such scientific inquiry, even that conducted in private institutes. Leading the attack was a parliamentarian and vulgar antisemite from Karl Lueger's Christian Social Party, Josef Gregorig. He called for a flat-out ban on all medical research. The antisemitic reactionaries charged modern scientists with being magicians, carrying on germ research in order to practice "alchemy" by becoming rich through the fame they cultivated from their discoveries. To do so, modern doctors conspired in "secret groups." At the forefront of this conspiracy were "Jewish doctors whose usurious spirit should be opposed not

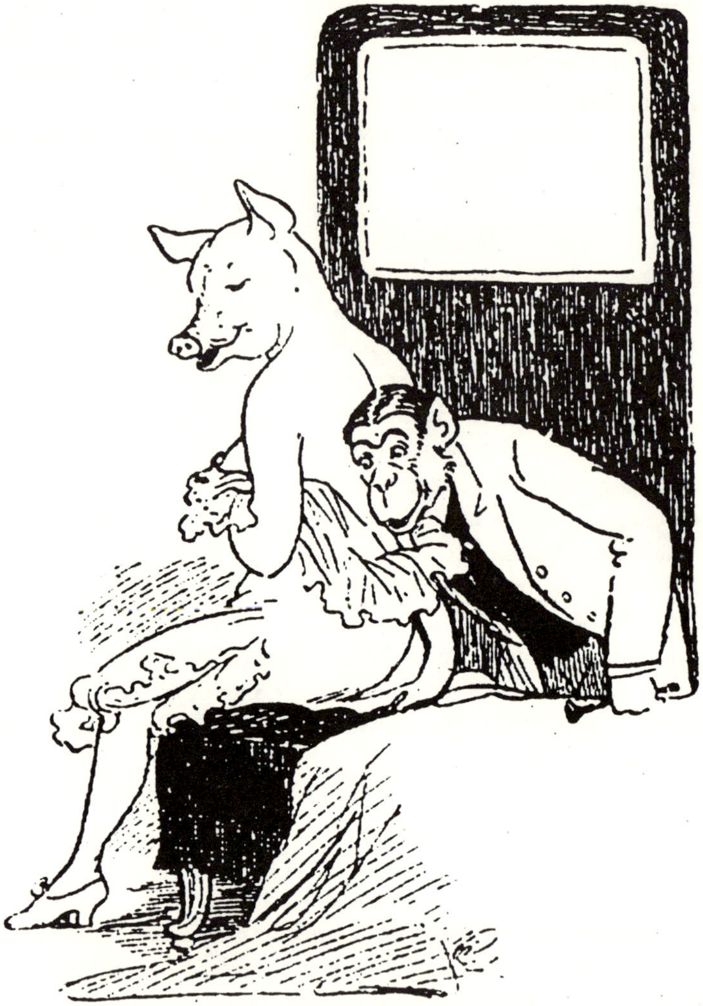

FIGURE 13. In this 1920 illustration from *Das deutsche Witzblatt*, entitled "Consultation," a Jewish doctor represented as an ape examines the scantily clad Christian patient, a woman with a pig's head. After informing her that she has a heart problem, the doctor prescribes that she take up nude dancing. Telling her that she could make a career of it, and assuring her an audience, the Jewish doctor is cast into the role of procurer as he informs her (in the caption, not shown here), "My friends don't eat pork, but they like to look at it." Source: Eduard Fuchs, *Die Juden in der Karikatur: Ein Beitrag zur Kulturgeschichte* (Munich, 1921).

just out of the material interests of Christian physicians, but out of the moral interests of the entire [medical] profession."[97]

Another antisemitic newspaper declared, "What Virchow is to Berlin, Nothnagel is to Vienna. Presumptuous, arrogant, liberal . . . he is naturally a protector of Jews, together with whom he kills poor animals in his clinic in order to torture them."[98] Disdain for medical specialization and modern research, a loathing of liberal politics, fear of the deliberate spread of contagion by Jews, and disgust with philosemitism all became ingredients in an intoxicating brew of hatred that fortified the ambitions of antisemitic propagandists.

World War I witnessed the entire German medical profession, from students to distinguished professors, rally to the call of national duty.[99] The overall impact of the war was that it brutalized many physicians to a point that they abandoned compassion, very often leading them to a crude Darwinian view of life and a subsequent affiliation with right-wing political causes. Also, the intensely hierarchical character and militaristic caste that medicine in the empire had displayed was reinforced by the war experience. Finally, of all the medical specialties, surgery emerged from the war as the most celebrated. The surgeon was akin to the soldier in that he carried out his duty amid the bloody and appalling conditions of the trenches. Thus, surgery was viewed as an especially masculine medical undertaking, whereas other "Jewish" specialties such as internal medicine, dermatology, ophthalmology, urology, and psychiatry were feminized.[100]

Naturally, Jews fared poorly in the post-war gendering of German medicine. In addition to the general feminization of the Jewish male (discussed in Chapter 4), during World War I, Jews were identified by enemies on the right as shirkers and war profiteers, and Jewish doctors were devalued. There were fewer surgeons among them, their specialties were considered unheroic, and they were tarred with the conspiratorial brush that painted all Jews as responsible for Germany's defeat.[101]

After the war, radical antisemitism became a constitutive force in German political and cultural life.[102] Born amid the impact of military defeat and left-wing revolution, the Weimar Republic was beset by political, social, economic, and cultural crises that made it an especially weak and fragile political organism from the beginning. For German doctors in the Weimar Republic, the economic outlook was precarious. Sharing the generic difficulties of readjusting to post-war society common to all veterans, German physicians were confronted with professional overcrowding, insufficient numbers of patients, an intergenerational battle between younger and older physicians scrambling for those patients, and a decline in earnings. The impact of this immediate crisis, combined with the fact of long-term hostility to Jews in German medicine, caused German doctors to become the most easily and eagerly nazified of any professional group. It is estimated that around 50 percent of all German doctors became members of the Nazi Party.[103]

All the ancient ideas about the medical malfeasance of Jewish doctors, which became part of the stock-in-trade arsenal of nineteenth-century Volkish antisemites, later occupied a significant place in the canon of Nazi beliefs.[104] The persecution of Jewish doctors by the Third Reich has been well documented by historians.[105] My aim is not to recall the details of Nazi policy but merely to outline the process that brought to an end the history of Jewish medical practice in Germany.[106] Above all, the goal of this chapter has been to suggest that German resentment over the success of Jewish doctors and the discrimination and then outright persecution they suffered at the hands of the Nazis was not something that was created de novo by Hitler. Rather, Nazi policy must be seen in the larger context of the place of Jews in German medicine and the vociferous campaign that was mounted against them at the end of the nineteenth century. Finally, the economic distress experienced in Germany from 1928 to 1932 saw the average annual taxable income of physicians decline by 34 percent. German doctors seized the opportunity to plunder afforded by Hitler's accession to power.

On April 5, 1933, Hitler met with Alfons Stauder, the elected head of Germany's two most important medical associations, the Hartmannbund and the German Medical Association. At the meeting, Stauder pledged to the chancellor the loyalty of the nation's doctors, promising him that they were determined to do their bit to build "an authentic racial community (*einer wahren Volksgemeinschaft*) based on the ideas of the National Socialist seizure of power (*nationale Erhebung*)." He also explained to Hitler the economic hardships physicians experienced, and the advantages to be accrued from the dismissal of Jewish doctors. For his part, Hitler responded by laying out his vision for the purification, both physical and intellectual, of the German people. This, he claimed, would come about with the "removal of the Jewish influence on the nation's cultural and intellectual life." The results of the meeting were soon published on the front page of Nazi Germany's leading nontechnical medical journal, the *Deutsches Ärzteblatt*. The promise of economic spoils to come in the wake of the "removal of Jewish influence" met with resounding editorial approval: "The Chancellor recognized the economic distress and hardship often existing in the medical community and especially among its young doctors. By energetic actions to remove racially

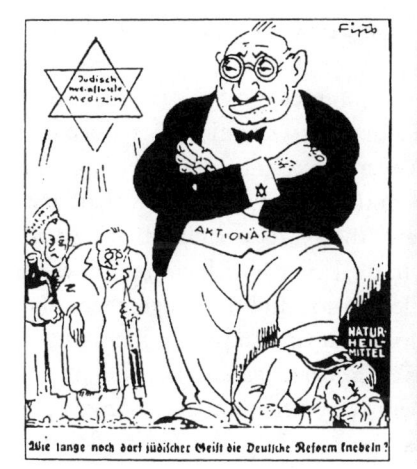

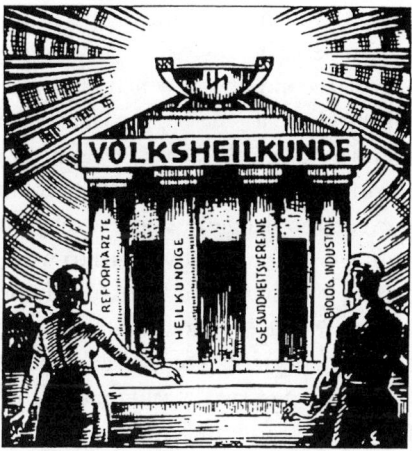

FIGURE 14. These two illustrations appeared in the Nazi periodical *Deutsche Volksgesundheit aus Blut und Boden* (1934). Left: A corpulent Jewish doctor with the word "Stockholder" on his vest, a reference to the fact that ever since the Middle Ages, Jewish doctors in Germany had been accused of practicing medicine for financial gain. The result of the alleged commercialization of medicine by the Jews was that innocent Germans were crushed underfoot, as is the Nazi preference for "Natural Healing," the words that appear above the head of the German. On the left are two aged, university-trained Jewish doctors, and above them a Star of David containing the words "Jewish influenced medicine." Right: A Nazi building with the words "People's Medicine" emblazoned on the front. Before this temple stand two healthy Germans, warmed by the liberating rays of "Natural Healing." Source: Courtesy of the Institute for the History of Medicine of the Robert Bosch Foundation, Stuttgart.

alien elements, employment opportunities and a space to exist must be generated for these young Germans."[107] Within one year, the income of German physicians had risen 11.3 percent. By 1934 their annual taxable income had increased by 25 percent.[108] Persecution paid off.

Essentially, the program of National Socialist discrimination against Jewish doctors occurred in three stages. In the first phase, beginning with the Nazi assumption of power in 1933, Jewish physicians were expelled from the national insurance scheme and were replaced with "Aryan" doctors who had long sought a way into the system. This essentially signaled the end of financially viable Jewish medical practices, because Jewish physicians were largely restricted to treating Jews. The Nuremberg Laws of 1935 further contributed to the miserable lot of Jewish physicians in that the Reich Physicians' Ordinance forbade the licensing of any new doctors of full or partial Jewish descent.

The second phase, which began in the summer of 1938, saw the decertification of all Jewish physicians. The aim was to significantly reduce the number of Jewish doctors treating the ever decreasing and increasingly ill Jewish population. In order to maintain minimum standards of hygiene and prevent the dangerous spread of disease, the Nazis permitted very small numbers of Jewish physicians to work in the larger Jewish communities of Berlin, Hamburg, and Frankfurt. In order to more fully humiliate them, the Nazis forbade Jews to call themselves "physicians," compelling them to use the more degrading term, "sick-treaters" (*Krankenbehändler*).

Following Kristallnacht, in November 1938, when hundreds of Jews were beaten and thousands more suffered psychological trauma, Jewish doctors were simply unable to provide sufficient care for their co-religionists. In 1933 there were approximately 5,500 Jewish doctors in Germany. Owing to emigration, forced retirement, incarceration, suicide, death, and murder, the number of Jewish physicians remaining in Germany by early 1939 was a mere 285. German Jewry was dying.

In the final phase, which covered the war years, health care for Jews was confined to the few remaining Jewish hospitals the Nazis had permitted to remain open.[109] Eventually, even these institutions, with the exception of the Jewish Hospital in Berlin, were closed down and the staffs, together with their patients, were deported to ghettos and death camps in the East. There, until their own deaths, Jewish doctors and nurses continued to administer treatment to the sick and dying Jews as best they could.

# CONCLUSION

As part of their war of extermination against European Jewry, the Nazis obliterated the prolonged and intense German Jewish involvement with medicine. Never to be recaptured, the historical moment had passed, and the intimate relationship, once so intense, had come to an end. Stretching from the Middle Ages to the Holocaust, the Jewish engagement with medicine was truly reflective of Jewish life and values. Because Judaism regards the physical and mental well-being of its adherents as a sine qua non of a religiously fulfilled and fulfilling experience, the sages of antiquity saw the doctor as playing a vital role. For this reason, physicians had long been esteemed figures in Jewish society, and the eagerness with which their services were sought — an oft-attested-to Jewish characteristic — was regarded as an expression of the fundamental tenets of Judaism. In fact, the cultural and social world of the Jewish people was dominated by a sense that the doctor was an asset to society, and a partner of God.

Yet in a truly symbiotic way, medicine was not only reflective of Jewish ideals, but also came to shape the Jewish value system. In Germany, the first Jewish intellectuals to reject a life of Torah study chose instead the practice of medicine. In so doing, they positioned themselves, if only initially in their own minds, in opposition to the army of Jewish lay health care providers. Although no more capable of effecting cures than the average *feldsher*, these men — who eschewed Hebrew incantations, the use of amulets, and folk practices — thus rendered those who did employ them as the bearers of superstition. Consequently, the turn to medicine betokened the emergence of the modern Jew with critical sensibilities. As an exponent of science and its epistemological underpinnings, the Jewish doctor was a harbinger of modernity.

As such, he was always potentially subversive of tradition. Therefore, Jewish communal elders in seventeenth-century Germany were not alto-

## CONCLUSION

gether wrong to suspect physicians of spreading modern ideas to their patients. To alter religious practice was to undermine it and along with it, the very political system that made Jewish society function. And so it was for this reason that physicians were prohibited from serving as lay leaders on communal boards until they were advanced in years.

With the eventual breakdown of traditional Jewish society in Germany in the eighteenth century, it became impossible for the leadership to unilaterally prevent change. Instead, change would have to be sanctioned or rejected by the people. The initial fears of the leadership were justified when, during the *Haskalah* and just beyond, doctors did indeed advocate changes to Jewish ritual based on reasons grounded in medical science. Although suggestions to forestall burial for a period of seventy-two hours met with stern rejection, as did the nineteenth-century proposal from a small number of Jews that animals be stunned prior to slaughter, other innovations such as the abolition of unmediated *metsitsah* became standard for the performance of *brit milah*. Thus did Jewish physicians play an important role in the debates over and the process of the modernization and secularization of German Jewry.

Just as their early modern forerunners had turned to medicine in order to seek a nonrabbinic path to communal honor, the sons of fin-de-siècle Jewish merchants became doctors partly in order to achieve a distinctly modern form of respectability. In so doing they positioned themselves to ride the wave of honor and prestige that modern society accords science and scientists. "Not everything was ideal in Imperial Germany," recalled the German Jewish geneticist Richard Goldschmidt, "but certainly science and its makers were ranked near the top of society."[1] And in Germany, which was preeminent in most branches of medicine at the turn of the twentieth century, the Jews were successful and ubiquitous.

An important handful could even enjoy international fame. Although all the Nobel Prizes and other honors for medicine received by German Jews had been won because the recipients were brilliant scientists and not because of anything to do with their Jewishness, German Jewry celebrated their achievements. The accolades bestowed upon the laureates were interpreted as acclamation for German Jewish civilization itself. Similarly, medicine helped inculcate among German Jewry a self-confidence that was sustaining and energizing.

Moreover, medicine helped facilitate the project of Jewish embourgeoisement. Despite the increasing economic hardships faced by German doctors, medicine continued to enable the upward mobility of Jews. Re-

## CONCLUSION

spected by their patients, and financially comfortable, Jewish physicians were able to live the German Jewish dream. That is to say, they would be accorded their due as practitioners of a universal art, for medicine was seen as one of the most promising avenues for Jews who sought so valiantly to be accepted as good Germans and good Europeans. In this way, they could, to paraphrase a contemporary appellation, be "German scientists of the Mosaic persuasion." Thus even when used for the most parochial of causes, such as justifying Jewish ritual, medicine was regarded by Jewish physicians at the time as an expression of a universal truth. Consequently, they tended to see themselves as citizens of the world and not, as Freud had said in another context, as participants in a "Jewish national affair."

But all Jews who practiced medicine in modern Germany, whether as a personal means to economic security or for the greater Jewish good, by working in a Jewish hospital, researching Jewish pathologies, or defending Jewish ritual, were indeed participants in a Jewish national affair. Most overtly, some Jews used medicine to promote political agendas that were distinctly products of the modern age.

Beginning in the eighteenth century, medicine was harnessed to the quest for civic emancipation. To sustain their own ideological and propagandistic needs, some *maskilic* physicians ridiculed a host of Jewish behaviors that they declared unhealthy. They were also among the first doctors to manufacture the stereotype of Jews as being at medical risk—despite the absence of any real evidence proving that Jews were less healthy than non-Jews. Similarly, at the end of the nineteenth century, although medical opinion almost unanimously concurred that Jews were less ravaged by disease than were their non-Jewish neighbors, Jews and non-Jews representing a host of political persuasions constructed an elaborate and, one might say, enduring image of diaspora Jews as weak and unhealthy.

It is ironic and instructive that the Zionists, like the maskilim before them, also tended to manufacture an image of Jews as sickly and in need of regeneration. This impulse is not, therefore, the consequence of something inherent or peculiar to Zionist thinking. Rather, it is a measure of the deep-rooted nature of the stereotype. Maskilim and Zionists diagnosed the Jewish condition similarly, although, to be sure, they offered radically different prescriptions for cure. Yet even they were joined by representatives from the assimilationist camp. In 1897, industrialist Walter Rathenau exhorted Jews to "look at yourselves in the mirror! This is the first step toward self-criticism. . . . As soon as you have recognized your unathletic build, your narrow shoulders, your clumsy feet, your sloppy roundish shape, you will

## CONCLUSION

resolve to dedicate a few generations to the renewal of your outer appearance."[2] It is testament to the malleability of medical discourse that representatives of Jewish political camps so far removed from one another could reach such fundamental agreement on the Jewish body.

All this has had important consequences for both Israeli politics and culture. The impact of the stereotype that began to be created in the eighteenth century is still very much with us, and continues to shape an important part of the Israel–Diaspora relationship in myriad cultural, psychological, economic, and political ways. The modern physical and psychological self-image of Jews both inside and outside Israel has been conditioned by the way competing Jewish ideologies have made use of medicine ever since the Haskalah.

More than just an objective-scientific undertaking, as doctors a century ago would have seen it, medicine also proved a worthy weapon of defense against those who sought to degrade Judaism. In the face of rising antisemitism in the late nineteenth century, Jewish doctors rallied to the cause, defending Judaism in ways starkly different, but equally impassioned and vigorous as medieval rabbis engaged in religious disputations. The specifically Jewish intellectual framework within which pre-modern Jewish physicians operated had certainly weakened in the modern age, its place having been taken by new Jewish concerns, ones spurred on by antisemitism, Jewish nationalism, professional identity, secularization, modernization, and embourgeoisement. It was these new interests and concerns that emerged to underpin the work of German Jewish doctors well into the twentieth century.

Following World War II, the focal points of Jewish life have become Israel and the United States. Consequently, those are the two countries with the greatest number of Jewish doctors, and where the majority of research into "Jewish" diseases take place. But in those countries, the historical context is so very different from what we have described as having taken place in Germany that it would be wrong to say the story we have told here merely continues in these new venues. To be sure, there are points of connection, but what is absent is the political and cultural dimension that determined the history of Jewish medicine in Germany.

For example, a preference for Jewish physicians by the lay and clerical elite does not characterize Gentile values and desires in the United States, and medicine is not a means to attain a sense of belonging for Jews in America. No longer shut out of the establishment, Jews can express their devoted citizenship through high-level participation in the political and military life of the United States in ways that were unimaginable in German-speaking Europe. Needless to say, this situation is even truer in Israel, where medicine—while a highly desirable occupation for one's children and is thus in keeping with age-old values—is a pursuit completely removed from questions involving Jewish identity, citizenship, and belonging.

This book has attempted to address the observation of nineteenth-century Scottish philosopher William Hamilton that "philosophy and medicine have been always too much viewed independently of each other." My aim has been to identify an episode in the history of medicine and in Jewish history when medicine and philosophy (read ideology or ethnicity) were indeed codependents. That is to say, that by studying the role of medicine among the Jews of Germany, and the attitudes of Germans toward Jewish physicians, we are afforded revealing insights into the subjective nature of medicine, and the social and perceptual space occupied by Jews in German society. For example, we have been able to note the impact of religion and nationalism on medicine. In both the medieval and modern periods, first in the name of Christianity and later in that of Aryan Germanism, Jewish doctors were reviled. In 1938 the rabid Nazi Julius Streicher published the following poem in his newspaper, *Der Stürmer*. In it, older anti-Judaism and modern racist antisemitism come together in an unholy union of hate aimed at the German Jewish physician:

> Den Judenarzt im deutschen Land
> hat uns der Teufel hergesandt.
> Und wie der Teufel schändet er
> die deutsche Frau, die deutsche Ehr.
> Das deutsche Volk wird nicht gesunden,
> wenn es nicht bald den Weg gefunden
> zu deutscher Heilkunst, deutschem Sinn,
> zum deutschen Arzte fürderhin.[3]

[The Jewish doctor in Germany has been sent to us by the Devil.
And just as the Devil endangers, so does the Jewish doctor damage German women and German honor.
The German people will not be made well unless they soon find a way to German medicine, German thinking, and German doctors.]

In the end, it was such magical thinking that prevailed in Germany, unleashing a murderous antisemitism that had been informed by biological notions drawn from modern medicine. Moreover, physicians played a central role in the Holocaust. And yet that story does not conclude with the

## CONCLUSION

destruction of the Third Reich in 1945. Seeking desperately to ensure the good name of German medicine, the country's post-war medical establishment still refuses to come to terms with its Nazi past.[4] Those German physicians who have called for an accounting of this have been subjected to scorn and ostracism at the hands of the German Physicians' Chamber, the leading professional organization of its kind. In contrast, Nazi physicians were reintegrated into post-war German society, often going on to enjoy prestigious careers. Of the some 200,000 physicians in Germany today, only about 300 are Jewish. All that remains of this once intimate relationship is its history.

# NOTES

### INTRODUCTION

1. Judith Walzer Leavitt, "Medicine in Context: A Review Essay of the History of Medicine," *American Historical Review* 95 (1990): 1471–1484.
2. For modern German-speaking Europe, Sander Gilman's foundational work stands out as an exception to the norm.
3. Howard Eilberg-Schwartz, *People of the Body: Jews and Judaism from an Embodied Perspective* (Albany: State University of New York Press, 1992).
4. Heinrich Loewe, *Die Juden in der katholischen Legende* (Berlin: Jüdischer Verlag, 1912), 31. There is a large literature on Jews and hemorrhoids, wherein their proclivity to the disorder was first established in the Middle Ages and repeated into the twentieth century. For the medieval period, the charge needs to be seen in the larger context of claims that Jews used blood for ritual purposes. See H. Kroner, "Die Hämorrhoiden in der Medizin des XII. und XIII. Jahrhunderts," *Janus* 16 (1911): 441–456, 644–718; Julius Aronius, *Regesten zur Geschichte der Juden im fränkischen und deutschen Reiche bis zum Jahre 1273* (Hildesheim: Georg Olms, 1970), no. 728; Joshua Trachtenberg, *Devil and the Jews: The Medieval Conception of the Jew and Its Relation to Modern Anti-Semitism* (Philadelphia: Jewish Publication Society, 1983), 140–155; Harry Friedenwald, *Jews and Medicine* vol. 2 (Baltimore: Johns Hopkins University Press, 1944), 527; H. J. Zimmels, *Magicians, Theologians and Doctors: Studies in Folk-Medicine and Folklore as Reflected in the Rabbinical Responsa, 12th–19th Centuries* (London: E. Goldston, 1952), 91–92; Peter Biller, "Views of Jews from Paris Around 1300: Christian or Scientific?" *Studies in Church History* 29 (1992): 187–207. For modern claims see Elcan Isaac Wolf, *Von den Krankheiten der Juden* (Mannheim: C.F. Schwann, 1777), 84; Maurice Fishberg, *The Jews: A Study of Race and Environment* (New York: Walter Scott Publishing, 1911), 305; Julius Moses Gutmann, *Über den heutigen Stand der Rasse- und Krankheitsfrage der Juden* (Munich: Rudolph Müller & Steinicke, 1920), 38; and Samuel Weissenberg, "Zur Sozialbiologie und Sozialhygiene der Juden," *Archiv für Rassen- und Gesellschaftsbiologie* 19 (1927): 410.

5. Mental illness, diabetes, and alcoholism are dealt with in detail in chapters four and five below. On cancer and the Jews in European medical literature before World War II see the entry "Cancer" by Maurice Fishberg in *The Jewish Encyclopedia* (New York: Funk and Wagnalls, 1904), 3: 529–531; Adolf Theilhaber, "Zur Lehre von der Entstehung der Uterustumoren," *Münchener medizinische Wochenschrift* 56 (1909): 1272–1273; Felix Theilhaber, "Zur Lehre von dem Zusammenhang der sozialen Stellung und der Rasse mit der Entstehung der Uteruscarcinome." (Inaugural dissertation. Munich: K.K. Ludwigs-Maximilians Universität, 1910); Sigismund Peller, "Über Krebssterblichkeit der Juden," *Zeitschrift für Krebsforschung* 34 (1931): 128–147; Maurice Sorsby, *Cancer and Race: A Study of the Incidence of Cancer Among Jews* (London: John Bale, Sons & Danielsson, 1931); I. Davidsohn, "Cancer Among Jews," *Medical Leaves* 2 (1939): 19–27; and Sander L. Gilman, *Freud, Race and Gender* (Princeton: Princeton University Press, 1993), 169–179.

6. See John Efron, *Defenders of the Race: Jewish Doctors and Race Science in Fin-de-Siècle Europe* (New Haven: Yale University Press, 1994); and Sander Gilman, *The Jews' Body* (New York: Routledge, 1991).

7. Anonymous, "Was und wie im Judenthume reformirt werden soll," *Allgemeine Zeitung des Judentums* 9, 21 (1845): 309–311.

8. A. D. Gordon, "People and Labor," in *The Zionist Idea,* ed. Arthur Hertzberg (New York: Atheneum, 1984), 372–374.

9. See Joachim Doron, "Rassenbewusstsein und naturwissenschaftliches Denken im deutschen Zionismus während der wilhelminischen Ära," *Jahrbuch des Instituts für deutsche Geschichte* 9 (1980): 389–427.

10. See the programmatic speech by Max Mandelstamm, "Rede Dr. Max Mandelstamms," *Die Welt* 4, 35 (1900): 1–7; Siegmund Kornfeld, "Die jüdischen Aerzte und der Zionismus," *Die Welt* 5, 16 (1901): 1–3; Balduin Groller, "Die körperliche Minderwertigkeit der Juden," *Die Welt* 5, 16 (1901): 3–5; Karl Jeremias, "Die körperliche Minderwertigkeit der Juden," *Die Welt* 5, 18 (1901): 3–5. For the use of metaphors drawn from contemporary psychiatry, see Leon Pinsker, *Auto-Emancipation* (New York: Federation of American Zionists, 1916); and Hans-Peter Söder, "Disease and Health as Contexts of Modernity: Max Nordau as a Critic of Fin-de-Siècle Modernism," *German Studies Review,* 14, 3 (1991): 473–487.

11. David Biale, *Power and Powerlessness in Jewish History* (New York: Schocken, 1986); Ezra Mendelsohn, *On Modern Jewish Politics* (New York: Oxford University Press, 1993); Alan Dowty, *The Jewish State: A Century Later* (Berkeley: University of California Press, 1998), 20.

12. Thorstein Veblen, "The Intellectual Pre-eminence of Jews in Modern Europe," in *The Portable Veblen,* ed. Max Lerner (New York: Viking Press, 1950), 467–479. The quotations appear on pp. 474–475. For a general appraisal of Jewish scientific success at the turn of the century see Siegmund Kaznelson, ed., *Juden*

*im deutschen Kulturbereich; Ein Sammelwerk,* 2nd ed. (Berlin: Jüdischer Verlag, 1959); Lewis Samuel Feuer, *The Scientific Intellectual: The Psychological and Sociological Origins of Modern Science* (New York: Basic Books, 1963); David Preston, "Science, Society, and the German Jews: 1870–1933" (Ph.D. Diss., University of Illinois at Urbana-Champaign, 1971); David Nachmannsohn, *German-Jewish Pioneers in Science, 1900–1933: Highlights in Atomic Physics, Chemistry, and Biochemistry* (New York: Springer-Verlag, 1979); and Shulamit Volkov, "Juden als wissenschaftliche 'Mandarine' im Kaiserreich und in der Weimarer Republik," *Archiv für Sozialgeschichte* 37 (1997): 1–18.
13. Quoted in Saul Friedländer, *Nazi Germany and the Jews: The Years of Persecution, 1933–1939,* vol. 1 (New York: Harper Collins, 1997), 226.
14. Robert N. Proctor, *Racial Hygiene: Medicine Under the Nazis* (Cambridge: Harvard University Press, 1988), 251–281.
15. I. J. Singer, *The Family Carnovsky* (New York: Harrow Books, 1973), 75.
16. Friedländer, *Nazi Germany and the Jews,* 226.

## CHAPTER 1. EMERGENCE OF THE MEDIEVAL JEWISH PHYSICIAN

1. On the theology of healing in Judaism see Immanuel Jakabovits, *Jewish Medical Ethics* (New York: Bloch, 1959); Julius Preuss, *Biblical and Talmudic Medicine,* trans. and ed., Fred Rosner (Northvale, NJ: Jason Aronson, 1993); Samuel S. Kottek, "Healing in Jewish Law and Lore" in *Jews and Medicine: Religion, Culture, Science,* ed. Natalia Berger (Tel Aviv: Beth Hatefutsoth, 1995), 33–43; David Margalith, "The Ideal Doctor as Depicted in Ancient Hebrew Writings," *Journal of the History of Medicine* 12, 1 (1957): 37–41; and J. David Bleich, "The Obligation to Heal in the Judaic Tradition: A Comparative Analysis," *Proceedings of the Association of Orthodox Jewish Scientists* 6 (1980): 11–64.
2. Joseph Shatzmiller, *Jews, Medicine, and Medieval Society* (Berkeley: University of California Press, 1994), 1. Shatzmiller claims that medicine as an occupation was second only to money-lending among medieval Jews.
3. See Samuel J. Kottek, "Concepts of Disease in the Talmud," *Koroth* 9, 1–2 (1985): 7–33.
4. Don Bates, ed., *Knowledge and Scholarly Medical Traditions* (Cambridge: Cambridge University Press, 1995). In this volume, which examines the Galenic, Chinese, and Ayurvedic scholarly medical traditions, the contribution of Jews to medical knowledge is not mentioned.
5. Historians contest the date and even place of publication, and there is a rather large literature on the origins of the book. The historiographical debate is summarized in Elinor Lieber, "Asaf's 'Book of Medicines': A Hebrew Encyclopedia of Greek and Jewish Medicine, Possibly Compiled in Byzantium on an Indian Model," *Dumbarton Oaks Papers* 38 (1984): 233–249.
6. See Moritz Steinschneider, *Die hebraeischen Übersetzungen des Mittelalters und*

*die Juden als Dolmetscher* (Berlin: Kommissionsverlag des Bibliographischen Bureaus, 1893), 672–673.

7. K. Codell Carter, "An Illustration of the Religious Foundations of Talmudic Medicine: Tractate Megillah Fol. 27b-28a," *Koroth* 9, 1–2 (1985): 92–98; Avraham Steinberg, "The Contribution of Rabbinic Law to the Understanding of Talmudic Medical Data," *Koroth* 9, 1–2 (1985): 60–72.

8. Quoted in Elliot N. Dorff, "The Jewish Tradition," in *Caring and Curing: Health and Medicine in the Western Religious Traditions,* ed. Ronald L. Numbers and Darrel W. Amundsen (New York: Macmillan, 1986), 21. On Maimonides see David B. Ruderman, *Jewish Thought and Scientific Discovery in Early Modern Europe* (New Haven: Yale University Press, 1995), 29–33.

9. Relative to the amount of historical information on medicine and the Jews in Southern Europe, there is a dearth concerning medicine and the Jews in Germany. See, however, Samuel Krauss, *Geschichte der jüdischen Aerzte vom frühesten Mittelalter bis zur Gleichberechtigung* (Vienna: A.S. Bettelheim-Stiftung, 1930); Jacob Shatzmiller, "Doctors and Medical Practice in Germany around the Year 1200: The Evidence of Sefer Hasidim," *Journal of Jewish Studies* 33 (1982): 583–593; Jacob Shatzmiller, "Doctors and Medical Practice in Germany around the Year 1200: The Evidence of *Sefer Asaph,*" *Proceedings of the American Academy for Jewish Research* 50 (1983):149–164; Moses Alter Spira, "Meilensteine zur Geschichte der jüdischen Ärzte in Deutschland," in *Melemata. Festschrift für Werner Leibbrand zum 70. Geburtstag,* ed. Joseph Schumacher (Mannheim: Mannheimer Grossdruckerei, 1967), 149–158; Peter Assion, "Jakob von Landshut: Zur Geschichte der jüdischen Ärzte in Deutschland," *Sudhoffs Archiv für Wissenschaftsgeschichte* 53, 3 (1969): 270–291; and for England see Cecil Roth, "Jewish Physicians in Medieval England" in *Essays and Portraits in Anglo-Jewish History,* ed. Cecil Roth (Philadelphia: Jewish Publication Society of America, 1962), 46–51.

10. Nancy G. Siraisi, *Medieval and Early Renaissance Medicine: An Introduction to Knowledge and Practice* (Chicago: University of Chicago Press, 1990), 10–13.

11. Max Meyerhof, "Medieval Jewish Physicians in the Near East, from Arabic Sources" in *Studies in Medieval Arabic Medicine,* ed. Penelope Johnstone (London: Valiorum Reprints, 1984), 432–460.

12. Shlomo Dov Goitein, "The Medical Profession in the Light of the Cairo Geniza Documents," *Hebrew Union College Annual* 34 (1963), 181.

13. There is an extensive literature on Maimonides' medical opinions. See the bibliography in Heinrich Schipperges, *Krankheit und Gesundheit bei Maimonides* (Berlin: Springer, 1996), 99–105; and Fred Rosner, *Medicine in the Mishneh Torah of Maimonides* (New York: Ktav, 1984).

14. Despite this fact, there is a glaring absence of references to Jews in the contemporary historiography on the epistemology of medicine. An explanation for this may come from Faith Wallis' general understanding of medieval medical

texts: "Although the great translation movement of the eleventh and twelfth centuries was motivated by a quest for the important texts of Antiquity, even these texts, and *a fortiori* the Arabic works that came in their wake, could never rise higher than the rank of plain texts in the value system of the medieval West" (Wallis, "Texts and Epistemology in Early Medieval Medicine," in *Knowledge and Scholarly Medical Traditions*, ed. Don Bates, 125).

15. Heinrich Schipperges, *Die Assimilation der Arabischen Medizin durch das Lateinische Mittelalter* (Wiesbaden: Franz Steiner, 1964), 127–129.

16. On the development of Hebrew as a language of medical instruction see Süssmann Muntner, *Le-korot ha-leshon ha-Ivrit ki-sefat ha-limud be-hokhmat ha-refuah* (Jerusalem: Leshonenu, 1940). The great enterprise of Jewish translation had ceased by the early part of the thirteenth century. See Shatzmiller, *Jews, Medicine, and Medieval Society*, 38–55, who also has an insightful discussion on the economics of the Hebrew translation project.

17. See Vern L. Bullough, *The Development of Medicine as a Profession* (New York: Hafner, 1966), esp. 93–111; Siraisi, *Medicine*, esp. 13–47. The expression "medicalization of society" is Shatzmiller's *Jews, Medicine, and Medieval Society*, 1–13.

18. Luis García-Ballester, Lola Ferre, and Eduard Feliu, "Jewish Appreciation of Fourteenth-Century Scholastic Medicine," *Osiris* 6 second series (1990): 85–117, esp. 94.

19. Geoffrey Chaucer, *The Prologue to the Canterbury Tales*, trans. Nevill Coghill (Salisbury: Perdix Press, 1984), 50–52.

20. BT Sanhedrin 17b.

21. Cecil Roth, "The Qualification of Jewish Physicians in the Middle Ages," *Speculum* 28 (1953): 834–843; and Shatzmiller, *Jews, Medicine, and Medieval Society*, 23–24.

22. See Shai Sholovitz, "The Image and Status of the Jewish Physician: A Reflection from Jewish Sources," *Koroth* 8 (1984): 463–466; Volker Zimmermann, "Jüdische Ärzte und ihre Beiträge zur Heilkunde des Spätmittelalters," *Koroth* 8 (1985): 245–254; and Volker Zimmermann, "Jüdische Ärzte und ihre Leistungen in der Medizin des Mittelalters," *Würzburger medizinhistorische Mitteilungen* 8 (1990): 201–205.

23. See H. J. Zimmels, *Magicians, Theologians and Doctors: Studies in Folk-medicine and Folk-lore as Reflected in the Rabbinical Responsa 12th–19th Centuries* (London: Edward Goldston & Son, 1952). Zimmels' sources make clear that the currency of medical knowledge among rabbis and doctors was widely circulated.

24. See Edwin Mendelssohn, *The Popes' Jewish Doctors 492–1655 CE* (Lauderhill, FL, n.p., 1991); Isak Münz, *Die jüdischen Aerzte im Mittelalter: Ein Beitrag zur Kulturgeschichte des Mittelalters* (Frankfurt am Main: J. Kauffmann, 1922), 101–102; Simon Scherbel, *Jüdische Ärzte und ihr Einfluss auf das Judentum* (Berlin: J. Singer, 1905), 51; Martin Gumpert and Alfred Joseph, "Medizin" in *Juden im deutschen Kulturbereich: Ein Sammelwerk*, ed. Siegmund Kaznelson (Berlin:

Jüdischer Verlag, 1959), 461; Louis Falstein, ed., *The Martyrdom of Jewish Physicians in Poland* (New York: Exposition Press, 1963), 5–11; and Shatzmiller, *Jews, Medicine, and Medieval Society,* 94.

25. *Jüdisches Lexikon,* vol. 4 (Berlin: Jüdischer Verlag, 1930), 35.

26. Joseph Shatzmiller, "On Becoming a Jewish Doctor in the High Middle Ages," *Sefarad* 43 (1983): 239.

27. See Monica Green, "Women's Medical Practice and Health Care in Medieval Europe," in *Sisters and Workers in the Middle Ages,* ed. Judith M. Bennett, Elizabeth A. Clark, et al. (Chicago: University of Chicago Press, 1989), 39–78. For the numbers, see pp. 45–51.

28. Kallmorgen, *Heilkunde in Frankfurt am Main,* 134.

29. Friedenwald, *Jews and Medicine,* 217.

30. Walther Schönfeld, *Frauen in der abendländischen Heilkunde vom klassischen Altertum bis zum Ausgang des 19. Jahrhunderts* (Stuttgart: Ferdinand Enke, 1947), 75.

31. Münz, *Die jüdischen Ärzte im Mittelalter,* 56–57. On Morada, see Moritz Güdemann, *Geschichte des Erziehungswesens und der Cultur der Juden in Deutschland,* vol. 3 (Vienna: Alfred Hölder, 1888), 113.

32. Interestingly enough, medieval Jewish alchemists were also prized by their Christian counterparts because of their facility with the holy tongue, and the perception of it as esoteric. See Rafael Patai, *The Jewish Alchemists: A History and Sourcebook* (Princeton: Princeton University Press, 1994), 155–156.

33. Quoted in Nicoline Hortzitz, *Der Judenarzt: Historische und sprachliche Untersuchungen zur Diskriminierung eines Berufsstands in der frühen Neuzeit* (Heidelberg: Universitätsverlag C. Winter, 1994), 14.

34. Günther Dammann, *Die Juden in der Zauberkunst: Jüdische Zauberkunstler* (Berlin: n.p., 1933).

35. Walter Scott, *Ivanhoe* (New York: Pocket Library, 1959), 282. I am grateful to Adam Burrows for bringing this reference to my attention.

36. Quoted in Joshua Trachtenberg, *The Devil and the Jews: The Medieval Conception of the Jew and Its Relation to Modern Anti-Semitism* (Philadelphia: Jewish Publication Society, 1983), 65–66.

37. Herman Pollack, *Jewish Folkways in Germanic Lands (1648–1806)* (Cambridge, MA: MIT Press, 1971), 114–115.

38. See Max Grunwald, "Aus Hausapotheke und Hexenküche," *Mitteilungen zur jüdischen Volkskunde* 5, 1 (1900): 1–70; and Max Grunwald, "Aus Hausapotheke und Hexenküche," *Jahrbuch für jüdischen Volkskunde* (1923): 178–226.

39. Joshua Trachtenberg, *Jewish Magic and Superstition: A Study in Folk Religion* (Cleveland: Meridian Books, 1961), 202.

40. Sylvie Anne Goldberg, *Crossing the Jabbok: Illness and Death in Ashkenazi Judaism in Sixteenth through Nineteenth Century Prague* (Berkeley: University of California Press, 1996), 151–156.

41. Trachtenberg, *Jewish Magic and Superstition*, 196.
42. Trachtenberg, *Jewish Magic and Superstition*, 204–206; and Goldberg, *Crossing the Jabbok*, 161–162.
43. Trachtenberg, *Jewish Magic and Superstition*, 195–197, 202. On amulets see Theodore Schrire, *Hebrew Amulets: Their Decipherment and Interpretation* (London: Routledge and Kegan Paul, 1966); Samuel Weissenberg, "Südrussische Amulette," *Verhandlungen der Berliner Gesellschaft für Anthropologie, Ethnologie und Urgeschichte* (1897): 367–369.
44. See Süssmann Muntner, *Alilot el rofim ha-yehudim be-aspaklariya shel toldot ha-refuah* (Jerusalem: Weiss, 1953).
45. Solomon Grayzel, *The Church and the Jews in the XIIIth Century: A Study of Their Relations During the Years 1198–1254, Based on the Papal Letters and the Conciliar Decrees of the Period* (New York: Hermon Press, 1966), 74.
46. Philip Ziegler, *The Black Death* (New York: John Day, 1969), 97–109.
47. Trachtenberg, *Devil and the Jews*, 99. Similar sentiments were heard in the supposedly more tolerant Islamic East. In the thirteenth century, the intemperate al-Jaubari declared: "Their [the Jews'] common people are connected with the apothecary business. . . . They adulterate all the drugs and while nobody pays attention, sell them to the people. . . . Among them are the naturalist physicians, most infidel and hypocritical. They have secrets unknown to anyone else, how to make the distant near and how to make the strong weak. If one wishes to heal a man . . . he will effect it in a couple of days; but if he wants to play a trick on him, he will first neglect to maintain the strength of the patient until it diminishes; then he will prescribe an effective medicine for him for three days, after which he will cause the patient to suffer from some other malady; and so on, thus reaping a rich harvest from the patient." See Moshe Perlmann, "Notes on the Position of Jewish Physicians in Medieval Muslim Countries," *Israel Oriental Studies* 2 (1972): 315–319.
48. Johannes Eck, *Ains Jüden büechlins verlegung* (Ingoldstadt: Alexander Weissenhorn, 1542), Fiiij.
49. Quoted in Leon Poliakov, *The History of Anti-Semitism: From the Time of Christ to the Court Jews* I (New York: Schocken, n.d.), 147.
50. Christopher Marlowe, *The Jew of Malta*, ed. T. W. Craik (London: Ernest Benn, 1979), 46; Bernard Glassman, *Antisemitic Stereotypes Without Jews: Images of Jews in England 1290–1700* (Detroit: Wayne State University Press, 1975), 65–66. On Elizabethan attitudes toward Jews, see the superb study by James S. Shapiro, *Shakespeare and the Jews* (New York: Columbia University Press, 1996).
51. Eliakim Carmoly, "Die jüdischen Aerzte aus Frankfurts Vergangenheit," *Der israelitische Volkslehrer* 6 (1856), 112. Already in the thirteenth century, Alfonso X of Castile had decreed that Christians were not to consume any prescription prepared by a Jew, though a Christian apothecary was permitted to fill the prescription of a Jewish doctor. Michael R. McVaugh, *Medicine Before the Plague:*

*Practitioners and Their Patients in the Crown of Aragon, 1285–1345* (Cambridge: Cambridge University Press, 1993), 59. On pharmacy among the Jews in Central Europe, see Lavoslav Glesinger, "Beiträge zur Geschichte der Pharmazie bei den Juden," *Monatsschrift für Geschichte und Wissenschaft des Judentums* 82, 2 (1938): 111–130; Lavoslav Glesinger, "Weitere Beiträge zur Geschichte der Pharmazie bei den Juden," *Monatsschrift für Geschichte und Wissenschaft des Judentums* 82, 6 (1938): 417–422; and Bruno Kisch, "History of the Jewish Pharmacy (Judenapotheke) in Prague," *Historia Judaica* 8, 2 (1946): 149–180.

52. Otto Stobbe, *Die Juden in Deutschland während des Mittelalters in politischer, socialer und rechtlicher Beziehung* (Braunschweig: C.A. Schwetschke, 1886), 180–181.
53. The quotation reads: "*Es sei besser mit Christo gestorben, als per Juden-Dr. mit dem Teufel gesund worden.*" See Krauss, *Geschichte der jüdischen Aerzte*, 56.
54. Ruderman, *Jewish Thought*, 285–289.
55. Eliakim Carmoly, *History of the Jewish Physicians* (Baltimore: J. Murphy, 1845), 37.
56. Jaime I. Tourtoulon, "Zur Geschichte der Juden in Spanien," *Monatsschrift für Geschichte und Wissenschaft des Judentums* 33 (1884): 501.
57. Yosef Hayim Yerushalmi, *From Spanish Court to Italian Ghetto: Isaac Cardoso. A Study in Seventeenth-Century Marranism and Jewish Apologetics* (Seattle: University of Washington Press, 1981), 70–72; Yosef Kaplan, "Jews and Judaism in the Political and Social Thought of Spain in the Sixteenth and Seventeenth Centuries," in *Antisemitism Through the Ages,* ed. Shmuel Almog (Oxford: Pergamon Press, 1989), 153–160; and Ruderman, *Jewish Thought*, 273–309.
58. Diego Gracia Guillén, "Judaism, Medicine, and the Inquisitorial Mind in Sixteenth-Century Spain," in *The Spanish Inquisition and the Inquisitorial Mind*, ed. Angel Alcala (Highland Lakes, NJ: Atlantic Research and Publications, 1987), 375–400. The quotation appears on p. 375.
59. On the connection between early modern Spanish and Nazi antisemitism see Yosef Hayim Yerushalmi, *Assimilation and Racial Anti-Semitism: The Iberian and the German Models.* Leo Baeck Memorial Lecture, no. 26 (1982).
60. For example, see the extended study of the de Castro family of Hamburg, and other physicians of Sephardic origin in Germany by Meyer Kayserling, "Zur Geschichte der jüdischen Aerzte," *Monatsschrift für Geschichte und Wissenschaft des Judentums* 7 (1858): 393–395; 8 (1859): 161–170, 330–339; 9 (1860): 92–98; 10 (1861): 38–40; 11 (1862): 350–353; 12 (1863): 182–183; 17 (1868): 151–152, 185–188.
61. Harry Friedenwald, *The Jews and Medicine: Essays II* (Baltimore: Johns Hopkins University Press, 1944. Reprint. 1967), 701–771. On Turkey see, Isaac Münz, *Die jüdischen Ärzte im Mittelalter. Ein Beitrag zur Kulturgeschichte des Mittelalters* (Frankfurt: J. Kauffmann, 1922), 71–78; Bernard Lewis, "The Privilege Granted by Mehmet II to His Physician," *Bulletin of the School of Oriental and African Studies* 14 (1952): 550–563; and Uriel Heyd, "Moses Hamon, Chief Jewish Physician to Sultan Süleyman the Magnificent," *Oriens* 16 (1963): 152–

170. Heyd notes that Jewish women with medical knowledge gained free access to the ladies of the harem and the Sultan's family, thus developing their own sources of influence at court. On Holland, see Hindle S. Hes, *Jewish Physicians in the Netherlands 1600–1940* (Assen: Van Gorcum, 1980). For Poland see Majer Balaban, *Juedische Aerzte und Apotheker aus Italien und Spanien in XVI. und XVII. Jahrhundert in Krakau* (Czernowitz: Buckdruckerei Gutenberg, 1912).
62. Friedenwald, *The Jews and Medicine: Essays II*, 551–612.
63. For what follows on Italy, I rely principally on David B. Ruderman, "The Impact of Science on Jewish Culture and Society in Venice (With Special Reference to Jewish Graduates of Padua's Medical School)," in *Essential Papers on Jewish Culture in Renaissance and Baroque Italy*, ed. David B. Ruderman (New York: New York University Press, 1992), 520–521. For an intimate portrait of an Italian Jewish physician of the Renaissance, see David B. Ruderman, *Kabbalah, Magic, and Science: The Cultural Universe of a Sixteenth-Century Jewish Physician* (Cambridge, MA: Harvard University Press, 1988). On Padua's medical school see Jerome J. Bylebyl, "The School of Padua: Humanistic Medicine in the Sixteenth Century," in *Health, Medicine, and Mortality in the Sixteenth Century*, ed. Charles Webster (Cambridge: Cambridge University Press, 1979), 335–370.
64. See Ruderman, *Jewish Thought*, 109; Jacob Shatzky, "On Jewish Medical Students of Padua," *Journal of the History of Medicine* 5 (1950): 444–447; and N. M. Gelber, "On the History of Jewish Doctors in Poland in the 18th Century" in *Shai le-Yishayahu* [jubilee volume in honor of Isaiah Wolfsberg] [Hebrew] (Tel Aviv: Ha-Merkaz le-Tarbut shel ha-Poel ha-Mizrachi, 1956), 347–371.
65. Ruderman, *Jewish Thought*, 113–114.
66. Ruderman, *Jewish Thought*, 105. The figure of 320 represents a sharp increase from the 29 Jewish students who studied medicine at Padua between 1520 and 1605.
67. Ruderman, "Impact of Science on Jewish Culture," 521–522.
68. Quoted in Ruderman, "Impact of Science on Jewish Culture," 535.
69. Ruderman, "Impact of Science on Jewish Culture," 536.
70. David B. Ruderman, "Science, Medicine and Jewish Culture in Early Modern Europe" (reprint of Spiegel Lecture in European Jewish History, Tel Aviv University, 1987), 17–18. Most recently, Ruderman has persuasively argued for the enduring and transformative impact on Jewish culture of both Isserles' and especially the Maharal's views of nature and science by their having demanded the inclusion of the study of nature in the Central and Eastern European Jewish curriculum. Especially crucial was their having sundered the link between physics and metaphysics. See Ruderman, *Jewish Thought*, 54–99. For more on science among Jews in Central and Eastern Europe in the early modern period see David E. Fishman, *Russia's First Modern Jews: The Jews of Shklov* (New York:

New York University Press, 1995); Joseph M. Davis, "Rabbi Yom Tov Lipman Heller, Joseph ben Isaac ha-Levi, and Rationalism in Ashkenazic Culture, 1550–1650" (Ph.D. Diss., Harvard University, 1990); and Andre Neher, *Jewish Thought and the Scientific Revolution of the Sixteenth Century: David Gans (1541–1613) and His Times* (Oxford: Oxford University Press, 1986).

71. On del Bene and Figo see Ruderman, *Jewish Thought*, 185–212.
72. Carmoly, "Frankfurts Vergangenheit," 111.

### CHAPTER 2. JEWISH PHYSICIANS: IN AND OUT OF THE GERMAN GHETTO

1. Archbishop Arno's Jewish doctor is mentioned in Julius Aronius, *Regesten zur Geschichte der Juden im fränkischen und deutschen Reiche bis zum Jahre 1273* (Hildesheim: Georg Olms, 1970), 29–30. More generally, on medieval Jewish doctors in Germany see Krauss, *Geschichte der jüdischen Aerzte*, 26–39.
2. Joseph Shatzmiller suggests the international dimensions of medieval Jewish medicine in his "Doctors and Medical Practice in Germany around the Year 1200: The Evidence of *Sefer Asaph*," *Proceedings of the American Academy of Jewish Research* 50 (1983): 149–164. On Jewish medical dynasties in Germany see, for example, David Kaufmann, "Hundert Jahre aus einer Familie Jüdischer Aerzte—Sr. Leo, dr. Jakob, dr. Isak, dr. Wold Winkler," *Allgemeine Zeitung des Judentums* 52 (1890): 468–471; and H. Schultze, "Geschichte der Familie Wallich," *Monatsschrift für Geschichte und Wissenschaft des Judentums* 49 (1905): 57–77, 183–192, 272–285, 450–458.
3. Shatzmiller, "*Sefer Asaph*," 152.
4. Shatzmiller, "*Sefer Asaph*," 163.
5. For what follows, I rely principally on Joseph Shatzmiller, "Doctors and Medical Practice in Germany around the Year 1200: The Evidence of *Sefer Hasidim*," *Journal of Jewish Studies* 33 (1982): 583–593.
6. The two examples are to be found in Shatzmiller, "Doctors and Medical Practice in Germany," 593.
7. H. J. Zimmels, *Magicians, Theologians and Doctors: Studies in Folk-Medicine and Folk-Lore as Reflected in the Rabbinical Responsa 12th–19th Centuries* (London: Goldston, 1952) 140–141.
8. On the complementarity of mysticism and science in the Italian setting, see Ruderman, *Kabbalah, Magic, and Science*.
9. J. E. Scherer, *Die Rechtsverhältnisse der Juden in den deutsch-österreichischen Ländern* (Leipzig: Duncker & Humblot, 1901), 41. Scherer lists synods and church councils between the years 692 and 1434 at which it was declared and reiterated that Christians were not to seek medical attention from Jews, nor take their medicines. This particular rule was changed from time to time. For example, in 1090, in the charter granted by Emperor Henry IV to the Jewish community of Speyer confirming the rights and privileges granted to the Jews in 1084,

article 14 reads: "... [the Jews] have the right to sell their wine and their dyes and *their medicines* to Christians" [my italics]. See Robert Chazan, *Church State and Jew in the Middle Ages* (West Orange, NJ: Behrman House, 1980), 62.

10. On the Christian body see Caroline Walker Bynum, *Holy Feast and Holy Fast: The Religious Significance of Food to Medieval Women* (Berkeley: University of California Press, 1987); Caroline Walker Bynum, *Fragmentation and Redemption: Essays on Gender and the Human Body in Medieval Religion* (New York: Zone Books, 1991); and Frank Bottomley, *Attitudes Toward the Body in Western Christendom* (London: Lepus Books, 1979).

11. See Ernst Königer, *Aus der Geschichte der Heilkunst. Von Ärzten, Badern und Chirurgen* (Munich: Prestel, 1958), 15; Hans Christoffel, "Grundzüge der Uroskopie," *Gesnerus* 10 (1953): 89–122; Walter Wüthrich, *Die Harnschau und ihr Verschwinden* (Zurich: Juris Verlag, 1967); Friedrich von Zglinicki, *Die Uroskopie in der bildenden Kunst: Eine kunst- und medizinhistorische Untersuchung über die Harnschau* (Darmstadt: Ernst Giebeler, 1982); and Thomas Schlich, "Das Uringlas als Erkennungsmerkmal des gelehrten Arztes. Harndiagnostik und ärztlicher Stand im Mittelalter," *Spektrum der Nephrologie* 5 (1992): 3–9. German-language urine-inspection manuals were also published for the benefit of surgeons who had not had university training and could not read Latin. See Ortrun Riha and Wiltrud Fischer, "Harndiagnostik bei Isaak Judaeus, Gilles des Corbeil und Ortolf von Baierland," *Sudhoffs Archiv* 72 (1988): 212–224.

12. Yehoshua O. Leibowitz, "Town Physicians in Jewish Social History," in *International Symposium on Society, Medicine and Law. Jerusalem, March 1972* (Amsterdam: Elsevier Scientific Publishing, 1973), 117–124.

13. The names of others are to be found in Krauss, *Geschichte der jüdischen Aerzte*, 31–32. On Jacob of Strasbourg and other references to the history of Jewish medical practice in Frankfurt, see Wilhelm Kallmorgen, *Siebenhundert Jahre Heilkunde in Frankfurt am Main* (Franfurt am Main: Moritz Diesterweg, 1936), 133–138.

14. On medieval clerical attitudes toward Jewish physicians see Ludwig Kotelmann, *Gesundheitspflege im Mittelalter. Kulturgeschichtliche Studien nach Predigten des 13., 14. und 15 Jahrhunderts* (Hamburg: Voss, 1890), 193–195.

15. K. Baas, "Jüdische Hospitäler im Mittelalter," *Monatsschrift für Geschichte und Wissenschaft des Judentums* (new edition) 21 (1913): 452–460; and Alexander Philipsborn, "The Jewish Hospitals in Germany," *Leo Baeck Institute Yearbook* 4 (1959): 220–234.

16. Jacob R. Marcus, *Communal Sick-Care in the German Ghetto* (Cincinnati: Hebrew Union College Press, 1947), 6–9.

17. For an example of the fund-raising concerns and measures adopted by an Ashkenazic community concerning the ill among them, see the Amsterdam Broadside, January 3, 1801, written in Judeo-German and reprinted in Marcus, *Communal Sick-Care*, 235–237.

18. Benjamin Hirsch Auerbach, *Geschichte der israelitischen Gemeinde Halberstadt* (Halberstadt: H. Meyer, 1866), 203.
19. See Richard Landau, *Geschichte der jüdischen Ärzte* (Berlin: S. Karger, 1895), 109–110.
20. In the seventeenth century, independent Jewish physicians were to be found in many places, among them Frankfurt am Main, Hamburg-Altona, Mannheim, and Prague.
21. Johann Hermann Baas, *Die geschichtliche Entwicklung des ärztlichen Standes und der medizinischen Wissenschaft* (Wiesbaden: Martin Sändig, 1967), 255.
22. Marcus, *Communal Sick-Care*, 246.
23. Louis Lewin, "Jüdische Aerzte in Grosspolen," *Jahrbuch der jüdisch-literarischen Gesellschaft* 9 (1911): 409–410; Louis Lewin, *Geschichte der Juden in Lissa* (Pinne: N. Gundermann, 1904), 156.
24. Marcus, *Communal Sick-Care*, 28–29.
25. Louis Lewin, *Geschichte der israelitischen Kranken-Verpflegungs-Anstalt und Beerdigungs-Gesellschaft zu Breslau, 1726–1926* (Breslau: T. Schatzky, 1926), 113–114; and Marcus' translation of the contract, *Communal Sick-Care*, 242–244.
26. M. Horovitz, "Jüdische Aerzte in Frankfurt a.M.," *Beilage zum Jahresbericht der israelitische Religionsschule* (1886), 27; Isidor Kracauer, *Geschichte der Juden in Frankfurt am Main (1150–1824)*, vol. 2 (Frankfurt am Main: I. Kauffmann, 1925–1927), 266; and Marcus, *Communal Sick-Care*, 29–32. On the role of the *parnas* and the structure of the community councils see Jacob Katz, *Tradition and Crisis: Jewish Society at the End of the Middle Ages* (New York: Schocken, 1993), 68–71.
27. For general background see Mary Lindemann, *Medicine and Society in Early Modern Europe* (Cambridge: Cambridge University Press, 1999).
28. David Ruderman has been the most forceful proponent of this view. See his *Jewish Thought*. In addition, see Eliot Horowitz, "The Eve of Circumcision: A Chapter in the History of Jewish Nightlife," in *Essential Papers on Jewish Culture in Renaissance and Baroque Italy*, ed. David B. Ruderman (New York: New York University Press, 1992), 554–588; and Eliot Horowitz, "Coffee-Houses and Nocturnal Rituals of Early Modern Jewry," *Association for Jewish Studies Review* 14 (1989): 17–46.
29. David E. Fishman, "Science, Enlightenment and Rabbinic Culture in Belorussian Jewry: 1772–1804" (Ph.D. Diss., Columbia University, 1985), 16. For what follows, I rely principally on Fishman and the following works: Emanuel Ringelblum, *Kapitln geshikhte fun amolikn yidishn leben in Poyln* [Yiddish] (Buenos Aires: Tsentral farband fun poylishe Yidn in Argentina, 1953), 183–386; N. M. Gelber, "Jewish Doctors in Poland," in *Jewish Physicians in Poland*, ed. Louis Falstein, 3–48; P. Kon, "Eyner fun di ershter yidishe doktoyrim in Vilne," *YIVO Bleter* 1 (1931), 53–61.

30. Fishman, "Science, Enlightenment and Rabbinic Culture," 24.
31. Lewin, "Jüdische Aerzte," 383–393.
32. Ignazy Shipper, *Kulturgeshikhte fun di Yidn in Poyln beysen Mitelalter* (Warsaw: Ch. Bzshoza, 1926), 194–196.
33. Fishman, "Science, Enlightenment and Rabbinic Culture," 27. On the activities of *shtadlanim* in the important community of Posen, see Louis Lewin, "Der Schtadlan im Posener Ghetto," in *Festschrift zum achtzigsten Geburtstage ... Wolf Feilchenfeld*, ed. Bernhard Koenigsberger and Moritz Silberberg (Pleschen-Schrimm: n.p., 1907), 31–39.
34. Fishman, "Science, Enlightenment and Rabbinic Culture," 28.
35. Jacob Katz, *With My Own Eyes: The Autobiography of an Historian* (Hanover, NH: University Press of New England, 1995), 11.
36. Lewin, "Jüdische Aerzte," 393. On the *shtadlan* see Katz, *Tradition and Crisis*, 71–72.
37. For general restrictions on Jews attending concerts, plays, and operas in the early eighteenth century, see Max Grunwald, "Luxusverbot der Dreigemeinden (Hamburg-Altona-Wandsbeck) aus dem Jahre 1715," *Jahrbuch für jüdische Volkskunde* (1923): 227–234.
38. Jonathan I. Israel, *European Jewry in the Age of Mercantilism 1550–1750* (Oxford: Clarendon Press, 1991), 205.
39. See Yitzhak Baer, *Das Protokollbuch der Landjudenschaft des Herzogtums Kleve* (Berlin: C.A. Schwetschke, 1922), 89.
40. Selma Stern, *The Court Jew: A Contribution to the History of Absolutism in Europe* (New Brunswick, NJ: Transaction Books, 1985); Israel, *European Jewry*, 123–144; and Vivian B. Mann and Richard I. Cohen, eds., *From Court Jews to the Rothschilds, 1600–1800: Art, Power, Patronage* (New York: Prestel, 1996).
41. Born in Metz, Gomperz was the scion of a family who had been Court Jews, and he was the son of the doctor of the Jewish community in Prague, Salman Gomperz. Monika Richarz, *Der Eintritt der Juden in die akademischen Berufe* (Tübingen: J.C.B. Mohr, 1974), 41–42.
42. Louis Lewin, "Die jüdischen Studenten an der Universität Frankfurt a.O.," *Jahrbuch der jüdisch-literarischen Gesellschaft* 14 (1921): 232.
43. Richarz, *Eintritt der Juden*, 29.
44. Calculated from the international list of Jewish medical graduates in Manfred Komorowski, *Bio-bibliographisches Verzeichnis jüdischer Doktoren im 17. und 18. Jahrhundert* (Munich: K.G. Saur, 1991), 33–38.
45. On the early modern history of Jewish doctors in Austria see Samuel Krauss, "Medicine Among the Jews of Austria," [Hebrew] *Koroth* 5, 9–10 (1971): 703–706.
46. Siegfried J. Plaschkes, "Die Ersten jüdischen Ärzte der Wiener Universität und ihre Schicksale," *Bulletin des Leo Baeck Instituts* 5 (1962): 202–204.

47. For the earlier period, see Yehoshua O. Leibowitz, "Historical Aspects of the Persecution of Jewish Physicians (in the late Middle Ages)," [Hebrew] *Dapim Refuim* 12 (1953): 75–79.
48. Heiko Oberman, "Three Sixteenth-Century Attitudes to Judaism: Reuchlin, Erasmus and Luther," in *Jewish Thought in the Sixteenth Century,* ed. Bernard Dov Cooperman (Cambridge, MA: Harvard University Press, 1983), 326. For a fuller discussion see also Oberman's *The Roots of Antisemitism: In the Age of Renaissance and Reformation* (Philadelphia: Fortress, 1984).
49. In Padua, Jews paid higher tuition, and upon graduation they were required to provide Christian students with 170 pounds of sweet meats (Ruderman, *Jewish Thought,* 110). In the seventeenth century, approximately three diatribes against the Jewish doctor were written in Poland. But coming nearly a century after the German texts, they are thoroughly derivative, lacking all originality. See Falstein, ed., *Jewish Physicians in Poland,* 11–12.
50. "Da steht das ganze Programm der Hitler-Zeit schon!" The quotation appears in Albert H. Friedlander, "Martin Luther und wir Juden," in *Die Juden und Martin Luther—Martin Luther und die Juden,* ed. Heinz Kremers (Neukirchen-Vluyn: Neukirchener Verlag, 1985), 289–300.
51. Carter Lindberg, "Tainted Greatness: Luther's Attitudes Toward Judaism and Their Reception," in *Tainted Greatness: Antisemitism and Cultural Heroes,* ed. Nancy A. Harrowitz (Philadelphia: Temple University Press, 1994), 26.
52. Many older titles, such as *Labyrinthus Medicorum,* are a difficult mix of Latin and German and consequently appear without parenthetical English translations. Wherever possible, however, I do provide translations. Paracelsus, *Theophrastus Paracelsus Werke,* vol. 2 (Basel: Schwabe, 1965), 443–444. On Paracelsus' antisemitism see Udo Benzenhöfer and Karin Finsterbusch, "Antijudaismus in den medizinisch-naturwissenschaftlichen und philosophischen Schriften des Paracelsus," *Sudhoffs Archiv* 81, 2 (1997): 129–138; and Fridolf Kudlien, "Some Interpretative Remarks on the Antisemitism of Paracelsus," in *Science, Medicine, and Society in the Renaissance: Essays in Honor of Walter Pagel,* vol. 1, ed. Allen G. Debus (New York: Science History Publications, 1972), 121–126.
53. The quotation appears in Harry Friedenwald, *The Jews and Medicine: Essays,* vol. 1 (Baltimore: Johns Hopkins University Press, 1944), 48–49.
54. Philipp Begardi, *Index Sanitatis* (Worms: Sebastian Wagner, 1539), xiii–xiv.
55. Begardi, *Index Sanitatis,* xxiii.
56. Begardi, *Index Sanitatis,* xxiiib.
57. Robert Jütte, "Contacts at the Bedside: Jewish Physicians and Their Christian Patients," in *In and Out of the Ghetto: Jewish-Gentile Relations in Late Medieval and Early Modern Germany,* ed. R. Po-chia Hsia and Hartmut Lehmann (Cambridge: Cambridge University Press, 1995), 139.
58. Begardi, *Index Sanitatis,* xxiiib.

59. Begardi, *Index Sanitatis,* xxiv–xxivb.
60. Martin Luther, *Martin Luthers Werke. Kritische Gesamtausgabe. Tischreden,* vol. 4 (Weimar: Hermann Böhlaus, 1916), nr. 4485., 338. There is an extensive literature on Luther's attitudes toward Jews and Judaism. See the above-noted excellent collection of essays in Kremers, ed., *Die Juden und Martin Luther.*
61. See the exhibition catalogue by Marcia Reines Josephy, *Magic and Superstition in the Jewish Tradition* (Chicago: Spertus College of Judaica Press, 1975).
62. Luther, *Martin Luthers Werke,* nr. 4195. The quotation also appears in R. Po-chia Hsia, *The Myth of Ritual Murder: Jews and Magic in Reformation Germany* (New Haven: Yale University Press, 1988), 132.
63. The quotation appears on pp. 87–88 of the article by Steven Rowan, "Luther, Bucer and Eck on the Jews," *Sixteenth Century Journal* 16, 1 (1985): 79–90.
64. Johannes Eck, *Ains Jüden büechelins verlegung* (Ingolstadt: Alexander Weißenhorn), Fiiij.
65. Adam Lonicer, *Kreuterbuch* (Frankfurt am Main: Matthäus Wagner, 1679), introduction.
66. Hortzitz, *Der Judenarzt,* 65.
67. Ludwig von Hörnigk, *Medicaster Apella oder Juden Artzt* (Strasbourg: Marx von der Heiden, 1631), 72.
68. Von Hörnigk, *Medicaster Apella,* 75–76.
69. Hortzitz, *Der Judenarzt,* 98–99.
70. Hortzitz, *Der Judenarzt,* 74.
71. Alfred Feilchenfeld, "Anfang und Blüthezeit der Portugiesengemeinde in Hamburg," *Zeitschrift für Hamburgische Geschichte* 10 (1899): 199–240. See also Max Grunwald, *Hamburgs deutsche Juden bis zur Auflösung der Dreigemeinden, 1811* (Hamburg: A. Janssen, 1904).
72. Hortzitz, *Der Judenarzt,* 76–80.
73. Johann Christoph Bitterkraut, *Wehmüthige Klag-Thränen der löblichen höchstbetrangten Artzney-Kunst* (Nuremberg: Michael and Johann Friedrich Endter, 1677), 301.
74. Hartwig von Hundt-Radowsky, *Judenspiegel. Ein Schand- und Sittengemälde alter und neuer Zeit* (Würzburg: Christian Schlagehart, 1819), esp. 126–128, on Jewish doctors and apothecaries.
75. Christian Treumundt, *Gewissen-loser Juden-Doctor* (Freyburg: n.p., 1698), 31, 52–54. He referred to the Jewish physician as a *Harn Prophet* (54).
76. Konrad Goehl and Gundolf Keil, "Eine Salzburger spätmittelhochdeutsche Stuhlschau," *Sudhoffs Archiv* 71 (1987): 113–115.
77. Siraisi, *Medieval and Early Renaissance Medicine,* 125.
78. Isaiah Shachar, *The Judensau: A Medieval Anti-Jewish Motif and Its History* (London: Warburg Institute, 1974); Eduard Fuchs, *Die Juden in der Karikatur: Ein Beitrag zur Kulturgeschichte* (Munich: Albert Langen, 1921), 114–123. In the me-

dieval cathedral at Freising, the inscription accompanying the depiction of the Judensau read: "As surely as the mouse never eats the cat, so surely can the Jew never a true Christian become." See Trachtenberg, *Devil and the Jews*, 218.
79. Treumundt, *Gewissen-loser Juden-Doctor*, 31.
80. Treumundt, *Gewissen-loser Juden-Doctor*, 33–35.
81. On *mauschel* see Sander L. Gilman, *Jewish Self-Hatred: Anti-Semitism and the Hidden Language of the Jews* (Baltimore: Johns Hopkins University Press, 1986), 139–148.
82. Treumundt, *Gewissen-loser Juden-Doctor*, 33. He even provides an example of a poorly spelled Latin prescription supposedly written by a Jewish doctor (35).
83. Johann Müller, *Judaismus oder Jüdenthum* (Hamburg: Jakob Rebenlein, 1644). The quotation appears in Hortzitz, *Der Judenarzt*, 87.
84. Johann Andreas Eisenmenger, *Entdecktes Judentum*, part II (Königsberg: n.p., 1711), 227–234. More generally on Eisenmenger see Jacob Katz, *From Prejudice to Destruction: Anti-Semitism, 1700–1933* (Cambridge: Harvard University Press, 1980), 13–22.
85. On sixteenth-century converts see Georg Hammann, "Konversionen deutscher und ungarischer Juden in der frühen Reformationszeit," *Zeitschrift für Kirchengeschichte* 39 (1970): 207–237; Hava Fraenkel-Goldschmidt, "On the Periphery of Jewish Society. Jewish Converts to Christianity in the Age of the Reformation," in *Tarbut ve-hevrah be-toldot Yisrael bi-Yeme-ha-benayim: kovets maamarim le zikhro shel Hayim Hillel Ben-Sasson*, ed. Menahem Ben-Sasson and Robert Bonfil (Jerusalem: Merkaz Zalman Shazar le-toldot Yisrael, 1989), 623–654; and Elisheva Carlebach, "Converts and Their Narratives in Early Modern Germany. The Case of Friedrich Albrecht Christiani," *Leo Baeck Institute Yearbook* 40 (1995), 65–83.
86. Stephen G. Burnett, "Distorted Mirrors: Antonius Margaritha, Johann Buxtorf and Christian Ethnographies of the Jews," *Sixteenth Century Journal* 25, 2 (1994): 275–287.
87. On Margaritha see Josef Mieses, *Die älteste gedruckte deutsche Übersetzung des jüdischen Gebetbuchs aus dem Jahre 1530 und ihr Autor Antonius Margaritha* (Vienna: W. Löwit, 1916); and Selma-Stern Taübler, *Josel of Rosheim, Commander of Jewry in the Holy Roman Empire of the German Nation,* trans. Gertrude Hirschler (Philadelphia: Jewish Publication Society, 1965), 98–103.
88. Ironically, it was Margaritha who had committed treason by denouncing the Jewish community of Regensburg to the authorities even prior to his conversion to Catholicism in 1522.
89. Antonio Margaritha, *Der gantz jüdisch Glaub* (Augspurg: Heynrich Steyner, 1530), Giiij.
90. Margaritha, *Der gantz jüdisch Glaub*, H.
91. Margaritha, *Der gantz jüdisch Glaub*, H.
92. David Khvolson, *Die Blutanklage und sonstige mittelalterliche Beschuldigungen*

*der Juden* (Frankfurt am Main: J. Kauffmann, 1901); and Hermann L. Strack, *The Jew and Human Sacrifice: Human Blood and Jewish Ritual* (London: Cope and Fenwick, 1909); and the recent collection, Rainer Erb, ed., *Die Legende vom Ritualmord: Zur Geschichte der Blutbeschuldigung gegen Juden* (Berlin: Metropol, 1993).

93. Hortzitz, *Der Judenarzt*, 62.
94. Samuel Friedrich Brenz, *Jüdischer abgestreiffter Schlangen-Balg* (Nuremberg: Balthasar Scherf, 1614), 22.
95. On Jewish use of Christian blood for medicinal purposes see Trachtenberg, *Devil and the Jews*, 140–155. The quotation appears on p. 152.
96. The text is partially reprinted in Harry Friedenwald, *The Jews and Medicine: Essays*, vol. 1 (Baltimore: Johns Hopkins University Press, 1944), 31–53. The quotation appears on p. 47.
97. Yerushalmi, *From Spanish Court to Italian Ghetto*, 416.
98. Salomon Zevi Hirsch, *Yudisher Teriyak* (Hanau: Eliyahu Zelikman Ulma, 1615), 1a and 36b. With utter contempt for Brentz, Hirsch begins most paragraphs with some variation of the phrase, "the apostate writes" [*der mumar shraibt*]. Hirsch's book also appeared in a very late Hebrew translation, entitled *Sefer marpe lashon* (Warsaw: Yitshak Goldman, 1873). See also Judah David Eisenstein, *Otsar Vikukhim* (Israel: n.p., 1969), 170–184, who offers a short introduction to the polemic and then exerpts from the 1873 Hebrew translation of *Yudisher Teriyak;* and *Allgemeine Zeitung des Judentums* nr. 23–24 (1846).
99. Within recent scholarship there has been a problematic attempt to valorize the popular and resistant qualities of pre-modern, "mass" Yiddish culture and thus distinguish it from the "elite" Hebrew dimensions of that same culture. This has been a most noticeable trend in the study of women's devotional literature. See Chava Weissler, "Women's Studies and Women's Prayers: Reconstructing the Religious History of Ashkenazic Women," *Jewish Social Studies* 1, 2 (1995): 28–47. For a brilliant discussion of the differences between early modern Hebrew and Yiddish versions of the same work and what those differences say about contemporary Jewish sensibilities, see Michael Stanislawski, "The Yiddish *Shevet Yehudah:* A Study in the 'Ashkenization' of a Spanish-Jewish Classic," in *Jewish History and Jewish Memory: Essays in Honor of Yosef Hayim Yerushalmi*, ed. Elisheva Carlebach, John M. Efron, and David N. Myers (Hanover, NH: University Press of New England, 1998), 134–149.
100. Hirsch, *Yudisher Teriyak*, 27.
101. Baas, *Entwicklung des ärztlichen Standes*, 258, 347.
102. See Charles E. McClelland, *State, Society and University in Germany, 1700–1914* (Cambridge: Cambridge University Press, 1980), 27–98.
103. Hans Rosenberg, *Bureaucracy, Aristocracy and Autocracy: The Prussian Experience, 1660–1815* (Cambridge, MA: Harvard University Press, 1958).
104. Richarz, *Eintritt der Juden*, 24.

105. On the changing nature of German medical education in the nineteenth century see Arleen Marcia Tuchman, *Science, Medicine, and the State in Germany: The Case of Baden, 1815–1871* (New York: Oxford University Press, 1993).
106. On eighteenth-century developments see Thomas Hoyt Broman, "University Reform in Medical Thought at the End of the Eighteenth Century," *Osiris* 5 (1989): 36–53.
107. Theodor Puschmann, *Geschichte des Medicinischen Unterrichts* (Leipzig: Veit, 1889), 325. See also E. Th. Nauck, "Die Zahl der Medizinstudenten deutscher Hochschulen im 14. bis 18. Jahrhundert," *Sudhoffs Archiv für Geschichte der Medizin und der Naturwissenschaften* 38, 2 (1954): 175–186.
108. See Krauss, *Geschichte der jüdischen Aerzte*, 82; and Richarz, *Eintritt der Juden*, 42.
109. In his diary, Von Humboldt reported positively that the spirit of enlightenment was beginning to make itself felt, for in addition to Hamburg, a Protestant named Heinse also graduated that day from Mainz, a Catholic university. Adolf Kober, "Rheinische Judendoktoren, vornehmlich des 17. und 18. Jahrhunderts" in *Festschrift zum 75 jährigen Bestehen des jüdisch-theologischen Seminars*, vol. 2 (Breslau: M. & H. Marcus, 1929), 191–194.
110. Richarz, *Eintritt der Juden*, 43.
111. See Louis Lewin, "Die Jüdische Studenten," 220. This statement on Polish tolerance needs to be qualified, for Polish polemicists also produced diatribes against Jewish doctors, though they were few in number and entirely derivative of the earlier German materials. For example, in a book on the plague by the seventeenth-century Catholic physician from Kalish, Sebastian Sleszkowski, the author claimed that Jewish doctors sought to poison their Christian patients and that "the epidemic spread [in Poland] only because of the complaisant attitude of the government toward the Jews. This was the cause of the Divine punishment." Also, when the economic interests of Christian physicians were threatened, Polish authorities were known to step in to assist them. One such occasion occurred on June 20, 1780, in the city of Posen, when the magistrate forbad Jewish doctors from treating Christian patients. Louis Lewin, "Jüdische Aerzte," 402–404.
112. Richarz, *Eintritt der Juden*, 46 and 178. Komorowski provides names of about 235 Jewish university graduates as well as biographical material on them. See his *Bio-bibliographisches Verzeichnis*, 40–80. But his, like other such lists, are incomplete in that they provide information about Jews only at the institutions they most frequented, and not every university at which they studied. In addition, Komorowski also fails to mention, for example, the well-known Moishe Marcuze of Königsberg. On Marcuze, see Chapter 3 of this book.
113. Ute Frevert, "Gesellschaftsstruktur und politische Veränderungsfaktoren in Deutschland um 1800—das klassische beispiel Preußen," in *Bürgerliche Gesellschaft in Deutschland*, ed. Lutz Niethammer (Frankfurt: Fischer, 1990), 41–51.

114. David Sorkin, *The Transformation of German Jewry, 1780–1840* (New York: Oxford University Press, 1987), 14. For a treatment of the Jewish entrance into the *Bildungsbürgertum* in the nineteenth century see the essays by Shulamit Volkov, Moshe Zimmermann, and Stefi-Jersch-Wenzel in *Bürgertum im 19. Jahrhundert. Deutschland im europaischen Vergleich,* ed. Jürgen Kocha, vol. 2 (Munich: Deutscher Taschenbuch Verlag, 1988), 343–420.
115. The expression is from Sorkin, *Transformation of German Jewry,* 17.
116. George L. Mosse, *German Jews Beyond Judaism* (Bloomington: Indiana University Press, 1985), 4.
117. On medicine in the eighteenth century, see Erwin H. Ackerknecht, *A Short History of Medicine* (Baltimore: Johns Hopkins University Press, 1992), 128–144.
118. George L. Mosse, *Confronting the Nation: Jewish and Western Nationalism* (Hanover, NH: University Press of New England, 1993), 121.

## CHAPTER 3. *HASKALAH* AND HEALING

1. Ismar Elbogen and Eleanore Sterling, *Die Geschichte der Juden in Deutschland* (Frankfurt am Main: Athenäum, 1988), 153.
2. Naphtali Herz Wessely, *Divrei Shalom ve-Emet* (Warsaw: R. Yosef Haim Zabelinski, 1886), 4. By making specific mention of syntax and "purity of expression," Wessely was referring to the derided Judeo-German or Western Yiddish, the vernacular of eighteenth-century German Jews.
3. On the aims of the Jewish Enlightenment, see Jacob Katz, *Out of the Ghetto: The Social Background of Jewish Emancipation, 1770–1870* (New York: Schocken, 1978).
4. On the political aspects of the Haskalah see Sorkin, *Transformation of German Jewry,* esp. 63–78. Haskalah education is covered by Mordekhai Eliav, *Ha-Hinukh ha-Yehudi be-Germanyah bi-Yeme ha-Haskalah ve-ha-Emantsipatsiyah* (Jerusalem: Sivan, 1960). For a local study of Jewish education in the wake of the Jewish enlightenment and emancipation see Claudia Prestel, *Jüdisches Schul- und Erziehungswesen in Bayern, 1804–1933* (Göttingen: Vandenhoeck and Ruprecht, 1989), esp. 56–74.
5. David Sorkin, "From Context to Comparison: The German Haskalah and Reform Catholicism," *Tel Aviver Jahrbuch für deutsche Geschichte* 20 (1991): 23–24.
6. The term *Judaism* in this context should not be taken to mean only the religious culture of Ashkenazic Jewry. Rather, it should be interpreted as broadly as possible, to include all popular and mundane manifestations of that culture. The distinction I have drawn between religious and popular culture among premodern Jews is not an arbitrary one. Many of the complaints made about Jewish culture by the doctors discussed in this chapter refer, to a great extent, to lifestyles, occupations, foods, and so forth. These categories are very different from the ones described by, for example, Isadore Twersky in his important

essay on Jewish religious culture, "Talmudists, Philosophers, Kabbalists: The Quest for Spirituality in the Sixteenth Century," in *Jewish Thought in the Sixteenth Century,* ed. Bernard Dov Cooperman (Cambridge, MA: Harvard University Press, 1983), 431–459.

7. Steven M. Lowenstein, *The Berlin Jewish Community: Enlightenment, Family, and Crisis, 1770–1830* (New York: Oxford University Press, 1994), 142; Shmuel Feiner, "The Early Haskalah among Eighteenth Century Jewry" [Hebrew] *Tarbiz* 67, 2 (1998): 189–124.

8. Monika Richarz, "Soziale Voraussetzungen des Medizinstudiums von Juden im 18. und 19. Jahrhundert," in *Medizinische Bildung und Judentum,* ed. Albrecht Scholz and Caris-Petra Heidel (Dresden: DDP Goldenbogen, 1998), 9.

9. On this topic, see Dan Miron, *Ha-rofe ha-medumeh: Iyunim be-sifrut ha-yehudit ha-klasit* (Tel Aviv: Hakibbutz Hameuchad, 1995), 9–21.

10. Three versions of the play are extant. I have consulted Zalman Reisen in *Arkhiv far der geshikhte fun yidishn teater un drame* 1 (1930): 94–146.

11. Yitshak Erter, *Ha-tsofeh le-veit Yisrael* (Tel Aviv: Akhdut, 1945), 57.

12. On the development of Alsatian Jewry see Paula Hyman, *The Emancipation of the Jews of Alsace: Acculturation and Tradition in the Nineteenth Century* (New Haven: Yale University Press, 1991).

13. Arthur Hertzberg, *The French Enlightenment and the Jews* (New York: Columbia University Press, 1990), 129.

14. Hertzberg, *French Enlightenment,* 328–338.

15. Henri Baptiste Grégoire, *Essay on the Physical, Moral, and Political Reformation of the Jews* (London: C. Forster, Poultry, 1791), 43–56.

16. On France, see Harvey Mitchell and Samuel S. Kottek, "An Eighteenth-Century Medical View of the Diseases of the Jews in Northeastern France: Medical Anthropology and the Politics of Jewish Emancipation," *Bulletin of the History of Medicine* 67 (1993): 248–281. On Germany, see my *Defenders of the Race,* chapter 1.

17. Elcan Isaac Wolf, *Von den Krankheiten der Juden* (Mannheim: C.F. Schwann, 1777), 6. The page numbers of all further citations from this work will appear in parentheses in the chapter text.

18. On mental illness among Jews see Chapter 5 of this book.

19. The document is reprinted in Mitchell and Kottek, "Diseases of the Jews," 278.

20. See Israel Abrahams, *Jewish Life in the Middle Ages* (New York: Atheneum, 1985), 150–152; and Robert Bonfil, *Jewish Life in Renaissance Italy* (Berkeley: University of California Press, 1994), 245–246.

21. On the qualitative decline of diet in Europe see Massimo Montanari, *Der Hunger und der Überfluss: Kulturgeschichte der Ernährung in Europa* (Munich: C.H. Beck, 1993), 173–177; and Wilhelm Abel, *Stufen der Ernährung* (Göttingen: Vandenhoeck & Ruprecht, 1981), 32–64. For an example of anthropometric history that discusses the impact of nutritional status on human stature

in Central Europe see John Komlos, *Nutrition and Economic Development in the Eighteenth-Century Habsburg Monarchy* (Princeton: Princeton University Press, 1989), esp. 55–119. On the changing patterns of food consumption in the eighteenth century see Günter Wiegelmann, "Der Wandel von Speisen- und Tischkultur im 18. Jahrhundert," in *Unsere tägliche Kost: Studien zur Geschichte des Alltags,* ed. Hans J. Teuteberg and Günter Wiegelmann (Münster: F. Coppenrath, 1986), 335–344.

22. Hans J. Teuteberg, "The Diet as an Object of Historical Analysis in Germany," in *European Food History: A Research Review,* ed. Hans J. Teuteberg (Leicester: Leicester University Press, 1992), 119.

23. *Quaestiones Medicae* (Paris: Quillau, 1672–1733). The material, which is located in the Lilly Library at Indiana University, is described as: "A collection of medical disputations held before the Medical Faculty of Paris with praeces and respondens for each. On questions of the dietary and therapeutic uses of coffee, tea, chocolate, milk, beer, wine, spirits, bread, sugar, tobacco." I thank my colleague Arthur Field for his help with the Latin.

24. J. Worth Estes, "The Medical Properties of Food in the Eighteenth Century," *Journal of the History of Medicine and Allied Sciences* 51, 2 (1996): 127–154.

25. The first coffeehouse in Germany was opened by English merchants in Hamburg in 1677. Within ten years, Vienna, Nuremberg, Regensburg, and Cologne had similar establishments. During the eighteenth century their numbers continued to grow to the point that they became common fixtures in towns throughout the country. See Wiegelmann, "Der Wandel von Speisen," 339–340; Hans J. Teuteberg, "Kaffeetrinken sozialgeschichtlich betrachtet," *Scripta mercaturae* 14 (1981): 27–54; and Woodruff D. Smith, "From Coffeehouse to Parlour: The Consumption of Coffee, Tea, and Sugar in North-Western Europe in the Seventeenth and Eighteenth Centuries," in *Consuming Habits,* ed. Jordan Goodman, Paul E. Lovejoy, and Andrew Sherratt (London: Routledge, 1995), 148–169.

26. Hans J. Teuteberg, "Die Eingliederung des Kaffees in den täglichen Getränkekonsum," in *Unsere tägliche Kost,* 185–201, esp. 189–190, for eighteenth-century medical opinions of coffee; Günter Wiegelmann, "Zucker und Süßwaren im Zivilizationsprozeß der Neuzeit," in *Unsere tägliche Kost,* 135–152; Maguelonne Toussaint-Samat, *A History of Food* (Blackwell: Oxford, 1992), 549–591.

27. Quoted in Roman Sandgruber, "Nutrition in Austria in the Industrial Age" in *European Food History,* ed. H. J. Teuteberg, 147.

28. Mitchell and Kottek, "Diseases of the Jews," 277.

29. For the origins of the Central and Eastern European Jewish diet see John Cooper, *Eat and Be Satisfied: A Social History of Jewish Food* (Northvale, NJ: Jason Aronson, 1993), 79–89.

30. K. Y. Guggenheim, *Basic Issues in the History of Nutrition* (Jerusalem: Akademia University Press, 1990), 55–63.

31. On medical education in the eighteenth century see Puschmann, *Medicinischen Unterrichts,* 329–364. On the history of the study of respiration and calorimetry see Elmer Verner McCollum, *A History of Nutrition* (Boston: Houghton Mifflin, 1957), 115–133.
32. Hans J. Teuteberg and Günter Wiegelmann, *Der Wandel der Nahrungsgewohnheiten unter dem Einfluß der Industrialisierung* (Göttingen: Vandenhoeck & Ruprecht, 1972), 26.
33. See Hans Wiswe, *Kulturgeschichte der Kochkunst: Kochbücher und Rezepte aus zwei Jahrtausenden* (Munich: H. Moos, 1970).
34. Teuteberg and Wiegelmann, *Wandel der Nahrungsgewohnheiten,* 29.
35. Teuteberg and Wiegelmann, *Wandel der Nahrungsgewohnheiten,* 30–33; Otto Brunner, "Hausväterliteratur," in *Handwörterbuch der Sozialwissenschaften,* 5th ed. (Stuttgart: Gustav Fischer, 1956–1965), 92–93; Fritz Hartmann, "Hausvater und Hausmutter als Hausarzt in der Frühen Neuzeit: Hausgewalt und Gesundheitsfürsorge," in *Staat und Gesellschaft in Mittelalter und Früher Neuzeit: Gedenkschrift für Joachim Leuschner,* ed. Katharina Colberg, Hans-Heinrich Nolte, and Hans Obenaus (Göttingen: Vandenhoeck & Ruprecht, 1983), 151–175.
36. Teuteberg and Wiegelmann, *Wandel der Nahrungsgewohnheiten,* 33–43.
37. See Jacob Katz, *Tradition and Crisis: Jewish Society at the End of the Middle Ages,* trans. Bernard Dov Cooperman (New York: New York University Press, 1993), 156–169.
38. Bernadino Ramazzini, *Diseases of Workers,* trans. Wilmer Cave Wright (New York: Hafner, 1964), 287.
39. W. H. Bruford, *Germany in the Eighteenth Century: The Social Background of the Literary Revival* (Cambridge: Cambridge University Press, 1965), 106.
40. Rainer Erb, "Warum ist der Jude zum Ackerbürger nicht tauglich? Zur Geschichte eines antisemitischen Stereotyps," in *Antisemitismus und jüdische Geschichte,* ed. Rainer Erb and Michael Schmidt (Berlin: Wissenschaftlicher Autorenverlag, 1987), 99–120.
41. Interestingly, the cost for the book's printing was borne by a Polish magnate, Michael Bobrowski. Moishe Marcuze, *Seyfer Refues* (Poritsk: n.p., 1790), 3. The page numbers of all further citations from this work will appear in parentheses in the chapter text. On the book see also Chone Shmeruk, *Sifrut Yidish be-Polin* (Jerusalem: Magnes Press, 1981), 184–203; and Yehoshua Leibowitz, "Marcuze's Book of Medicine (1790) in Yiddish," [Hebrew] *Koroth* 4, 1–2 (1966): 3–10.
42. Lefin's translation appeared in two stages: a partial rendering in 1789, and then a complete version in 1794. Shmeruk, "Moishe Marcuze," 187–199. See also Shmeruk's original Yiddish version, "Moishe Marcuze fun Slonim un der makor fun zeyn bukh *Ezer Yisrael,*" in *Sefer Dov Sadan,* ed. Shmuel Verses, et al. (Jerusalem: Ha-Kibbutz ha-Meukhad, 1977), 361–382, esp. 365–377; and Leibowitz, "Marcuze's Book of Medicine," 8. Between 1761 and 1794 Tissot's phe-

nomenally successful book was translated into German, Italian, Spanish, English, Dutch, Hungarian, Danish, Swedish, Russian, and Polish.
43. Marcuze, *Seyfer Refues,* title page; also, on 98b, he again makes the similar claim that readers can ward off sickness by closely following his book.
44. Marcuze, *Seyfer Refues,* 57b. He is especially apologetic to his fellow scholars, pleading "I beg one hundred pardons if I should misuse even one word of Hebrew by mixing it with bad Yiddish."
45. There is no doubt about Marcuze's natural facility with Yiddish. An outstanding Yiddish philologist, Noah Prilutski, asserted that Marcuze was "versatile, learned, intelligent, a fine observer, and an *outstanding literary talent*" [my emphasis]. See Prilutski's, "A Yidishist fun 18ten yohrhundert," in his *Samelbikher far yidisher folklor, filologye un kultur-geshikhte* vol. 2 (Warsaw: Nayer Verlag, 1917), 7. Prilutski also applauds Marcuze's "natural, easy, popular and yet at the same time highly cultured style" (13). Elsewhere, he claims that "*Seyfer Refues* ought to be seen as the basis for a dictionary of modern Yiddish" (18). For Prilutski, the traces of German syntax in Marcuze's Yiddish are evidence that he may have come from Prussia (9–10). Nevertheless, *Seyfer Refues* has been of major significance in the field of Yiddish linguistics, precisely because Marcuze's syntax and vocabulary point away from Western Yiddish, or Judeo-German to Eastern, or Polish, Yiddish, marking a milestone in the development of Yiddish literature. See Mikhl I. Herzog, "Grammatical Features of Marcuze's *Seyfer Refues* (1790)," in *The Field of Yiddish,* ed. Uriel Weinreich (The Hague: Mouton, 1965), 49–62. Also, Yehoshua Leibowitz describes Marcuze's Yiddish as "juicy and in the Volhyian dialect." Leibowitz, "Marcuze's Book of Medicine," 3. Israel Zinberg says that Marcuze "undoubtedly deserves to have his name occupy an honored place in the history of modern Yiddish literature as one of the first authors who attempted to employ the folk-language, the 'jargon' so despised by all the maskilim and 'enlighteners,' as a secular, *literary* language." Israel Zinberg, *A History of Jewish Literature,* vol. 8 (Cleveland: Press of Case Western Reserve University, 1976), 154.
46. Hans-Jürgen Krüger, *Die Judenschaft von Königsberg in Preussen 1700–1812* (Marburg: Lahn, 1966), 57 and 91.
47. Marcuze states, "I came to you in Poland in my sixteenth year," 99. This means that he returned sixteen years prior to the publication of *Seyfer Refues*. This would put his arrival in Poland around 1774, at about the age of forty-seven.
48. Prilutski, "A Yidishist," 18–19.
49. Max Grunwald, "Bibliomantie und Gesundbeten," *Mitteilungen zur jüdischen Volkskunde* 10, 2 (1902): 81–98.
50. See, for example, the discussion of one such book by Jacob Shatzky, "*Sefer ha-Kheshek:* A Lost Medical Book of the 18th Century" [Yiddish], *YIVO Bleter* 6 (1932): 223–235.

51. Issachar Bär Teller, *Be'er Mayim Khayyim* (The wellspring of living waters), trans. Arthur Teller (New York: Tal Or Oth, 1988), n.p.
52. Teller in fact included Delmedigo's Hebrew translation of Hippocrates' aphorisms in *Be'er Mayim Khayyim*.
53. Ruderman, *Jewish Thought*, 233.
54. Both books were reprinted in 1712. Krauss, *Geschichte der jüdischen Aerzte*, 150; Lewin, "Jüdische Aerzte," 401; Falstein, ed., *Jewish Physicians in Poland*, 22–23.
55. Tobias Cohen, *Ma'aseh Tuviyyah* (Jerusalem: Bakal, 1976), 82.
56. Marcuze, *Seyfer Refues*, 82. On Cohen and his book see Ruderman, *Jewish Thought*, 229–255.
57. Landau, *Geschichte der jüdischen Ärzte*, 117.
58. *Sefer ha-Refues* (Jessnitz: Israel ben Abraham, 1722), 2a.
59. Paul Starr, *The Social Transformation of American Medicine: The Rise of a Sovereign Profession and the Making of a Vast Industry* (New York: Basic Books, 1982), 15; Eliot Friedson, *Profession of Medicine: A Study in the Sociology of Applied Knowledge* (New York: Dodd, Mead, 1970). For Germany, see Claudia Huerkamp, *Der Aufstieg der Ärzte im 19. Jahrhundert Vom gelehrten Stand zum professionellen Experten: Das Beispiel Preußens* (Göttingen: Vandenhoeck & Ruprecht, 1985).
60. On the rise of professionalization in Germany see Charles E. McClelland, *The German Experience of Professionalization: Modern Learned Professions and Their Organizations from the Early Nineteenth Century to the Hitler Era* (Cambridge: Cambridge University Press, 1991), esp. 38–40, on medicine. On France see Toby Gelfand, *Professionalizing Modern Medicine: Paris Surgeons and Medical Science and Institutions in the Eighteenth Century* (Westport, CT: Greenwood Press, 1980). On England see Roy Porter, *Health for Sale: Quackery in England, 1660–1850* (Manchester: Manchester University Press, 1989); and the insightful article by Margaret Pelling, "Medical Practice in Early Modern England: Trade or Profession?" in *The Professions in Early Modern England*, ed. Wilfrid Prest (London: Croom Helm, 1987), 90–128.
61. Charles E. McClelland, *State, Society, and University in Germany 1700–1914* (Cambridge: Cambridge University Press, 1980), 3.
62. Thomas H. Broman, *The Transformation of German Academic Medicine, 1750–1820* (Cambridge: Cambridge University Press, 1996).
63. R. Steven Turner, "The *Bildungsbürgertum* and the Learned Professions in Prussia, 1770–1830: The Origins of a Class," *Histoire Sociale/Social History* 13 (1980): 105–135.
64. Marcuze, *Seyfer Refues*, 110a–b. Also quoted in Zinberg, *Jewish Literature*, 165–166. Maimon's description of the *heder* appears in *Solomon Maimon: An Autobiography* (New York: Schocken, 1975), 11–12.
65. Quoted in Guy Williams, *The Age of Agony: The Art of Healing c. 1700–1800* (London: Constable, 1975), 24.

66. Marcus, *Communal Sick-Care*, 48–50.
67. Hilary Marland, ed., *The Art of Midwifery: Early Modern Midwives in Europe* (Routledge: London, 1993).
68. David Harley, "Provincial Midwives in England: Lancashire and Cheshire, 1660–1760," in *Art of Midwifery*, ed. H. Marland, 27–48.
69. Hilary Marland, "The '*burgerlijke*' Midwife: The *Stadsvroedvrouw* of Eighteenth-Century Holland," in *Art of Midwifery*, ed. H. Marland, 192–213.
70. Marcuze, *Seyfer Refues*, 76b–77.
71. Cohen, introduction to *Ma'aseh Tuviyyah*.
72. Edward Kossoy and Abraham Ohry, *The Feldshers: Medical, Sociological and Historical Aspects of Practitioners of Medicine with Below University Level Education* (Jerusalem: Magnes Press, 1992), 9–33. The quotation appears on p. 10.
73. Kossoy and Ohry, *The Feldshers*, 142–146.
74. *The Memoirs of Glückel of Hameln*, trans. Marvin Lowenthal (New York: Schocken, 1977), 146–152.
75. Janet M. Hartley, *Alexander I* (London: Longman, 1994), 132. The army was not to be used outside Poland.
76. Kossoy and Ohry, *The Feldshers*, 154–155.
77. Kossoy and Ohry, *The Feldshers*, 151.
78. Marcuze, *Seyfer Refues*, 122b–123; Zinberg, *Jewish Literature*, 157.
79. On Marcuze's personal experience with bloodletting see, *Seyfer Refues*, 93a–b. On the difficulty of distinguishing between academic and folk medicine see Mary Lindemann, *Health and Healing in Eighteenth-Century Germany* (Baltimore: Johns Hopkins University Press, 1996), 73–74; Ute Frevert, *Krankheit als politisches Problem, 1770–1880: Soziale Unterschichten in Preußen zwischen medizinisher Polizei und staatlicher Sozialversicherung* (Göttingen: Vandenhoeck & Ruprecht, 1984).
80. The best work on this subject pertains to England but is relevant to the context discussed here. See William F. Bynum and Roy Porter, eds., *Medical Fringe & Medical Orthodoxy, 1750–1850* (London: Croom Helm, 1987).
81. McClelland, *Experience of Professionalization*, 11–27.
82. See James C. Riley, *The Eighteenth-Century Campaign to Avoid Disease* (New York: St. Martin's Press, 1987). Foucault's expression appears in his *The Birth of the Clinic: An Archaeology of Medical Perception* (New York: Pantheon Books, 1973), 51.
83. Johann Peter Frank, "The People's Misery: Mother of Diseases," trans. and introduction Henry E. Sigerist, *Bulletin of the History of Medicine* 9 (1941): 81–100.
84. Christian Barthel, *Medizinische Polizey und medizinische Aufklärung: Aspekte des öffentlichen Gesundheitsdiskurses im 18. Jahrhundert* (Frankfurt: Campus, 1989).
85. See the collection of essays in Andrew Cunningham and Roger French, eds., *The Medical Enlightenment of the Eighteenth Century* (Cambridge: Cambridge

University Press, 1990), especially the article by Roger French, "Sickness and the Soul: Stahl, Hoffmann and Sauvages on Pathology," 88–110. More generally for Germany see Arina Völker, ed., *Dixhuitieme: Zur Geschichte von Medizin und Naturwissenschaften im 18. Jahrhundert* (Halle: Martin-Luther-Universität, 1988).

86. The name *Baal Shem* means "Master of the (Divine) Name," and was the title awarded to a man who wrote amulets against diseases and evil spirits. On the founder of Hasidism see Moshe Rosman, *Founder of Hasidism: A Quest for the Historical Ba'al Shem Tov* (Berkeley: University of California Press, 1996); and Simon Dubnow, "The Beginnings: The Baal Shem Tov (Besht) and the Center in Podolia," in *Essential Papers on Hasidism: Origins to the Present*, ed. Gershon David Hundert (New York: New York University Press, 1991), 25–51.

87. Rabbi Nathan of Breslov, *Tsaddik: A Portrait of Rabbi Nachman*, trans. Avraham Greenbaum (Jerusalem: Breslov Research Institute, 1987), 83. Nevertheless, despite Reb Nachman's instruction, he himself visited a physician in Lvov in 1808, having contracted tuberculosis. He was also known to quote prominent physicians (407). According to Chone Shmeruk, Reb Nachman had also read *Seyfer Refues*. On the relation of Marcuze's book to Hasidism see Shmeruk, "Moishe Marcuze fun Slonim," 378–381. More generally, see David Margalith, "The Role of Medicine in the Hasidic Movement," *Koroth* [Hebrew] 1, 1–2 (1952): 31–37.

88. Dubnow explicitly addresses the importance of the faith healers in eighteenth-century Polish Jewish society, claiming not only that they filled an important void created by the absence of trained physicians but also that they were instrumental in disseminating knowledge of the Torah, and spreading Sabbateanism. Dubnow, "The Beginnings: The Baal Shem Tov," 31–32.

89. Marcus Herz, *Ha-Meassef* 7 (1790): 424; Herz was also the author of another physician's prayer, which dated from 1783, and which he attributed to Maimonides. See also Fred Rosner, "The Physician's Prayer Attributed to Moses Maimonides," *Bulletin of the History of Medicine* 41 (1967): 440–454. On the variety of medical practices and the range of practitioners offering their services in eighteenth-century Germany see Lindemann, *Health and Healing*, 144–235.

90. Ernst Frankel, "David Friedländer und seine Zeit," *Zeitschrift für die Geschichte der Juden in Deutschland* 6 (1935): 65–77. On Friedländer and his role in the fight for Jewish emancipation and promotion of Haskalah see Michael Meyer, *The Origins of the Modern Jew: Jewish Identity and European Culture in Germany, 1749–1824* (Detroit: Wayne State University Press, 1967), 57–84.

91. For an analysis of Herz's activities in these two areas, see Martin L. Davies, *Identity or History? Marcus Herz and the End of the Enlightenment* (Detroit: Wayne State University Press, 1995).

92. Brigitte Ibing, "Markus Herz: A Biographical Study," *Koroth* 9, 1–2 (1985): 114.
93. Wolfram Kaiser and Arina Völker, "Berolina iubilans: Berliner Ärzte als hallesche Doktoranden (V). Markus Herz (1747–1803) und die Berliner jüdischen Ärzte," *Zeitschrift für die gesamte innere Medizin* 42 (1987): 618–623.
94. For the influence of German intellectuals on Jewish reformers, see Michael Meyer, "Reform Jewish Thinkers and Their German Intellectual Context," in *The Jewish Response to German Culture: From the Enlightenment to the Second World War*, ed. Jehuda Reinharz and Walter Schatzberg (Hanover, NH: University Press of New England, 1985), 64–84.
95. Of course, in the 1760s and 1770s Moses Mendelssohn, David Friedländer, the Meyer family, and Markus Levin had already opened their homes to Christian intellectuals and nobles.
96. Davies, *Identity or History?* 7.
97. Quoted in Deborah Hertz, *Jewish High Society in Old Regime Berlin* (New Haven: Yale University Press, 1988), 100.
98. "Ich kenne manchen orthodoxen Juden, der, als er aus Herz Physik kam, die Lehre von den Wundern zu bezweifeln anfing." Wolf Davidson, *Ueber die bürgerliche Verbesserung der Juden* (Berlin: Ernst Felisch, 1798), 94. On Wolf, about whom almost nothing is known, see Meyer, *Origins of the Modern Jew*, 74–75.
99. For a view of Herz's reputation among the contemporary Jewish intelligentsia, see his necrology, "Biographie des Herrn Marcus Herz," *Sulamith* 2 (1811): 77–97.
100. The traditional interpretation of the affair is in Katz, *Out of the Ghetto*, 150–151.
101. Ingrid Stoessel, *Scheintod und Todesangst: Äußerungsformen der Angst in ihren geschichtlichen Wandlungen* (17.-20. Jahrhundert) (Cologne: Instituts für Geschichte der Medizin der Universität Köln), 5 and 9.
102. Martin Patak, *Die Angst vor dem Scheintod in der zweiten Hälfte des 18. Jahrhunderts* (Zurich: Juris Verlag, 1967).
103. Marielene Putscher, *Geschichte der medizinischen Abbildung* vol. 2 (Munich: H. Moos, 1972).
104. Carolyn Walker Bynum, *The Resurrection of the Body in Western Christianity, 200–1336* (New York: Columbia University Press, 1995), 58.
105. See Peter Hanns Reill, "Death, Dying and Resurrection in Late Enlightenment Science and Culture," in *Wissenschaft als kulturelle Praxis, 1750–1900*, ed. Hans Erich Bödeker et al. (Göttingen: Vandenhoeck & Ruprecht), 255–274; Philip Aries, *The Hour of Our Death* (New York: Random House, 1982), 396–406; and Sean M. Quinlan, "Apparent Death in Eighteenth-Century France and England," *French History* 9, 2 (1995): 27–47; William Tebb, *Premature Burial and How It Can Be Prevented* (London: S. Sonnenschein, 1905). No less fearful than Europeans were Americans, whose fright at the prospect of premature interment was given eloquent expression in the nineteenth-century Gothic thriller by Edgar Allen Poe, "The Premature Burial."

106. Stoessel, *Scheintod und Todesangst*, 6; Ariès, *Hour of Our Death*, 403–404.
107. For the medical dimension of *Scheintod* see Margarit Augener, *Scheintod als medizinisches Problem im 18. Jahrhundert* (Medical dissertation: University of Kiel, 1965); and Juliane Brigitte Spengler, *Über die ärztliche Leichenschau— Gedanken zur Vermeidung fehlerhafter Feststellung des Todes* (Medical dissertation: University of Tübingen, 1978).
108. R. V. Lee, "Cardiopulmonary Resuscitation in the Eighteenth Century: A Historical Perspective on the Present Practice," *Journal of the History of Medicine* 27 (1972): 418–433; Elizabeth M. France, "Some Eighteenth Century Authorities on Resuscitation," *Anaesthesia* 30 (1975): 530–538; and D. Dünschel, "Berichte von Wiederbelebungsmaßnahmen im 18. und 19. Jahrhundert," *Clio Medica* 12, 2/3 (1977): 173–184.
109. For eighteenth-century examples see Anton Wilhelm Plaz, "Von der Notwendigkeit die Kennzeichen des Todes genau zu Untersuchen," in *Medicinisch-gerichtliche Beobachtungen nebst ihrer Beurtheilung*, vol. 3, ed. Christian Ludwig Schweickhard (Strassburg: n.p., 1789), 222–234; and Johann Daniel Metzger, *Über die Kennzeichen des Todes und den auf die Ungewißheit derselben gegründeten Vorschlag Leichenhäuser zu errichten* (Königsberg: n.p., 1792).
110. Stoessel, *Scheintod und Todesangst*, 31; and Elizabeth H. Thomson, "The Role of Physicians in the Humane Societies of the Eighteenth Century," *Bulletin of the History of Medicine* 37 (1963): 43–51.
111. In Central Europe, in 1756, Gerard van Swieten, court physician to Empress Maria Theresa, suggested that a waiting period of two days be instituted before permitting burial to take place. In addition, he proposed that morgues be established in order to watch over the presumed dead, to ensure that they had really expired. His proposals were later adopted in many parts of Germany. See Erna Lesky, "Van Swieten über Kriterien des Todes," *Wiener klinische Wochenschrift* 84, 15 (1972): 244–245.
112. This is based on the biblical command of Deut. 21:22–23.
113. The duke's order appears in *Ha-Meassef* 7 (1794), 155–158. See also the letter from the Schwerin community in Moses Mendelssohn, *Gesammelte Schriften* 16 (Berlin: Akademie Verlag, 1929), 154–155.
114. For a detailed account of the burial controversy see Sigfried Silberstein, "Mendelssohn und Mecklenburg," *Zeitschrift für die Geschichte der Juden in Deutschland* 1, 3 (1929): 233–244; and 1, 4 (1930): 275–290; Alexander Altmann, *Moses Mendelssohn: A Biographical Study* (Philadelphia: Jewish Publication Society, 1973), 288–294; Samuel S. Kottek, "The Controversy Concerning Early Burial," *Jewish Medical Ethics* 1, 1 (1988): 31–33; and for a general discussion of Jewish approaches to death in the modern period see the excellent study by Michael Edward Panitz, "Modernity and Mortality: The Transformation of Central European Jewish Responses to Death, 1750–1850" (Ph.D. dissertation, Jewish Theological Seminary, 1989).

115. See Anonymous, "Auszug eines Briefes von einem Juden an seinen Freund einen Christen," *Ha-Meassef* (1784): 15–18.
116. In 1786, Euchel applied for a lectureship in Hebrew at the University of Königsberg and was supported warmly in this endeavor by Kant. The university rejected Euchel's application because of his refusal to convert to Protestantism.
117. Zinberg, *Jewish Literature*, 135.
118. Moshe Pelli, *The Age of Haskalah: Studies in Hebrew Literature of the Enlightenment in Germany* (Leiden: Brill, 1979), 210; and Max Grunwald, ed., *Die Hygiene der Juden* (Dresden: Verlag der Historischen Abteilung der Internationalem Hygiene-Austellung, 1911), 269.
119. Ludwig Geiger, "Markus Herz über die frühe Beerdigung der Juden," *Zeitschrift für die Geschichte der Juden in Deutschland* 4 (1890): 55–57. Also quoted in Davies, *Identity or History?*, 201. See also Ludwig Geiger, "Vor hundert Jahren: Mitteilungen aus der Geschichte der Juden Berlins," *Zeitschrift für die Geschichte der Juden in Deutschland* 3 (1889): 185–233.
120. Marcus Herz, *Über die frühe Beerdigung der Juden* (Berlin: Christian Friedrich Voss and Son, 1788), 30–32; and quoted in Falk Wiesemann, "Jewish Burials in Germany—Between Tradition, the Enlightenment and the Authorities," *Leo Baeck Institute Yearbook* 37 (1992), 21. The page numbers of all further citations from Herz's work will appear in parentheses in the chapter text.
121. Herz, *Beerdigung der Juden*, 36. Herz was somewhat unfair to Landau, one of the greatest rabbis of his generation. Recognized as a bold and often lenient interpreter of Jewish law, Landau was the first rabbi to sanction (with severe restrictions) autopsies.
122. Again, this aspect of the Haskalah criticism of traditional Jewish society must not be seen in isolation from general developments. In criticizing the qualifications of official Habsburg cadaver inspectors in Vienna, Gerard van Swieten described them as "great ignoramuses." But Herz excludes criticism of Christian authorities, choosing instead to praise them whenever possible. See Lesky, "Van Swieten," 244.
123. Marcus, *Communal Sick-Care*, 96–97.
124. Hertz, *Jewish High Society*, 99.
125. Despite losing the battle over delaying burial, Jewish advocates of the practice continued to wage their campaign into the nineteenth century, specifically calling on physicians to advocate for the building of mortuaries. "Ueber Scheintod und Leichenhäuser," *Allgemeine Zeitung des Judentums* 1, 58 and 59 (1837): 227 and 238–239.
126. Jacob Marx, *Ueber die Beerdigung der Todten* (Hannover: Schmidt, 1788), 13–20. The page numbers of all further citations from this work will appear in parentheses in the chapter text.
127. See Barbara Suchy, *Lexikographie und Juden im 18. Jahrhundert: Die Darstellung von Juden und Judentum in den englischen, französischen und deutschen*

*Lexika und Enzyklopädien im Zeitalter der Aufklärung* (Cologne: Böhlau, 1979), 240.

128. Johann Georg Krünitz, *Oekonomische Encyklopädie, oder allgemeines System der Staats-Stadt-Haus- und Landwirtschaft*, vol. 31 (Berlin: Joachim Pauli, 1784), 604.

129. Henri Baptiste Grégoire, *Essai sur la régénération physique, morale et politique des Juifs* (Paris: Flammarion, 1988).

## CHAPTER 4. THE JEWISH BODY DEGENERATE?

1. The literature on this topic is very large. See, for example, Nancy Stepan, *The Idea of Race in Science: Great Britain 1800–1960* (London: Macmillan Press, 1982); George L. Mosse, *Toward the Final Solution: A History of European Racism* (Madison: University of Wisconsin Press, 1985); and for a discussion of the links between race and gender see Sandra Harding, ed., *The Racial Economy of Science: Toward a Democratic Future* (Bloomington: Indiana University Press, 1993). On the relation of science and medicine to issues of gender see Ludmilla Jordanova, *Sexual Visions: Images of Gender in Science and Medicine between the Eighteenth and Twentieth Centuries* (Madison: University of Wisconsin Press, 1989).

2. See the entry "Expectation of Life," in the *Jewish Encyclopaedia*, vol. 5, 306–308. In addition, see John Stockton Hough, "Longevity and Other Biostatic Peculiarities of the Jewish Race," *Medical Record* 8 (1873): 241–244.

3. Aharon Appelfeld, *The Retreat* (New York: E.P. Dutton, 1984), 103.

4. See Sander Gilman, *The Jews' Body* (New York: Routledge, 1991).

5. Christina von Braun, "Und der Feind ist Fleisch geworden: Der rassistische Antisemitismus," in *Der ewige Judenhass: Christlicher Antijudaismus, Deutschnationale Judenfeindlichkeit, Rassistischer Antisemitismus,* ed. Christina von Braun and Ludger Heid (Stuttgart and Bonn: Burg Verlag, 1990), 149–213.

6. P. M. S. Clark and L. J. Kricka, *Medical Consequences of Alcohol Abuse* (Chichester: Ellis Horwood, 1980); Wolfgang Schmidt, "Effects of Alcohol Consumption on Health," *Journal of Public Health Policy* 25, 1–2 (1980): 25–40; C. Samuel Mullin, *The Medical Consequences of Chronic Alcohol Abuse* (Boston: Division of Alcoholism, Massachusetts Dept. of Public Health, 1980).

7. See Barry Glassner and Bruce Berg, "How Jews Avoid Alcohol Problems," *American Sociological Review* 45, 4 (1980): 647–664.

8. Sheldon C. Seller, "Alcohol Abuse in the Old Testament," *Alcohol and Alcoholism* 20, 1 (1985): 69–76. The quotation appears on p. 69. See also Samuel S. Kottek, "'Do Not Drink Wine or Strong Drink': Alcohol and Responsibility in Ancient Jewish Sources," *Medicine and Law* 8 (1989): 255–259.

9. R. F. Bales, "Cultural Differences in Rates of Alcoholism," *Quarterly Journal of Studies on Alcohol* 6 (1946): 480–499; David G. Mandelbaum, "Alcohol and Culture," *Current Anthropology* 6, 3 (1965): 281–288; and A. M. Greeley, W. M. McCready, and G. Theisen, *Ethnic Drinking Subcultures* (New York: Praeger, 1979).

10. Charles Snyder, *Alcohol and the Jews* (New Haven: Yale University Press, 1958), 5.
11. Hugo Hoppe, *Krankheiten und Sterblichkeit bei Juden und Nichtjuden: Mit besonderer Berücksichtigung der Alkoholfrage* (Berlin: S. Calvary, 1903), 44.
12. William M. Feldman, "Racial Aspects of Alcoholism," *British Journal of Inebriety* 21, 1 (1923): 7.
13. Robin Room, "Cultural Contingencies of Alcoholism: Variations Between and Within Nineteenth-Century Urban Ethnic Groups in Alcohol-Related Death Rates," *Journal of Health and Social Behavior* 9 (1968): 99–113. See the entry "Alcoholism," by William S. Gottheil, in the *Jewish Encyclopedia* (New York: Funk and Wagnalls, 1904), 1, 334; Nathan Glazer, "Why Jews Stay Sober," *Commentary* 13 (1952): 183–184; Arthur Ruppin, *The Jews in the Modern World* (London: Macmillan, 1934), 264.
14. On the immunity of Jews to certain diseases see Maurice Fishberg, "Die angebliche Rassen-Immunität der Juden," *Zeitschrift für Demographie und Statistik der Juden* 4, 12 (1908): 177–188; and Samuel Weissenberg, "Das verhalten der Juden gegen ansteckende Krankheiten," *Zeitschrift für Demographie und Statistik der Juden* 7, 10 (1911): 137–146; J. S. Billings, *Vital Statistics of the Jews in the United States* (Washington: Census Bulletin, No. 19), Dec. 30, 1890; Emil Bogen, "Diseases among the Jews," *Medical Leaves* 5 (1943): 151–159; W. Cohn, "Sterblichkeitsverhältnisse der Stadt Posen," *Vierteljahrsschrift für Gerichtliche Medicin* (1869): 268–285; Augustus A. Eshner, "Krankheits- und Sterblichkeitsstatistik der Juden," *Ost und West* 1, 6 (1901): 434–438; Maurice Fishberg, "The Comparative Pathology of the Jews," *New York Medical Journal* 13 (1901): 537–543, and 14 (1901): 576–582. See the entry "Morbidity," by Fishberg, in the *Jewish Encyclopedia*, vol. 9, 1–7. Eduard Glatter, "Das Racenmoment in seinem Einfluss auf Erkrankungen," *Vierteljahrsschrift für gerichtliche und öffentliche Medicin* 25 (1864): 38–49; and Leo Sofer, "Zur Biologie und Pathologie der jüdischen Rasse," *Zeitschrift für Demographie und Statistik der Juden* 2, 6 (1906): 85–92.
15. See the following studies: "Discussion sur la Pathologie de la Race Juive," *Bulletin de l'Académie de Médicine de Paris* 26 (1891): 238–241; Alexander Pilcz, "Geistesstörungen bei den Juden," *Wiener klinische Rundschau* 47 (1901): 888–890, and 48 (1901): 908–910; Max Sichel, "Über die Geistesstörungen bei den Juden," *Neurologisches Centralblatt* 27 (1908): 357; Fishberg, *The Jews,* 273–274, 329; and Heinrich Singer, *Allgemeine und spezielle Krankheitslehre der Juden* (Leipzig: Benno Konegen, 1904), 110.
16. Immanuel Kant, *Anthropology from a Pragmatic Point of View,* trans. Mary J. Gregor (The Hague: Martinus Nijhoff, 1974), 47.
17. J. McGonegal, "The Role of Sanction in Drinking Behavior," *Quarterly Journal of Studies in Alcohol* 33 (1972): 692–697.
18. Fishberg, *The Jews,* 275.
19. For then current opinion on the congenital predisposition or aversion of various peoples to excess consumption of alcohol and drugs, see Harry Campbell,

"The Craving for Stimulants," *British Journal of Inebriety* 4, 1 (1906–07): 4–35; Harry Campbell, "The Pathology and Treatment of Morphia Addiction," *British Journal of Inebriety* 20, 4 (1923): 147–168; and Charles F. Harford, "Racial Psychology in Relation to Alcoholism, especially with reference to the Coloured Races," *British Journal of Inebriety* 19, 4 (1922): 153–164.

20. Norman Shanks Kerr, *Inebriety, or, Narcomania: Its Etiology, Pathology, Treatment and Jurisprudence* (London: H.K. Lewis, 1894), 169–170.

21. George Archdall Reid, *Alcoholism, a Study in Heredity* (London: Bailliere, Tindall & Cox, 1902), 100, 117–118. Other proponents of the Darwinian thesis include John Berry Haycraft, *Darwinism and Race Progress* (London: S. Sonnenschein, 1895); and Frederick Webb Headly, *Problems of Evolution* (London: Duckworth, 1900).

22. William Z. Ripley, *Races of Europe* (New York: D. Appleton, 1899), 384–385.

23. Joseph Jacobs, *Studies in Jewish Statistics: Social, Vital and Anthropometric* (London: D. Nutt, 1891), vii.

24. Fishberg, *The Jews*, 259.

25. Fishberg, *The Jews*, 265.

26. James Samuelson, *A History of Drink: A Review, Social, Scientific, and Political* (London: Trübner & Co., 1880), 70–71.

27. Karl Kautsky, *Are the Jews a Race?* (New York: International Publishers, 1926), 131–133.

28. Ruppin, *Modern World*, 264.

29. Fishberg, *The Jews*, 276.

30. Hugo Hoppe, "Die Kriminalität der Juden und der Alkohol," *Zeitschrift für Demographie und Statistik der Juden* 3, 4 (1907): 56. See also Sander L. Gilman, *The Case of Sigmund Freud: Medicine and Identity at the Fin-de-Siècle* (Baltimore: Johns Hopkins University Press, 1993), 169–215.

31. Fishberg, *The Jews*, 276.

32. Emile Durkheim, *Suicide* (Glencoe, IL: Free Press, 1951), 152–170.

33. L. Cheinisse, "Die Rassenpathologie und der Alkoholismus bei den Juden," *Zeitschrift für Demographie und Statistik der Juden* 6, 1 (1910): 1–8.

34. Pierre Birnbaum, *Anti-semitism in France: A Political History from Leon Blum to the Present* (Oxford: Oxford University Press, 1992), 133–135.

35. Glazer, "Why Jews Stay Sober," 185–186. For a more historicist explanation of the Jewish aversion to drunkenness see Mark Keller, "The Great Jewish Drink Mystery," *British Journal of Addiction to Alcohol and Other Drugs* 64, 3 (1970): 287–295.

36. Three studies suggest an increase in drinking among Jews, but all are of questionable value given the biased sampling data upon which the findings are based. See M. M. Glatt, "Jewish Alcoholics and Addicts in the London Area," *Mental Health and Society* 2 (1975): 168–174; n.a., "Jews and Alcoholism: No Cultural Immunity Found," *Medical World News* (June 26 1978): 17–21; and

Sheila B. Blume and D. Dropkin, "The Jewish Alcoholic—An Unrecognized Minority," in *Alcoholism in the Jewish Community,* ed. A. Blaine (New York: Commission on Synagogue Relations, 1980), 123–133.

37. For example, see A. R. King, "The Alcohol Problem in Israel," *Quarterly Journal of Studies on Alcohol* 22 (1961): 321–324; Alan Apter et al., "Death Without Warning?: A Clinical Postmortem Study of Suicide in 43 Israeli Adolescent Males," *Archives of General Psychiatry* 50, 2 (1993): 138–142; Jeremy Kark et al., "Does Religious Observance Promote Health? Mortality in Secular versus Religious Kibbutzim in Israel," *American Journal of Public Health* 86, 3 (1996): 341–346; Giora Rahav, Deborah Hasin, and Andrea Paykin, "Drinking Patterns of Recent Russian Immigrants and Other Israelis: 1995 National Survey Results," *American Journal of Public Health* 89, 8 (1999): 1212–1216; M. E. Chafetz and H. W. Demone, *Alcoholism and Society* (New York: Oxford University Press, 1962); Wolfgang Schmidt and Robert E. Popham, "Impressions of Jewish Alcoholics," *Journal of Studies on Alcohol* 37, 7 (1976): 931–939. Ira Rosenwaike and Katherine Hempstead, "Differential Mortality by Ethnicity: Foreign-Born Irish, Italians and Jews in New York City, 1979–1981," *Social Science and Medicine* 29, 7 (1989): 885–889; Itzhak Levav et al., "Vulnerability of Jews to Affective Disorders," *American Journal of Psychiatry* 154, 7 (1997): 941–947.

38. J. McGonegal, "The Role of Sanction in Drinking Behavior," *Quarterly Journal of Studies on Alcoholism* 33 (1972): 692–697; Suzanne Bainwol and Charles F. Gressard, "The Incidence of Jewish Alcoholism: A Review of the Literature," *Journal of Drug Education* 15, 3 (1985): 217–224. See also the interesting characterizations by Jews as to who is an alcoholic in Barry Glassner and Bruce Berg, "Social Locations and Interpretations: How Jews Define Alcoholism," *Journal of Studies on Alcohol* 45, 1 (1984): 16–25. Glassner and Berg maintain that while the Orthodox tend to view an alcoholic as one who has a disease and is in need of help, Conservative and Reform Jews take an active dislike to alcoholics, exhibit less sympathy, and blame them for what they consider to be a moral failing.

39. On alcohol consumption see P. Sulkunen, "Drinking Patterns and the Level of Alcohol Consumption: An International Overview," in *Research Advances in Alcohol and Drug Problems,* vol. 3, ed. R. J. Gibbens et al. (New York: Wiley & Sons, 1976), 223–281.

40. Quoted in Hoppe, *Krankheiten und Sterblichkeit,* 1.

41. Evyatar Friesel, *Atlas of Modern Jewish History* (New York: Oxford University Press, 1990), 15.

42. Wilhelm Carl de Neufville, *Lebensdauer und Todesursachen zwei und zwanzig verschiedener Stände und Gewerbe nebst vergleichender Statistik der christlichen und israelitischen Bevölkerung Frankfurts* (Frankfurt: J.D. Sauerlander, 1855), 116; Benjamin Ward Richardson, *Diseases of Modern Life* (New York: D. Appelton, 1880), 20; Luigi Silvagni, "La Patologia comparata negli Ebrei," *Revista Critica*

*di Clinica Medico* 35 (1901): 619; J. S. Billings, *Vital Statistics of the Jews in the United States*: 11–12; and Ripley, *The Races of Europe,* 383.

43. Fishberg, *The Jews,* 255–259; Hoffmann, "The Jew as a Life Risk," *The Spectator* (1895): 222–224, 233–234; Moses Julius Gutmann, *Über den heutigen Stand der Rasse- und Krankheitsfrage der Juden* (Munich: Rudolph Müller & Steinicke, 1920), 27; Maretzki, "Die Gesundheitsverhältnisse der Juden," in *Statistik der Juden* (Berlin: Jüdischer Verlag, 1918), 125.

44. Cesare Lombroso, *Der Antisemitismus und die Juden im Lichte der modernen Wissenschaft* (Leipzig: Georg H. Wigand, 1894), 95; Hoppe, *Krankheiten und Sterblichkeit,* 9; David L. Ransel, "Infant-Care Cultures in the Russian Empire," in *Russia's Women: Accommodation, Resistance, Transformation,* ed. Barbara Evans Clements, Barbara Alpern Engel, and Christine D. Worobec (Berkeley: University of California Press, 1991), 113–132. The figures for Russian deaths appear on pp. 114 and 123. The infant mortality rate for the Moslems of the empire was 166 deaths per 1,000.

45. Lombroso, *Antisemitismus,* 97; A. Goldscheider, "Die Entwicklung der jüdischen Bevölkerung Preussens im 19. Jahrhundert," *Zeitschrift für Demographie und Statistik der Juden* 2 (1907): 70–75. See also, *Zeitschrift für Demographie und Statistik der Juden* 1, 8 (1905): 15; Elias Auerbach, "Die Sterblichkeit der Juden in Budapest 1901–1905," *Zeitschrift für Demographie und Statistik der Juden* 4, 10 (1908): 152; and the *Minutes of Evidence Taken Before the Royal Commission on Alien Immigration* (1902–03), 11–17, 21, 214, 749–57, 3,960. F. G. Hoffmann, "Expectation of Life," in *Jewish Encyclopedia,* vol. 5, 306–308. For the 1920s see Ruppin, *Modern World,* 87–88.

46. Anonymous, "Die Gesundheitsverhältnisse der Juden," *Die Welt* 14, 25 (1910): 614.

47. Anatole Leroy-Beaulieu, *Israel among the Nations: A Study of the Jews and Anti-semitism* (New York: G.P. Putnam's Sons, 1895), 155.

48. Fishberg, *The Jews,* 228–229; and Richard Andree, *Zur Volkskunde der Juden* (Bielefeld and Leipzig: Velhagen & Klasing, 1881), 70–80; Felix Theilhaber, *Der Untergang der deutschen Juden: Eine volkswirtschaftliche Studie* (Berlin: Jüdischer Verlag, 1921). On Theilhaber see my *Defenders of the Race,* 141–153; Friesel, *Atlas,* 20–21; Ruppin, *Modern World,* 72.

49. Usiel O. Schmelz, "Die demographische Entwicklung der Juden in Deutschland von der Mitte des. 19. Jahrhunderts bis 1933," *Zeitschrift für Bevölkerungswissenschaft* 8 (1982): 62.

50. Eliyahu Brodna, "Muters, Git di brust eyere zoigkinder!" [Yiddish] *Folksgezunt* 8, 5 (1930): 41–42, and *Folksgezunt* 8, 7 (1930): 58–59; Usiel O. Schmelz, *Infant and Early Childhood Mortality among the Jews of the Diaspora* (Jerusalem: Institute of Contemporary Jewry, 1971). For comparative figures for breast-feeding in the United States see Robert Morse Woodbury, "Causal Factors in Infant Mortality," United States Children's Bureau Publication, no. 142 (Washington,

DC: Government Printing Office, 1925). In nineteenth-century Russian village life, children were breast-fed for only about a year and a half. But in summer, when they went to work in the fields, Russian women, if they nursed at all, did so only early in the morning and late at night. Very often infants were put at risk by being given solid food within days of being born. See Ransel, "Infant Care-Cultures," 117.

51. Marion Kaplan, *The Making of the Jewish Middle Class: Women, Family, and Identity in Imperial Germany* (New York: Oxford University Press, 1991), 157; Anonymous, *Zeitschrift für Demographie und Statistik der Juden* (January–April, 1923): 17. In 1907, statistics indicate, 18 percent of Jewish women in Germany were gainfully employed as compared to 31 percent of non-Jewish women. Kaplan is correct to point out that much Jewish women's work went "unrecognized" in official statistics. Among many other activities, women worked in the family shop, keeping the books and delivering merchandise. Because a considerable number of the 18 percent of Jewish working women were Eastern European immigrants, the percentage of native-born, German Jewish paid workers was even smaller. Kaplan, 153–157 and 284, fn. 26.

52. Martin Engländer, *Die auffallend häufigen Krankheitserscheinungen der jüdischen Rasse* (Vienna: J.L. Pollack, 1902), 13.

53. Uriah Zevi Engelman, "Sources of Jewish Statistics," in *The Jews: Their History, Culture, and Religion,* vol. 2, ed. Louis Finkelstein (New York: Harper & Brothers, 1949), 1192.

54. Salo Wittmayer Baron, *A Social and Religious History of the Jews,* vol. 2 (New York: Columbia University Press, 1937), 266.

55. Jacobs, *Studies in Jewish Statistics,* vii.

56. B. Baneth, "Das jüdische Ritualgesetz in hygienischer Beleuchtung," in *Die Hygiene der Juden,* ed. Max Grunwald (Dresden: Historischen Abteilung der Internationalen Hygiene-Ausstellung, 1911), 75–79.

57. Nathan Reich, "The Economic Structure of Modern Jewry," in *The Jews: Their History,* vol. 2, ed. Louis Finkelstein (New York: Schocken Books, 1970), 1239–1266.

58. For Germany, see Jacob Toury, "Der Eintritt der Juden ins deutsche Bürgertum," in *Das Judentum in der deutschen Umwelt, 1800–1850,* ed. Hans Liebeschütz and Arnold Paucker (Tübingen: J.C.B. Mohr, 1977), 139–242; Jacob Toury, *Soziale und politische Geschichte der Juden in Deutschland, 1847–1871* (Düsseldorf: Droste, 1977), 114 and 277; Monika Richarz, "Jewish Social Mobility in Germany during the Time of Emancipation," *Leo Baeck Institute Yearbook* 20 (1975): 69–77; Steven M. Loewenstein, "The Pace of Modernization of German Jewry in the Nineteenth Century," *Leo Baeck Institute Yearbook* 21 (1976): 41–56; Avraham Barkai, "The German Jews at the Start of Industrialization—Structural Change and Mobility, 1835–1860," in *Revolution and Evolution: 1848 in German-Jewish History,* ed. Werner E. Mosse, Arnold Paucker, Reinhard Rürup (Tü-

bingen: J.C.B. Mohr, 1981), 123–149; Lawrence Schofer, "Emancipation and Population Change," in *Revolution and Evolution,* ed. Werner E. Mosse et al., 63–89. See also David Sorkin, *The Transformation of German Jewry, 1780–1840* (New York: Oxford University Press, 1987), 107–123.

59. Lara V. Marks, *Model Mothers: Jewish Mothers and Maternity Provision in East London, 1870–1939* (Oxford: Clarendon Press, 1994).

60. Ransel, "Infant Care-Cultures," 116–121. Ransel makes the case that Muslims, who also lived in close proximity to Russians, enjoyed far lower infant mortality rates. See also David L. Ransel, "Mothering, Medicine, and Infant Mortality in Russia: Some Comparisons" (Occasional Paper #236, Kennan Institute for Advanced Russian Studies, The Woodrow Wilson Center for Scholars, 1990).

61. Mark Zborowski and Elizabeth Herzog, *Life Is with People: The Culture of the Shtetl* (New York: Schocken, 1962), 323–329.

62. See Samuel Weissenberg, "Kinderfreud und -leid bei den südrussischen Juden," *Globus* 83, 20 (1903): 315–320; and Samuel Weissenberg, "Das neugeborene Kind bei den südrussischen Juden," *Globus* 93, 6 (1908): 85–88.

63. Odin W. Anderson, "Infant Mortality and Social and Cultural Factors: Historical Trends and Current Patterns," in *Patients, Physicians, and Illness,* ed. Egbert G. Jaco (Glencoe, IL: Free Press, 1958), 23; and quoted in Raphael Patai, *The Jewish Mind* (New York: Charles Scribner's Sons, 1977), 412.

64. Alice Goldstein, Susan C. Watkins, and Ann R. Spector, "Childhood Health-Care Practices among Italians and Jews in the United States, 1910–1940," *Health Transition Review* 4, 1 (April 1994): 54–62; Gretchen A. Condran and Ellen A. Kramarow, "Child Mortality among Jewish Immigrants to the United States," *Journal of Interdisciplinary History* 22, 2 (Autumn 1991): 223–254; and Sidney H. Croog, "Ethnic Origins, Educational Level, and Responses to a Health Questionnaire," *Human Organization* 20, 2 (Summer 1961): 65–69.

65. David Mechanic, "Religion, Religiosity, and Illness Behavior: The Special Case of the Jews," *Human Organization* 22, 3 (1963): 206.

66. Mark Zborowski, "Cultural Components in Responses to Pain," in *Patients, Physicians, and Illness,* 256–268. The quotation appears on p. 267.

67. For details see Chapter 7. In Hungary, 48.3 percent of all physicians were Jews; in Budapest specifically, they constituted 60 percent of doctors. See Michael K. Silber, ed., *Jews in the Hungarian Economy, 1760–1945* (Jerusalem: Magnes Press, 1992), 4.

68. Samuel Weissenberg, "Krankheit und Tod bei den südrissischen Juden," 41, 23 *Globus* (1907): 357; and Samuel Weissenberg, "Südrussische Amulette," *Verhandlungen der Berliner Gesellschaft für Anthropologie, Ethnologie und Urgeschichte* (1897): 367–369.

69. Samuel Weissenberg, "Zur Sozialbiologie und Sozialhygiene der Juden," *Archiv für Rassen- und Gesellschaftsbiologie* 19, 4 (1927): 402–418, esp. 408.

70. Johannes Lange, "Ueber manisch-depressives Irresein bei Juden," *Münchener Medizinische Wochenschrift* 42 (1921): 1357–1359, esp. 1359.
71. Mechanic, "Religion, Religiosity, and Illness," 203–206.
72. Bogen, "Diseases among the Jews," 155.
73. Patai, *The Jewish Mind*, 413.
74. See Frank Ryan, *Tuberculosis: The Greatest Story Never Told* (Bromsgrove, England: Swift Publishers, 1992); Roy Porter, "The Case of Consumption," in *Understanding Catastrophe*, ed. Janine Bourriau (Cambridge: Cambridge University Press, 1992), 179–203; Barbara Bates, *Bargaining for a Life: A Social History of Tuberculosis, 1876–1938* (Philadelphia: University of Pennsylvania Press, 1992); F. B. Smith, *The Retreat of Tuberculosis, 1850–1950* (London: Croom Helm, 1988); Peter Reinicke, *Tuberkulosefürsorge: Der Kampf gegen eine Geißel der Menschheit dargestellt am Beispiel Berlins 1895–1945* (Weinheim: Oterstudien Verlag, 1988); and Richard Bochalli, *Die Entwicklung der Tuberkuloseforschung in der Zeit von 1878–1958* (Stuttgart: Georg Thieme, 1958).
75. Jeffrey Meyers, *Disease and the Novel, 1880–1960* (New York: St. Martin's Press, 1985); and Brigitte Schader, *Schwindsucht — Zur Darstellung einer tödlichen Krankheit in der deutschen Literatur vom poetischen Realismus zur Moderne* (Frankfurt am Main: Peter Lang, 1987).
76. Carl Hart, *Die mechanische Disposition zur Lungenspitzen zur Erkrankung an tuberkulöser Phthise* (Stuttgart: Ferdinand Enke, 1906); Carl Hart and Paul Georg Otto Harrass, *Der Thorax phthisicus* (Stuttgart: Ferdinand Enke, 1908); and Carl Hart, "Thoraxbau und Tuberkulose Lungenphthise," *Beihefte zur medizinishen Klinik* 8 (1912): 275–302.
77. Fishberg, *The Jews*, 286. The thoracic profile of Jews was of great significance in the late nineteenth century. Large-scale measuring of Jews was undertaken by the armies of various European nations in order to determine if Jews were fit to serve. Military service, a marker of national acceptance, was of decisive importance to Jews in their quest for integration at the state level.
78. Singer, *Krankheitslehre der Juden*, 75.
79. Fishberg, *The Jews*, 286–287.
80. See Jean-Christian Boudin, *Traité de Géographie et de statistique médicales et des maladies endémiques*, vol. 2 (Paris: J.B. Balliere & Sons, 1857), 141; Maurice Fishberg, "The Infrequency of Tuberculosis among the Jews," *American Medicine* 3 (Nov. 2, 1901): 695–698; Schamschen Kreinermann, *Über das Verhalten der Lungentuberkulose bei Juden* (Basel: Benno Schwabe, 1915); and Alfred von Sokolowski, "Kommen die Lungenschwindsucht und einige andere Krankheiten der Atmensorgane häufiger bei der jüdischen als bei der christlichen Bevölkerung vor?" *Zeitschrift für Tuberculose* 19, 2 (1912): 143–163.
81. See Glatter, "Das Racenmoment," 25 (1864): 38–49; John S. Billings, "Vital Statistics of the Jews," *North American Review* 76 (January 1891): 78–79; Fishberg, "Tuberculosis among Jews," *American Medicine* (Nov. 2, 1901): 695–699.

82. For Vienna, see Siegfried Rosenfeld, "Die Sterblichkeit der Juden in Wien und die Ursachen der jüdischen Mindersterblichkeit," *Archiv für Rassen- und Gesellschaftsbiologie* 4, 1 (1907): 47–62, and 4, 2 (1907): 189–200. The figures appear on p. 52. On Budapest, see Auerbach, "Juden in Budapest," *Zeitschrift für Demographie und Statistik der Juden* 4, 10 (1908): 145–158, and 4, 11 (1908): 161–168. Budapest was a site of considerable statistics gathering. See the anonymous report, "Todesursachen der Juden und Christen in Budapest im Jahre 1902," *Zeitschrift für Demographie und Statistik der Juden* 1, 11 (1905): 13–14, wherein the greater infrequency of tuberculosis among Jews is confirmed, while their greater propensity for cancer, heart, and neurological disorders is attested to; and Josef von Körösy, "Einfluss der Confession, beziehungsweise der Race auf die Todesursachen," in *Die Sterblichkeit der Haupt- und Residenzstadt Budapest in den Jahren 1886–1890 und deren Ursachen,* ed. Josef von Körösy (Berlin: Puttkammer und Mühlbrecht, 1898), 49.

83. Woods Hutchinson, "Varieties of Tuberculosis According to Race and Social Condition," *New York Medical Journal* 86, 14 (1907): 624–629, and 86, 15 (1907): 671–767; Franz Koch, "Tuberkulose und Rasse," *Zeitschrift für Tuberkulose* 16 (1910): 82–86; Hermann Schelenz, "Immunität der Juden gegen Schwindsucht," *Generalanzeiger für die gesamten Interessen des Judentums* 40 (1910); Francis P. McCarthy, "The Influence of Race in the Prevalence of Tuberculosis," *Boston Medical and Surgical Record* 166, 6 (1912): 207–211; and G. Selikin, "Die Tuberkulose unter den Schulkindern verschiedener Nationalitäten," *OSE Rundschau* 4, 12 (1929): 1–8.

84. Cesare Lombroso, *Der Antisemitismus und die Juden im Lichte der modernen Wissenschaft* (Leipzig: Georg H. Wigand, 1894), 104.

85. Fishberg, *The Jews,* 293.

86. Von Sokolowski, "Krankheiten der Atmensorgane," 155.

87. Von Sokolowski, "Krankheiten der Atmensorgane," 156.

88. Sokolowski, "Krankheiten der Atmensorgane," 156–157.

89. Kreinermann, *Lungentuberkulose bei Juden,* 21–22.

90. William Moses Feldman, "Tuberculosis and Alcoholism among Jews," *OSE Rundschau* 4, 7/8 (1929): 10–13.

91. Tostivint and Remlinger, "Note sur la Rareté de la Tuberculose chez les Israélites Tunisiens," *Revue d'hygiéne et de Police Sanitaire* 22 (1900): 984–986.

92. Henry Behrend, "Diseases Caught from Butcher's Meat," *Nineteenth Century* 26 (1889): 409–422. See the following on the dispute over Robert Koch's erroneous announcement in 1907 that bovine tuberculosis could not be transmitted to humans. Barbara Rosenkrantz, "The Trouble with Bovine Tuberculosis," *Bulletin of the History of Medicine* 59, 2 (1985): 155–175; H. Reimer, "Robert Koch und die Rindertuberkulose," *Zeitschrift für die Gesamte Hygiene* 28 (1982): 156–160.

93. Hugo Hoppe, "Die Tuberkulose unter den Juden in London," *Zeitschrift für Demographie und Statistik der Juden* 4, 8 (1908): 122–124.

94. I. M. Arluck and I. J. Winocouroff, "Zur Frage über die Ansteckung an Tuberkulose jüdischer Kinder während der Beschneidung," *Beiträge zur Klinik der Tuberkulose* 22, 3 (1912), supplementary volume: 341–349. On *metsitsah* see Chapter 6.
95. Sander Gilman, *Franz Kafka, the Jewish Patient* (London: Routledge, 1995), 33–36, 169–228.
96. See Clarence A. Lucas, *Tuberculosis and Diseases Caused by Immoral or Intemperate Habits* (Indianapolis: Bookwalter-Ball, 1920); and Jules Héricourt, *The Social Diseases: Tuberculosis, Syphilis, Alcoholism, Sterility,* trans. Bernard Miall (London: George Routledge and Sons, 1920).
97. Salcia Landmann, *Jüdische Witze* (Munich: DTV, 1997), 218.
98. See Thomas Tschoetschel, "Die Diskussion über die Häufigkeit von Krankheiten bei den Juden bis 1920" (Inaugural dissertation, Johannes Gutenberg-Universität, Mainz, 1990), 119.
99. John Rollo, *An Account of Two Cases of Diabetes Mellitus,* 2 vols. (London: T. Gillet, 1797); and Robert Watt, *Cases of Diabetes, Consumption &c.* (Edinburgh: Archibald Constable, 1808).
100. Joseph Seegen, *Der Diabetes mellitus* (Berlin: August Hirschwald, 1893), 125; Friedrich Theodor von Frerichs, *Über den Diabetes* (Berlin: August Hirschwald, 1884), 185; Wallach, "Notizen zur Diabetessterblichkeit in Frankfurt a.M.," *Deutsche medizinische Wochenschrift* 19 (1893): 779–780; Singer, *Krankheitslehre der Juden,* 81; Rudolf Eduard Külz, *Klinische Erfahrungen über Diabetes mellitus* (Jena: Th. Rumpf, 1899), 243; Georg Heimann, "Zur Verbreitung der Zuckerkrankheit im preussischen Staate," *Deutsche medizinische Wochenschrift* 26 (1900): 505.
101. See Gustave Lagneau, "A propos de l'hygiene et des maladies des juifs," *Le Semaine médicales* (1891): 366; and Jules Worms, "A propos de l'hygiene et des maladies des juifs," *Le Semaine médicales* (1891): 373.
102. Julius Rudisch, *Mount Sinai Hospital Reports* (1898–1899): 26–29.
103. Heinrich Stern, "The Mortality from Diabetes Mellitus in the City of New York (Manhattan and the Bronx) in 1899," *The Medical Record* 58 (1900): 766–774; H. Morrison, "A Statistical Study of the Mortality from Diabetes Mellitus in Boston from 1895 to 1913, with Special Reference to Its Occurrence among Jews," *Boston Medical Record and Surgical Journal* 175 (1916): 54–57. The citation appears on p. 54.
104. Carl von Noorden, *Die Zuckerkrankheit und ihre Behandlung* (Berlin: August Hirschwald, 1912), 56.
105. Carl von Noorden, "Ueber Diabetes mellitus," *Berliner klinische Wochenschrift* 37 (1900): 1118.
106. Felix Buschan, "Einfluß der Rasse auf die Form und Häufigkeit und die Formen der Geistes- und Nervenkrankheiten," *Allgemeine medicinische Central-Zeitung* 9 (1897): 104, 117, 131, 141–143, 156. In his work on Jews, Buschan argued that

the pathological peculiarities of Aryans and Semites were essentially different and incompatible. See his, "Einfluß der Rasse auf die Form und Häufigkeit pathologischer Veränderungen," *Globus* 67 (1895): 21–24, 43–47, 60–63, 76–80.

107. H. Morrison, "Diabetes Mellitus in Boston," 57.
108. Seegen, *Der Diabetes mellitus,* 125–126.
109. Bernhard Naunyn, "Der Diabetes mellitus," in Hermann Nothnagel, ed., *Specielle Pathologie und Therapie,* vol. 7, 1 (Vienna: A. Holder, 1898), 124.
110. Wilhelm Reutlinger, "Über die Häufigkeit der Verwandtenehen bei den Juden in Hohenzollern und über Untersuchungen bei den Deszendten aus jüdischen Verwandtenehen," *Archiv für Rassen- und Gesellschaftsbiologie* 14 (1922): 301–305. See also Joseph Jacobs, *Jewish Statistics,* 1–9. There he argues against there being any deleterious effects from the consanguineous marriage patterns of the Jews.
111. Stern, "Mortality from Diabetes Mellitus," 767.
112. Hoppe, *Krankheiten und Sterblichkeit,* 54–56.
113. Arnold Lorand, *Die Entstehung der Zuckerkrankheit und ihre Beziehung zu den Veränderungen der Blutgefässdrüsen* (Berlin: Hirschwald, 1903), 2.
114. Wilhelm Sternberg, *Die Judenkrankheit, die Zuckerkrankheit, eine Folge der rituellen Küche und orthodoxen Lebensweise der Juden?* (Mainz: Wirth, 1903), 10–11.
115. Felix Theilhaber, "Zur Sterblichkeit der Juden," *Zeitschrift für Demographie und Statistik der Juden* 5 (1909): 10.
116. Ottomar Rosenbach, "Zur Lehre vom Diabetes," *Deutsch medicinische Wochenschrift* 16 (1890): 649–651.
117. Arnold Pollatschek, "Zur Aetiologie des Diabetes mellitus," *Zeitschrift für klinische Medizin* 42 (1901): 478–482. Pollatschek's figures are on p. 481.
118. Carl Anton Ewald quoted in Tschoetschel, "Krankheiten bei den Juden," 138.
119. Pollatschek, "Zur Aetiologie," 479. Pollatschek was not without critics. See, for example, the terse reply of the Hungarian physician Arnold Lorand, who declared, "That there can be a contrary opinion is, to me, simply mysterious." Lorand, *Entstehung der Zuckerkrankheit,* 2; and Adolf Magnus-Levy's dismissal of Pollatschek's claim as "comical, a remarkable misjudgement of statistical interpretation." Adolf Magnus-Levy, "Diabetes Mellitus," in *Spezielle Pathologie und Therapie innerer Krankheiten,* vol. 1, ed. Friedrich S. Kraus and Theodor Brugsch (Berlin: Urban and Schwartzenberg, 1919), 40.
120. Dietrich von Engelhardt, ed., *Diabetes: Its Medical and Cultural History* (Berlin: Springer, 1989).
121. Joseph Jacobs, *Jewish Statistics: Social, Vital and Anthropometric* (London: D. Nutt, 1891), appendix, x.
122. Robert Saundby, "Diabetes Mellitus," in *A System of Medicine,* vol. 3, ed. Thomas Clifford Allbutt (New York: Macmillan, 1897), 197–198.
123. Elias Auerbach, "Die Sterblichkeit der Juden in Budapest 1901–1905," *Zeitschrift für Demographie und Statistik der Juden* 4, 10 (1908): 145–158; and *Zeitschrift für Demographie und Statistik der Juden* 4, 11 (1908): 161–168.

124. Hermann Eichhorst, *Handbuch der speziellen Pathologie und Therapie innerer Krankheiten für praktische Ärzte und Studirende*, vol. 5 (Vienna: Urban & Schwarzenberg, 1895), 136.
125. *Jewish Encyclopedia*, 4: 554.
126. Singer, *Krankheitslehre der Juden*, 83.
127. Both quotations appear in Fishberg, *The Jews*, 300–301.
128. H. L. Eisenstadt, "Methoden und Ergebnisse der jüdischen Krankheitsstatistik," *Zeitschrift für Psychotherapie und medizinische Psychologie* 7 (1916–1919): 128–154. The quotations appear on pp. 137–138.
129. Engländer, *Krankheitserscheinungen*, 36–37.
130. Engländer, *Krankheitserscheinungen*, 38.
131. Singer, *Krankheitslehre der Juden*, 83–84. A variation on this theme comes from Wilhelm Sternberg. He claimed that Jews, both Orthodox and non-Orthodox, had a preference for fatty foods. Given that alcohol abuse had not destroyed their palate, Jews tended "all the more towards things with the opposite taste—sweets and fats." Sternberg, *Die Judenkrankheit*, 62.
132. Maurice Fishberg in his entry, "Diabetes," in *Jewish Encyclopedia* 4: 556.
133. Singer, *Krankheitslehre der Juden*, 83.
134. Anatole Leroy-Beaulieu, *Israel among the Nations: A Study of the Jews and Antisemitism*, trans. Frances Hellman (New York: Putnam's, 1895), 163–164.
135. By contrast, Hermann Zondek, the German Jewish physician, remarked on the excessive alcohol consumption of Jewish students while he was at the University of Göttingen. See his memoirs, *Auf Festem Fusse: Errinerungen eines jüdischen Klinikers* (Stuttgart: Deutsche Verlags-Anstalt, 1973), 27.
136. Arthur Ruppin, *Tagebücher, Briefe, Erinnerungen* (Königstein/Ts.: Jüdischer Verlag Athenäum, 1985), 105–106.
137. Appelfeld, *The Retreat*, 104.
138. Von Noorden, *Die Zuckerkrankheit*, 246.
139. Fishberg, *The Jews*, 299–300.
140. Cynthia Russett, *Sexual Science: The Victorian Construction of Womanhood* (Cambridge, MA: Harvard University Press, 1989). See the standard nineteenth-century anthropological treatments of women's craniometry and brain studies, such as J. McGrigor Allan, "On the Real Differences in the Minds of Men and Women," *Journal of the Anthropological Society of London* 7 (1869): cxcv–ccviii; John Cleland, "An Inquiry into the Variations of the Human Skull," *Philosophical Transactions, Royal Society* 89 (1870): 117–174; and Alexander Sutherland, "Woman's Brain," *Nineteenth Century* 47 (1900): 802–810. Twentieth-century sources include: Havelock Ellis, *Man and Woman: A Study of Secondary Sexual Characters* (London: A. & C. Black, 1926), esp. 106–107; Paul Möbius, *Über den physiologischen Schwachsinn des Weibes* (Munich: Matthes & Seitz, 1907); Viola Klein, *The Feminine Character: History of an Ideology* (London: Routledge & Kegan Paul, 1971); John S. Haller and Robin S. Haller, *The Physi-*

*cian and Sexuality in Victorian America* (Urbana: University of Illinois Press, 1974); Ludmilla Jordanova, *Sexual Visions: Images of Gender in Science and Medicine Between the Eighteenth and Twentieth Centuries* (New York: Harvester Wheatsheaf, 1989); and Barbara Duden, *The Woman Beneath the Skin: A Doctor's Patients in Eighteenth Century Germany* (Cambridge, MA: Harvard University Press, 1991).

141. Nancy A. Harrowitz, *Antisemitism, Misogyny, & the Logic of Cultural Difference: Cesare Lombroso & Matilde Serao* (Lincoln: University of Nebraska Press, 1994), 12–13.

142. For example, on the way the medical community studied homosexuals see Rainer Herrn, "On the History of Biological Theories of Homosexuality," *Journal of Homosexuality* 28, 1–2 (1995): 31–56.

143. Theodore Porter, *The Rise of Statistical Thinking, 1820–1900* (Princeton: Princeton University Press, 1986).

144. See Jay Geller, "(G)nos(e)ology: The Cultural Construction of the Other," in *People of the Body: Jews and Judaism from an Embodied Perspective*, ed. Howard Eilberg-Schwartz (Albany: State University of New York Press, 1992), 243–282; Ritchie Robertson, "Historicizing Weininger: The Nineteenth-Century German Image of the Feminized Jew," in *Modernity, Culture and "the Jew,"* ed. Bryan Cheyette and Laura Marcus (Stanford: Stanford University Press, 1998), 23–39.

145. Quoted in Sander L. Gilman, "Psychoanalysis and Anti-Semitism: Tainted Greatness in a Professional Context," in *Tainted Greatness; Antisemitism and Cultural Heroes*, ed. Nancy A. Harrowitz (Philadelphia: Temple University Press, 1994), 94–95.

146. Adolf Jellinek, *Der jüdische Stamm. Ethnographische Studien* (Vienna: Herzfeld and Bauer, 1869), 89–97.

147. Dennis B. Klein, *Jewish Origins of the Psychoanalytic Movement* (Chicago: University of Chicago Press, 1985), 171.

148. Otto Weininger, *Sex and Character* (London: W. Heineman, 1910), 312.

149. Jacques Le Rider, *Der Fall Otto Weininger: Wurzeln des Antifeminismus und Antisemitismus*, trans. Dieter Hornig (Vienna: Löcker Verlag, 1985); Christina von Braun, "'Der Jude' und 'Das Weib': Zwei Stereotypen des 'Anderen' in der Moderne," *Metis* 2 (1992): 6–28; and Christina von Braun, "Antisemitismus und Mysogynie: Von Zusammenhang zweier Erscheinungen," in *Von einer Welt in die Andere: Jüdinnen im 19. und 20. Jahrhundert*, ed. Jutta Dick and Barbara Hahn (Vienna: Verlag Christian Brandstätter, 1993), 179–196. Nancy Harrowitz has, with justification, pointed out that the Italian Jewish criminologist, Cesare Lombroso, earlier "set the stage for Weininger's reception," in his separate and highly jaundiced studies of women and Jews. Harrowitz, *Cultural Difference*, 73.

150. Sander L. Gilman, "Otto Weininger and Sigmund Freud: Race and Gender in the Shaping of Psychoanalysis," in *Jews and Gender: Responses to Otto Weininger,*

ed. Nancy A. Harrowitz and Barbara Hyams (Philadelphia: Temple University Press, 1995), 103–120.
151. Weininger, *Sex and Character*, 316. See Wagner's essay *Das Judentum in der Musik*, wherein he claimed that in lieu of inherent genius, the Jews had developed imitative powers that permitted them to mimic European culture but never really contribute to it in their own right. Richard Wagner, *Wagner's Prose Works*, trans. William Ashton Ellis, vol. 3 (New York: Broude Brothers, 1966), 84. Also on Wagner's antisemitism see Marc A. Weiner, *Richard Wagner and the Antisemitic Imagination* (Lincoln: University of Nebraska Press, 1995).
152. Weininger, *Sex and Character*, 309.
153. Klaus Hödl, *Die Pathologisierung des jüdischen Körpers: Antisemitismus, Geschlecht und Medizin im Fin-de-Siècle* (Vienna: Picus, 1998), esp. 164–232; and Daniel Boyarin, *Unheroic Conduct: The Rise of Heterosexuality and the Invention of the Jewish Man* (Berkeley: University of California Press, 1997), 210. As this applies to France, see Christopher E. Forth, "Intellectuals, Crowds and the Body Politics of the Dreyfus Affair," *Historical Reflections/Reflexions Historique* 24, 1 (1998): 63–91.
154. Uta Gerhardt, *Ideas about Illness: An Intellectual and Political History of Medical Sociology* (New York: New York University Press, 1989).
155. Michel Foucault, *The Birth of the Clinic: An Archaeology of Medical Perception* (New York: Pantheon, 1973).
156. Gilman, *Freud, Race and Gender*, 21.
157. John Hoberman, "Otto Weininger and the Critique of Jewish Masculinity," in *Jews and Gender: Responses to Otto Weininger*, ed. N. A. Harrowitz and B. Hyams, 142–143.
158. Max Nordau "Muskeljudentum" in *Zionistische Schriften* (Berlin: Jüdischer Verlag, 1909), 379–381; Ludwig Werner, "Die jüdische Turnerschaft," *Die Welt* 8, 41 (1904): 5–7; George Eisen, "Zionism, Nationalism and the Emergence of the jüdische Turnerschaft," *Leo Baeck Institute Yearbook* 28 (1983): 247–262; David Biale, "Zionism as an Erotic Revolution," in *People of the Body*, ed. H. Eilberg-Schwartz, 283–307; and Michael Berkowitz, *Zionist Culture and West European Jewry Before the First World War* (Cambridge: Cambridge University Press, 1993), 105–109.

CHAPTER 5. PSYCHOPATHOLOGY OF EVERYDAY JEWISH LIFE

1. Kraus's remark about the press appears in his collection of aphorisms, *Beim Wort genommen* (Munich: Kösel, 1955), 223. More generally on Kraus see Harry Zohn, *Karl Kraus* (New York: Twayne, 1971). An abbreviated discussion of his Jewishness appears on pp. 35–41. On Kraus and his vehement opposition to psychoanalysis see Thomas Szasz, *Karl Kraus and the Soul Doctors: A Pioneer Critic and His Criticism of Psychiatry and Psychoanalysis* (Baton Rouge: Louisiana University Press, 1977).

NOTES TO PAGES 152-155

2. Heinrich Singer, *Allgemeine und spezielle Krankheitslehre der Juden* (Leipzig: Benno Konegen, 1906), 89.
3. Joseph Czermak, "Beitrag zur Statistik der Psychosen," *Allgemeine Zeitschrift für Psychiatrie* 15 (1858): 251–271.
4. Luigi Silvagni, "La Patologia comparata negli Ebrei," *Rivista Critica di Clinica Medica* 35 and 36 (1901): 618–622, 635–638. The quotation appears on p. 636.
5. Felix Theilhaber, *Der Untergang der deutschen Juden: Eine volkswirtschiftliche Studie* (Berlin: Jüdischer Verlag, 1921), 49.
6. Singer, *Krankheitslehre der Juden*, 89.
7. When the Second Reich was founded in 1871, the Jewish population of Prussia stood at 325,426, or 13.2% of the total population. By 1900, the total Jewish population had increased to 392,372 but had decreased in percentage terms to 11.4%. Theilhaber, *Untergang*, 53.
8. Singer, *Krankheitslehre der Juden*, 90–91.
9. Singer, *Krankheitslehre der Juden*, 89.
10. Ivan Sikorski and Maximoff, *Verhandlung des XII. internationalen medizinischen Kongresses* (1900), 251.
11. Anonymous, "Rasse und Geisteskrankungen," *Die Welt* 12, 42 (1908): 12–13.
12. Peter Swayles, "Freud, Katherina and the 'First Wild Analysis,'" in *Freud: Appraisals and Reappraisals*, vol. 3, ed. Paul Stepansky (Hillsdale, NJ: Analytic Press, 1988), 80–164, esp. 152, fn. 36.
13. Singer, *Krankheitslehre der Juden*, 88.
14. Johannes Lange, "Ueber manisch-depressives Irresein bei Juden," *Münchener medizinische Wochenschrift* 42 (October 1921): 1357–1359. The quotation appears on p. 1358.
15. Emil Kraepelin, *Psychiatrie: Ein Lehrbuch*, vol. 1 (Leipzig: Johann Ambrosius Barth, 1903), 106. For a fuller explanation of Kraepelin's degeneration theory see his "Zur Entartungsfrage," *Zentralblatt für Nervenheilkunde und Psychiatrie* 31 (Oct 1908): 745–749.
16. See also Alexander Pilcz, "Geistesstörungen bei den Juden," *Wiener klinische Rundschau* 15 (1901): 888–890, 908–910.
17. Richard von Krafft-Ebing, *Text-Book of Insanity*, trans. Charles Gilbert Chaddock (Philadelphia: F.A. Davis, 1904), 143. In keeping with the ambivalent attitude of the German medical profession toward Jews, Krafft-Ebing, despite his views, could treat individual Jews rather differently. In 1897, he, together with Hermann Nothnagel, head of the Division of Internal Medicine at the University of Vienna, proposed Sigmund Freud for the position of *Ausserordentlicher Professor*. Individual Jews were always more acceptable than Jews *en masse*.
18. Singer, *Krankheitslehre der Juden*, 91.
19. For nineteenth-century medical views of consanguineous marriage among Jews see my *Defenders of the Race*, 65–67.

20. Daniel Pick, *Faces of Degeneration: A European Disorder, c. 1848–c. 1918* (New York: Cambridge University Press, 1989).
21. Quoted in Sander L. Gilman, *Difference and Pathology: Stereotypes of Sexuality, Race, and Madness* (Ithaca: Cornell University Press, 1985), 155.
22. Engländer, *Krankheitserscheinungen der jüdischen Rasse*, 24–25.
23. Max Sichel, "Über die Geistesstörungen bei den Juden," *Neurologisches Centralblatt* 27 (1908): 360.
24. Leo Sofer, "Zur Biologie und Pathologie der jüdischen Rasse," *Zeitschrift für Demographie und Statistik der Juden* 2, 6 (1906): 89.
25. S. K., "Der Zionismus und die jüdische Nervosität," *Israelitisches Familienblatt* 20, 37 (1918): 1.
26. Erwin Ackerknecht, "Diathesis: The Word and the Concept in Medical History," *Bulletin of the History of Medicine* 56 (1982): 317–325.
27. Jean-Martin Charcot, *Leçons du Mardi à la Salpêtrière*, vol. 2 (Paris: Progrès médical, 1889), 11–12.
28. E. L. Freud, *Letters of Sigmund Freud*, trans. T. & J. Stern (New York: Basic Books, 1960), 210; and Larry Stewart, "Freud Before Oedipus: Race and Heredity in the Origins of Psychoanalysis," *Journal of the History of Biology* 9, 2 (1976): 215–228.
29. Specifically, Freud broke with Charcot's doctrine of the hereditary etiology of tabes dorsalis and general paralysis in patients with syphilis. In so doing he adhered to the opposing position of Alfred Fournier and Wilhelm Erb as developed in the mid-1880s. See Toby Gelfand, "Charcot's Response to Freud's Rebellion," *Journal of the History of Ideas* 50 (1989): 293–307. In the obituary, Freud noted: "So greatly did Charcot over-estimate heredity as a cause [of nervous diseases] that no loophole was left by which nervous disease could be acquired." Sigmund Freud, "Charcot," in *Sigmund Freud: Collected Papers*, vol. 1, ed. Ernest Jones (New York: Basic Books, 1961), 23.
30. On Freud's break with hereditarianism see Sander L. Gilman, *Difference and Pathology*, 204–216.
31. Toby Gelfand, "Sigmund-sur-Seine: Fathers and Brothers in Charcot's Paris," in *Freud and the History of Psychoanalysis*, ed. Toby Gelfand and John Kerr (Hillsdale, NJ: Analytic Press, 1992), 51.
32. Of course, a tiny minority among Jewish psychiatrists stressed the racial predisposition of the Jews to mental illness at the expense of an environmental explanation. For example, see the 1905 lecture entitled "Illness and Rates of Death among the Jews." The author, a Dr. M. Epstein, deemphasized the role of history and culture in the creation of the psychology of the Jew. Instead, focusing on inbreeding, he noted: "Their nervousness is a racial trait. It is a product of the selection process." The report on the lecture appears in the *Zeitschrift für Demographie und Statistik der Juden* 1, 5 (1905): 16.
33. On this point see Michael Marrus, *The Politics of Assimilation: The French Jewish*

*Community at the Time of the Dreyfus Affair* (Oxford: Oxford University Press, 1971).

34. Jan Goldstein, "The Wandering Jew and the Problem of Psychiatric Anti-semitism in Fin-de-Siècle France," *Journal of Contemporary History* 20, 4 (1985): 521–551.
35. On melancholy among Germans see Buschan, "Einfluß der Rasse," 23–24.
36. On various aspects of the Jewish experience at this time, see Werner Mosse and Arnold Paucker, eds., *Juden in wilhelminischen Deutschland 1890–1914* (Tübingen: J.C.B. Mohr, 1976).
37. Paul Weindling, *Health, Race and German Politics Between National Unification and Nazism, 1870–1945* (Cambridge: Cambridge University Press, 1989). See also Sheila Faith Weiss, *Race Hygiene and National Efficiency: The Eugenics of Wilhelm Schallmayer* (Berkeley: University of California Press, 1987).
38. George L. Mosse, *The Crisis of German Ideology: Intellectual Origins of the Third Reich* (New York: Grosset & Dunlap, 1964).
39. See George L. Mosse, *Toward the Final Solution: A History of European Racism* (Madison: University of Wisconsin Press, 1985); and my *Defenders of the Race*, esp. chapter 1.
40. Anonymous, "Die Disposition der Juden für Geistes- und Nervenkrankheiten," *Die Welt* 10, 16 (1906): 18.
41. On Wolf and his place within seventeenth- and eighteenth-century Jewish medical literature see M. Dienemann, "Hygiene der Juden im 17. und 18. Jahrhundert," in *Die Hygiene der Juden: Im Anschluss an die Internationale Hygiene-Ausstellung Dresden 1911*, ed. Max Grunwald (Dresden: Verlag der Historischen Abteilung der Internationalen Hygiene-Ausstellung, 1911), 265–267.
42. Wolf, *Von den Krankheiten der Juden*, 12–13.
43. *Moses Mendelssohn: Gesammelte Schriften Jubiläumsausgabe*, vol. 12, pt. 2, ed. Alexander Altmann (Stuttgart: Friedrich Frommann, 1976), 45.
44. Johann Auguste Schilling, *Psychiatrische Briefe oder die Irren, das Irresein und das Irrenhaus* (Augsburg: J.A. Schlosser, 1866), 53. Also on Mendelssohn's illness see Aron Brand-Auraban, "The Sickness of Moses Mendelssohn of Dessau," *Koroth* [Hebrew] 6, 7–8 (1974): 421–426.
45. Marcus Herz, *Über die frühe Beerdigung der Juden* (Berlin: Christian Friedrich Voss and Son, 1788), 3.
46. Cited in Ann E. Goldberg, "A Social Analysis of Insanity in Nineteenth-Century Germany: Sexuality, Delinquency and Anti-Semitism in the Records of the Eberbach Asylum" (Ph.D. dissertation, UCLA, 1992), 291.
47. Goldberg, "A Social Analysis of Insanity," 298–299.
48. Goldberg, "A Social Analysis of Insanity," 282–283.
49. Cecil Beadles, "The Insane Jew," *The Journal of Mental Science* 46, 195 (1900): 731–737.

50. Beadles, "The Insane Jew," 736.
51. Beadles, "The Insane Jew," 736.
52. Frank G. Hyde, "Notes on the Hebrew Insane," *American Journal of Insanity* 58 (1901–1902): 470.
53. Moritz Benedikt, "The Insane Jew: An Open Letter to Dr. C.F. Beadles," *The Journal of Mental Science* 47, 198 (1901): 505–506.
54. Benedikt, "The Insane Jew," 506.
55. Benedikt, "The Insane Jew," 506.
56. Benedikt, "The Insane Jew," 506; Anonymous, "Die Disposition der Juden," 18.
57. Benedikt, "The Insane Jew," 507.
58. Goerge Rosen, *Madness in Society: Chapters in the Historical Sociology of Mental Illness* (New York: Harper Torchbooks, 1969), 247–262.
59. Benedikt, "The Insane Jew," 509.
60. Maurice Fishberg, *The Jews,* 324–325.
61. Moritz Benedikt, "Der geisteskranke Jude," *Nord und Süd: Eine deutsche Monatsschrift* 167, 43 (1918): 266–267.
62. Benedikt, "Der geisteskranke Jude," 269.
63. Wolf, *Von den Krankheiten der Juden,* 12–13.
64. See Max Isidore Bodenheimer, *Wohin mit den russischen Juden? Syrien ein Zufluchtsort der russischen Juden* (Hamburg: Verlag des Deutsch Israelitischen Familienblattes, 1891); Jehuda Reinharz, *Fatherland or Promised Land: The Dilemma of the German Jew, 1893–1914* (Ann Arbor: University of Michigan Press, 1975), 90–101; and Stephen M. Poppel, *Zionism in Germany, 1897–1933: The Shaping of Jewish Identity* (Philadelphia: Jewish Publication Society, 1977), 2–32.
65. Benedikt, "Der geisteskranke Jude," 269–270.
66. Not only was it a barrier to integration, but Yiddish, because of its similarity to German, was regarded as a threat by German-speaking Jews, long sensitive to accusations of linguistic corruption. See Sander L. Gilman, *Jewish Self-Hatred Anti-Semitism and the Hidden Language of the Jews* (Baltimore: Johns Hopkins University Press, 1986).
67. Benedikt, "Der geisteskranke Jude," 270.
68. On the cult of the Eastern European Jew see Steven E. Aschheim, *Brothers and Strangers: The East European Jew in German and German-Jewish Consciousness, 1800–1923* (Madison: University of Wisconsin Press, 1982), 185–214.
69. The charge of hypochondria is one that does not occur with much frequency in the works of the younger generation of Jewish psychiatrists. By describing it as a malady specific to Eastern European Jewry, Oppenheim falls within that earlier trend of Jewish medicine that identified the traditionally Orthodox Jew as the psychopathological personality. Indeed, in 1777, Elcan Isaac Wolf had identified hypochondria, stomach disorders, and hemorrhoids, as the three most common ailments of adult Jews. Wolf, *Krankheiten,* 84.

70. Hermann Oppenheim, "Zur Psychopathologie und Nosologie der russisch-jüdischen Bevölkerung," *Journal für Psychologie und Neurologie* 13 (1908): 2–3.
71. Oppenheim, "Psychopathologie und Nosologie," 3.
72. Despite his faith in German civilization, Oppenheim himself was the victim of that country's institutional antisemitism. He had earned an international reputation based among other things on his widely translated *Lehrbuch der Nervenkrankheiten für Aerzte und Studierende* (1894), which became a standard textbook for neurologists throughout the world for decades. Despite a unanimous recommendation by the medical faculty of the University of Berlin that he be appointed to the chair of neurology, he was turned down by the Prussian government unless he accepted baptism. This he steadfastly refused to do. See *Jüdisches Lexikon*, vol. 4, 583–584.
73. Oppenheim, "Psychopathologie und Nosologie," 3.
74. Oppenheim, "Psychopathologie und Nosologie," 4. The view of the Eastern European Jew as constantly seeking multiple medical opinions is further confirmed by Hugo Hoppe, *Krankheiten und Sterblichkeit*, 26.
75. Oppenheim, "Psychopathologie und Nosologie," 5.
76. Engländer identified some of the more prevalent diseases among "ghetto Jews" such as: weak bone, muscular, and respiratory development, tuberculosis, trachoma, and myopia. Engländer, *Krankheitserscheinungen der jüdischen Rasse*, 11–12.
77. Quoted in Sander L. Gilman, *Freud, Race, and Gender* (Princeton: Princeton University Press, 1993), 95.
78. The two quotations appear in Kraus, *Beim Wort genommen*, 351 and 349.
79. Engländer, *Krankheitserscheinungen der jüdischen Rasse*, 12–13.
80. Engländer, *Krankheitserscheinungen der jüdischen Rasse*, 16.
81. Engländer, *Krankheitserscheinungen der jüdischen Rasse*, 17.
82. On the theory of degeneration as it permeated the discourse of science, art, and politics in the nineteenth century, see the collection of essays edited by J. Edward Chamberlain and Sander L. Gilman, *Degeneration: The Dark Side of Progress* (New York: Columbia University Press, 1985). See also Gunter Mann, "Dekadenz-Degeneration-Untergangsangst im Lichte der Biologie des 19. Jahrhunderts," *Medizinhistorisches Journal* 20, 1–2 (1985): 6–35.
83. Engländer, *Krankheitserscheinungen der jüdischen Rasse*, 29.
84. Leroy-Beaulieu, *Israel Among the Nations*, 168–169.
85. Fishberg, *The Jews*, 330–331.
86. Fritz Wittels, *Der Taufjude* (Vienna: M. Breitensteins Verlagsbuchhandlung, 1904), 6, 13–32. See also Dennis B. Klein, *Jewish Origins of the Psychoanalytic Movement* (Chicago: University of Chicago Press, 1985), 138–141. Wittels was uncompromising in his assessment of Austrian antisemitism and, according to Peter Gay, tended to project his feelings about it onto others. In December 1923 he sent Freud an advance copy of his Freud biography. Of Freud's early years,

Wittels wrote: "His fate as a Jew in the German cultural area made him sicken early with the feeling of inferiority, which no German Jew can escape." Gay maintains that Freud expressed his disapproval of Wittels' claim by annotating the margin with an "!" The exclamation mark, however, can just as easily be a sign of approval. See Peter Gay, *Freud: A Life for Our Time* (New York: Norton, 1988), 27.

87. Rank's essay appears in Klein, *Jewish Origins*, 170–173. The quotation appears on p. 171.
88. Quoted in Klein, *Jewish Origins*, 172.
89. Klein, *Jewish Origins*, 103–104.
90. See Gilman, *Difference and Pathology*, 159; and Manfred Bleuler, "Geschichte des Burghölzlis und der psychiatrischen Universitätsklinik," in *Zürcher Spitalgeschichte*, vol. 2 (Zurich: Regierungsrat des Kantons Zürich, 1951), 396.
91. Gilman, *Self-Hatred*, 294–295.
92. Published as *Die jüdische Nervosität: ihre Art, Entstehung und Bekämpfung* (Zurich: Speidel & Wurzel, 1918). All further page citations from this work appear in parentheses in the text.
93. Jizchok Taitz, *Psychosen und Neurosen bei Juden: Inaugural-Dissertation* (Basel: n.p., 1937), 28.
94. Max Sichel, "Paralyse der Juden in sexuologischer Beleuchtung," *Zeitschrift für Sexualwissenschaft* 6, 3 (1919): 98–104.
95. Freud expressed his belief in the relation between individual obsessions and organized religious practice when he wrote, "In view of these resemblances and analogies one might venture to regard the obsessional neurosis as a pathological counterpart to the formation of a religion, to describe this neurosis as a private religious system, and religion as a universal obsessional neurosis." See his "Obsessive Acts and Religious Practices" (1907) in *Sigmund Freud: Collected Papers*, vol. 2, ed. Ernest Jones (New York: Basic Books, 1961), 25–35. See also Freud's fuller exposition on religion in *The Future of an Illusion*, trans. and ed. James Strachey (New York: Norton, 1961).
96. Becker, *Die jüdische Nervosität*, 16–17.
97. Felix Resek, "Die judische Nervosität," *Der Israelit* 27 (1918): 2. See also Resek's "Die judische Nervosität," *Der Israelit* 12 (1918): 3–4, where he takes on a more pronounced Zionist and less religious tone, claiming that "Zionism would not only contribute a solution to the Jewish Question politically and socially, but eugenically as well — that is to say, in terms of racial improvement," p. 4.
98. Hermann Seckbach, "Die Nervenkranke," *Der Israelit* 1 (1919): 2–3.
99. Gershom Scholem, *From Berlin to Jerusalem: Memoirs of My Youth* (New York: Schocken Books, 1988), 156.
100. Franz G. Alexander and Sheldon T. Selesnick, *The History of Psychiatry: An Evaluation of Psychiatric Thought and Practice from Prehistoric Times to the Present* (New York: Harper and Row, 1966), 32.

101. Daniel Pasmanik, "Die Judenassimilation seit Mendelssohn," *Jüdischer Almanach 5670* (Vienna: Jüdischer Verlag, 1910): 50. See also his book, *Die Seele Israels: Zur Psychologie des Diasporajudenthums* (Cologne: Jüdischer Verlag, 1911).
102. Pasmanik, "Die Judenassimilation," 51.
103. Pasmanik, "Die Judenassimilation," 63–64.
104. The publication on Swiss Jews is "Über die Verbreitung der Geisteskrankungen bei den Juden in der Schweiz," *Israelitisches Wochenblatt für die Schweiz* 45 (1918): 6–7. Becker's proposals are "Das jüdische Nervensanatorium in Palästina," *Volk und Land* 17 (1919): 541–542; "Vegn farzorgen yidishe psikhishe kranke," [Yiddish] *Folksgezunt* 19 (1929): 350–351; and "Gaystikkranke Yidn in Poyln un di frage vegn oyfzikht iber zay," [Yiddish] in *Shriftn fun ersten landdoktoyrim fun "TOZ" 23–25 Juni 1928*, ed. Leon Wullman (Warsaw: Tsentrale fun "TOZ," 1929), 66–69.
105. Rafael Becker, "Ein Beitrag zur Frage der Verbreitung der Geisteskrankheiten bei den Juden in Polen," *OSE-Rundschau* 5, 1 (1930): 2–4; and Rafael Becker, "Die Geisteserkrankungen bei den Juden in Polen," *Allgemeine Zeitschrift für Psychiatrie* 96 (1932): 50. Heinrich Singer reported that of 3,200 patients at one German mental asylum there were 970 Jewish morphine addicts. See his *Krankheitslehre der Juden*, 92.
106. Becker, "Gaystikkranke Yidn in Poyln," 67.
107. Becker, "Die Geisteserkrankungen bei den Juden in Polen," 54.
108. Rafael Becker, "Di nerven-krankhaytn un der kamf kegn zay," [Yiddish] *Folksgezunt* 1 (1924): 13–16; Rafael Becker, "Gaystikkranke Yidn in Poyln," 68; and Rafael Becker, "Die Bedeutung der Rassenhygiene für die jüdische Familie," *Jüdische Familien-Forschung* 4, 1 (1928): 2–6. In the latter article, Becker accepted German serologist Hermann Rohleder's categories of "inferior individuals" who should be prevented from propagating. They were the mentally inferior, the physically inferior, and the socially inferior.
109. Yosef Hayim Yerushalmi, *Freud's Moses: Judaism Terminable and Interminable* (New Haven: Yale University Press, 1991), 10.

CHAPTER 6. IN PRAISE OF JEWISH RITUAL

1. See Howard Eilberg-Schwartz, *The Savage in Judaism: An Anthropology of Israelite Religion and Ancient Judaism* (Bloomington: Indiana University Press, 1990), 31–48.
2. Jonathan M. Hess, "Johann David Michaelis and the Colonial Imaginary: Orientalism and the Emergence of Racial Antisemitism in Eighteenth-Century Germany," *Jewish Social Studies* 6, 2 (Summer 2000): 65; and Anna-Ruth Löwenbrück, *Judenfeindschaft im Zeitalter der Auflärung. Eine Studie zur Vorgeschichte des modernen Antisemitismus am Beispiel des Göttinger Theologen und Orientalisten Johann David Michaelis (1717–1791)* (Frankfurt am Main: Peter Lang, 1995).
3. Eilberg-Schwartz, ed., *People of the Body*, 4.

4. Immanuel Kant, *Religion Within the Limits of Reason Alone,* trans. Theodore M. Green and Hoyt H. Hudson (Chicago: Open Court, 1934), 116–120. On Kant's views of Jews and Judaism see Michael A. Meyer, "Reform Jewish Thinkers and Their German Intellectual Context," in *The Jewish Response to German Culture: From the Enlightenment to the Second World War,* ed. Jehuda Reinharz and Walter Schatzberg (Hanover, NH: University Press of New England, 1985), 64–84.
5. Susannah Heschel, *Abraham Geiger and the Jewish Jesus* (Chicago: University of Chicago Press, 1998), 9.
6. Heschel, *Abraham Geiger,* 15.
7. Susannah Heschel, "Nazifying Christian Theology: Walther Grundmann and the Institute for the Study and Eradication of Jewish Influence on German Church Life," *Church History* 63 (December 1994): 587–605; and Jost Hermand, *Old Dreams of a New Reich: Volkish Utopias and National Socialism* (Bloomington: Indiana University Press, 1992), 161–163.
8. Michael A. Meyer, "Should and Can an 'Antiquated' Religion Become Modern?" in *The Jews in European History,* ed. Wolfgang Beck (Cincinnati: Hebrew Union College Press, 1994), 57–72.
9. As an example see "Zur Sabbatfrage," *Allgemeine Zeitung des Judentums* 55, 23 (1891): 266–267.
10. See, e.g., the *Jewish Encyclopaedia,* 12 vols. (New York: Funk & Wagnalls, 1901–1906). On the aims of the editors of the *Jewish Encyclopedia* see Shuly Rubin Schwartz, *The Emergence of Jewish Scholarship in America: The Publication of the Jewish Encyclopedia* (Cincinnati: Hebrew Union College Press, 1991). Exemplary of the genre of works that assess the contribution, both religious and secular, of Judaism to western civilization is Joseph Jacobs, *Jewish Contributions to Civilization: An Estimate* (Philadelphia: Jewish Publication Society, 1945).
11. See, e.g., Adolf Harnack, *What Is Christianity?* (New York: Harper, 1957).
12. The quotation appears in Michael Friedländer, *The Jewish Religion* (London: Kegan Paul, Trench, Trübner, 1891), 455.
13. Max Marcuse, "Die christliche-jüdische Mischehe," *Sexual-Probleme* 7 (1912): 691–749, here 708.
14. On this development see Michael Meyer, *The Origins of the Modern Jew: Jewish Identity and European Culture in Germany, 1749–1824* (Detroit: Wayne State University Press, 1967); and Jacob Katz, *Out of the Ghetto: The Social Background of Jewish Emancipation 1770–1870* (Cambridge, MA: Harvard University Press, 1973).
15. Norbert Elias, *The History of Manners: The Civilizing Process,* vol. 1 (New York: Pantheon, 1982); and Norbert Elias, *Power and Civility: The Civilizing Process* (New York: Pantheon, 1983).
16. See the dissertation titles of Jewish physicians in Germany in Komorowski, *Biobibliographisches Verzeichnis.*

17. Francis Schiller, "The Earliest Account of Talmudic Medicine," *Koroth* 9 (1988): 255–261.
18. Azriel Shohat, *Im Hilufe Tekufot. Reshit Hahaskalah be-Yahadut Germanya* (Jerusalem: Bialik Institute, 1960), 207.
19. Schiller, "Talmudic Medicine," 258–259.
20. Rueben Josef Wunderbar, *Biblisch-talmudische Medicin: Staatsarzneikunde, gerichtliche Medicin und medicinische Polizei der alten Israeliten* (Riga and Leipzig: W.F. Häcker, 1865). The quotation is taken from the Foreword.
21. Wunderbar, *Biblisch-talmudische Medicin*, pt. I, II, 25.
22. Wunderbar, *Biblisch-talmudische Medicin*, pt. I, 28–29.
23. Wunderbar, *Biblisch-talmudische Medicin*, pt. II, 10–18.
24. See Thomas Schlich, "Medicalization and Secularization: The Jewish Ritual Bath as a Problem of Hygiene (Germany 1820s-1840s)," *Social History of Medicine* 8, 3 (1995): 423–442.
25. Wunderbar, *Biblisch-talmudische Medicin*, pt. IV, 18.
26. Wunderbar, *Biblisch-talmudische Medicin*, pt. IV, 28–30.
27. Wunderbar, *Biblisch-talmudische Medicin*, pt. IV, 34.
28. Wunderbar, *Biblisch-talmudische Medicin*, pt. IV, 26–27, 30.
29. On Nossig's political career see Ezra Mendelsohn, "From Assimilation to Zionism in Lvov: The Case of Alfred Nossig," *Slavonic and East European Review* 14, 117 (1971): 521–534; and Shmuel Almog, "Alfred Nossig: A Reappraisal," *Studies in Zionism* 7 (1983): 1–29.
30. Alfred Nossig, *Die Sozialhygiene der Juden und des altorientalischen Völkerkreises* (Stuttgart: Deutsche Verlags-Anstalt, 1894), 1–4. On Nossig's contribution to the discourse of social hygiene in Germany see Mitchell Hart, "Moses the Microbiologist: Judaism and Social Hygiene in the Work of Alfred Nossig," *Jewish Social Studies* 2, 1 (1995): 72–97.
31. Nossig, *Sozialhygiene der Juden*, 31–34, 67–68. By rejecting the religious dimension of Jewish law, Nossig was a maverick, but his impulse to read *halakha* as science was nevertheless part of the larger intellectual trend.
32. Alexander Rattray, *Divine Hygiene: Sanitary Science and Sanitarians of the Sacred Scriptures and Mosaic Code* vol. 2 (London: James Nisbet, 1903), 23.
33. Nossig, *Sozialhygiene der Juden*, 136–140.
34. Nossig, *Sozialhygiene der Juden*, 70–74.
35. Nossig, *Sozialhygiene der Juden*, 35–36.
36. On degeneration, see J. Edward Chamberlin and Sander L. Gilman, eds., *Degeneration: The Dark Side of Progress* (New York: Columbia University Press, 1985); and Daniel Pick, *Faces of Degeneration* (Cambridge, MA: Harvard University Press, 1989).
37. Several smaller and less distinguished attempts at such histories were made prior to Preuss, but none can compare in scope or comprehensiveness to his. Very often such works concentrated on one particular medical disorder or pro-

cedure and the relevant discussions pertaining to them in the Bible or Talmud. See the bibliography in Julius Preuss, *Biblical-Talmudic Medicine,* trans. Fred Rosner (Northvale, NJ: Jason Aronson, 1993), 583–596. See also the recent reprint of the 1903 study by Wilhelm Ebstein, *Die Medizin im neuen Testament und im Talmud* (Munich: Werner Fritsch, 1975), 316–328.
38. Preuss, *Biblical-Talmudic Medicine,* 1.
39. Preuss, *Biblical-Talmudic Medicine,* 8.
40. Preuss, *Biblical-Talmudic Medicine,* 4.
41. Steven M. Lowenstein, *The Mechanics of Social Change: Essays in the Social History of German Jewry* (Atlanta: Scholars Press, 1992); Michael A. Meyer, ed., *German-Jewish History in Modern Times,* vol. 2 (New York: Columbia University Press, 1996), 151–152; and Steven M. Lowenstein, "The Pace of Modernization of German Jewry in the Nineteenth Century," *Leo Baeck Institute Yearbook* 21 (1976): 41–56.
42. For a contemporary account of Jews eating in public places with Christians see Jacob Toury, "Der Eintritt der Juden ins deutsche Bürgertum," in *Das Judentum in der Deutschen Umwelt 1800–1850. Studien zur Frühgeschichte der Emanzipation,* ed. Hans Liebeschütz and Arnold Paucker (Tübingen: J.C.B. Mohr, 1977), 199.
43. On German antisemitism of the pre-emancipation era see Eleonore Sterling, *Judenhaß: Die Anfänge des politischen Antisemitismus in Deutschland 1815–1850* (Frankfurt am Main: Europäische Verlagsanstalt, 1969); Paul Lawrence Rose, *Revolutionary Antisemitism in Germany from Kant to Wagner* (Princeton: Princeton University Press, 1990).
44. See Elias Birkenstein, *Über die moralische Verbesserung der Juden nebst einer Entlarvung des Rabbinismus* (Marburg: J.E. Krieger, 1823), esp. 48–50, 98–107. For a view of the extent to which some Jews believed the dietary laws impinged on their ability to fully participate in the life of the nation, see the memorandum sent by 168 Breslau Jews to the 1845 rabbinical conference in Frankfurt, wherein they claimed that "the kitchen has become the refuge of religion." "Die zweite Rabbinerversammlung," *Allgemeine Zeitung des Judentums* 9 (1845): 449–459. The quotation appears on p. 458. Abraham Geiger said of the dietary laws that they were "inane, thereby so damaging to social life," quoted in Heschel, *Abraham Geiger,* 38.
45. For an abolitionist, see Adolf Wiener, *Die jüdische Speisegesetze nach ihren verschiedenen Gesichtspunkten* (Breslau: S. Schottlaender, 1895). A moderate reformist position was adopted by the German American rabbi Kaufmann Kohler. See his series of articles, "Die Speisegesetze," *Allgemeine Zeitung des Judentums* 59 (1895): 245–247, 257–259, 267–269. The retentionists are represented by Orthodoxy.
46. See Jacob Levinger, "Maimonides' Guide of the Perplexed on Forbidden Food in the Light of His Own Medical Opinion," in *Perspectives on Maimonides: Philo-*

*sophical and Historical Studies,* ed. Joel Kraemer (Oxford: Oxford University Press, 1991), 195–208.

47. See the excellent study by Thomas Schlich, "The Word of God and the Word of Science: Nutrition Science and the Jewish Dietary Laws in Germany, 1820–1920," in *The Science and Culture of Nutrition, 1840–1940,* ed. Harmke Kamminga and Andrew Cunningham (Atlanta: Wellcome Institute, 1995), 97–128.

48. Many Reform opponents of kashrut objected on the basis of this specific point, arguing that in the cool climate of Europe such considerations no longer applied.

49. Ironically, the medical community came to charge Jews with having a particular proclivity for diseases of the skin. See Fishberg, *The Jews,* 317–319.

50. Ignaz Kahn, *Ueber den medizinisch-polizeylichen Sinn der mosaischen Gesetze* (Augsburg: J.M. Hillenbrand, 1825), 7–16, 46–53.

51. "Diätätische Vorschriften des Pentatuech," *Der Israelit des neunzehnten Jahrhunderts* 2 (1840): 25–27, 29–30.

52. Schlich, "Nutrition Science," 108–109, 124.

53. F. "Ärztliche Besprechung der mosaischen Sanitätsgesetze. I. Die Speisegesetze," *Der Israelit des neunzehnten Jahrhunderts* 4 (1843): 211–213.

54. Maurice Fluegel, *Die mosaische Diät und Hygiene: Vom physiologischen und ethischen Standpunkte, und deren Resultat auf Körper und Geist* (Cincinnati: Bloch, 1881), 4.

55. Fluegel, *Die mosaische Diät und Hygiene,* 20–21.

56. Philipp Münz, *Handbuch der Ernährung für Gesunde und Magenkranke. Mit besonderer Berücksichtigung der jüdischen Speisegesetze* (Mainz: Johann Wirt, 1901), 133–135.

57. For other contemporary views on gastrointestinal disorders among Jews see Fishberg, *The Jews,* 309–310; and Tschoetschel, *Häufigkeit von Krankheiten,* 153–157.

58. Münz, *Handbuch der Ernährung,* 5–8.

59. Münz, *Handbuch der Ernährung,* 9.

60. The quotations appear in Münz, *Handbuch der Ernährung,* 11–12.

61. Münz, *Handbuch der Ernährung,* 17.

62. Münz, *Handbuch der Ernährung,* 14, 20–27, 58–59, 156–163.

63. Münz, *Handbuch der Ernährung,* 138–154.

64. Münz, *Handbuch der Ernährung,* 174–180.

65. Wilhelm Sternberg, *Die Judenkrankheit, die Zuckerkrankheit, eine Folge der rituellen Küche und orthodoxen Lebensweise der Juden?* (Mainz: Johann Wirth, 1903), 39.

66. Sternberg's views were greeted approvingly in the Zionist press. See Dr. K., "Eine Judenkrankheit," *Die Welt* 8, 4 (1904): 15.

67. Sternberg, *Die Judenkrankheit,* 43–46, 51. Further proof for this came when researchers in the late nineteenth century began large-scale studies on married

couples to see if diabetes was in any way contagious, or whether a shared environment, such as identical food consumption, led to the spouse of a diabetic contracting the disease. The studies proved that one could not "catch" diabetes. See Richard Schmitz, "Kann der Diabetes mellitus übertragen werden?" *Berliner klinische Wochenschrift* 27, 20 (1890): 449–451; and Bruno Oppler and C. Külz, "Ueber das Vorkommen von Diabetes mellitus bei Ehegatten (Uebertragbarkeit des Diabetes mellitus)," *Berliner klinische Wochenschrift* 33, 26 (1896): 583–586.

68. Sternberg, *Die Judenkrankheit*, 44.
69. Sternberg, *Die Judenkrankheit*, 62.
70. "Schalet is the food of Heaven, And the recipe was given, By the Lord himself to Moses, One fine day upon Mount Sinai, On the very spot where likewise, God revealed his moral doctrines, And the holy Ten Commandments, In the midst of flames and lightning. Schalet is God's bread of rapture, It's the kosher-type ambrosia that is catered straight from Heaven." Heinrich Heine, *Jewish Stories and Hebrew Melodies* (New York: Markus Wiener, 1987), 100–101.
71. See A. Levin, *Kriegszug gegen das Schächten* (Sagan: Schönborn, 1889).
72. T. B. Wood, J. Barcroft, and L. F. Newman, *The Jewish Method of Slaughtering Animals for Food: Joint Report* (London: I.W. Kahn, 1925); and Siegfried Lichtenstaeder, *Schächtfrage und Tierschutz: Ein Appell an Wahrheit und Gerechtigkeit* (Leipzig: Engel, 1929).
73. S. Lieben, "Ueber das Verhalten des Blutdruckes in den Hirngefäßen nach Durchschneidung des Halses (Schächtschnitt der Juden.)," *Monatshefte für praktische Tierheilkunde* 31 (1920): 481–496, esp. 492.
74. See the malicious attack by Ernst von Schwartz, *Das betäubungslose Schächten der Israeliten* (Konstanz: Ackermann, 1905).
75. Philip B. Benny, *The Shechita: The Jewish Mode of Slaughtering Cattle, and Its Advantages* (Sheffield: Loxley Brothers, 1875), 9. See also pp. 10–15 for a more detailed comparison of Jewish and non-Jewish methods of slaughter, in which the writer insists upon the absence of cruelty in the Jewish method.
76. "Die jüdische Schlachtmethode," *Allgemeine Zeitung des Judentums* 59 (1895): 222–223.
77. Hermann Engelbert, *Ist das Schlachten der Tiere nach jüdischem Ritus wirklich Tierquälerei?* (St. Gallen: Zollikoser, 1867).
78. Hermann Engelbert, *Das Schächten und die Bouterole* (St. Gallen: Zollikoser, 1876), 2.
79. The anti anti-*shehitah* campaign was organized by a rabbi and historian, Meyer Kayserling, who published the opinions of the experts in his volume, *Die rituale Schlachtfrage oder ist Schächten Tierquälerei?* (Aargau: Sauerländer, 1867).
80. Reprints of the expert testimonials are to be found in Engelbert, *Das Schächten*. The quotations come from pp. 13–29.
81. Engelbert, *Das Schächten*, 6–8.

82. The canton of Aargau was an exception and there, full emancipation came into effect only in 1879. Again, this came about largely because of the vigorous lobbying efforts of Meyer Kayserling.
83. Engelbert, *Das Schächten*, 11–12. Actually, religious liberty in Switzerland is qualified according to the wording of Article 50 in the Constitution. It reads, "The free exercise of acts of worship is guaranteed within the limits set by public order and morality."
84. See Leopold Stein's remarks in *Jüdische Stimmen gegen das Schächten ohne vorherige Betäubung* (Berlin: Berliner Tierschutz-Verein, n.d.), 10; and Jakob Stern, *Das Schächten: Streitschrift gegen den jüdischen Schlachtritus* (Leipzig: Kössling, 1883), 1–11.
85. Jeremiah J. Berman, *Shehitah: A Study in the Cultural and Social Life of the Jewish People* (New York: Bloch, 1941), 236–237.
86. To hold a national plebiscite required 50,000 signatures. The restrictionists were able to muster 82,000.
87. On the report sent by the Swiss consul in the United States to his government, see Isaac Dembo, *The Jewish Method of Slaughter* (London: Kegan Paul, Trench, Trübner, 1894), 48.
88. See the Swiss Constitution in Gisbert H. Flanz, ed., *Constitutions of the Countries of the World*, vol. 19 (Dobbs Ferry, NY: Oceana, 1995), n.p.
89. *American Hebrew* (December 15, 1893): 167–168.
90. Quoted in Berman, *Shehitah*, 238.
91. Mordechai Breuer, *Tradition Within Modernity: The Social History of Orthodox Jewry in Imperial Germany* (New York: Columbia University Press, 1992), 342.
92. "Die Petition der Tierschutzvereine im deutschen Reichstage," *Allgemeine Zeitung des Judentums* 51 (1887): 326–329.
93. Breuer, *Tradition Within Modernity*, 341–342.
94. Berman, *Shehitah*, 238–239. Saxony eventually repealed the ban against *shehitah* in 1910. See also the front-page article "Professor Carl Vogt über das Schächten" in the Orthodox periodical *Der Israelit* 33, 11 (1892): 197–199. Opposition to shehitah was also voiced in Hamburg, a host of locales in Prussia, and Braunschweig. See Friedrich Weichmann, *Das Schächten: (Das rituelle Schlachten bei den Juden)* (Leipzig: J.C. Hinrichs, 1899), 22–23.
95. Hirsch Hildesheimer, *Das Schächten: Eine vorläufige Auseinandersetzung* (Berlin: CV, 1905), 17–18.
96. Hildesheimer, *Das Schächten*, 18; and Isak Unna, *Tierschutz im Judentum* (Frankfurt: J. Kauffmann, 1928), 20–21.
97. *Gutachten über das jüdisch-rituelle Schlachtverfahren* (Berlin: Emil Apolant, 1894), 13. This was testimony that Virchow actually gave back in 1867, but he was called upon repeatedly over the years to bear witness, and he permitted his older remarks to be printed alongside his newer ones in all the collections of expert testimonials in which his opinions appear.

98. *Gutachten*, 23.
99. Dembo, *The Jewish Method of Slaughter*, 16–45. All further page references to this work are made in parentheses in the body of the text.
100. Confirming the view that bled meat keeps longer is the opinion of Dr. Max, "Ueber Fleischbeschau und die Notwendigkeit der Einführung für alles zur Nahrung für Menschen bestimmte Schlachtvieh vor und nach dem Schlachten," *Deutsche Vierteljahrsschrift für öffentliche Gesundheitspflege* 27 (1895): 492–526, esp. 508.
101. For a compilation of statements for and against shehitah, many of the latter blatant in their self-confessed antisemitism, see the collection edited by the Trier rabbi H. Ehrmann, *Thier-Schutz und Menschen-Trutz: Sämmtliche für und gegen das Schächten* (Frankfurt am Main: Kauffmann, 1885).
102. For a virulently antisemitic anti-shehitah tract see C. Bauwerker, *Das rituale Schächten der Israeliten im Lichte der Wissenschaft* (Kaiserslautern: n.p., 1882). See also the critical response to Bauwerker by Wilhelm Landsberg, *Das Rituelle Schächten der Israeliten im Lichte der Wahrheit* (Kaiserslautern: Eugen Crusius, 1882).
103. Ehrmann, *Thier-Schutz und Menschen-Trutz*, 4.
104. Ehrmann, *Thier-Schutz und Menschen-Trutz*, 10.
105. Eduard Biberfeld, *Halsschnitt, nicht Hirnzertrümmerung!* (Berlin: Louis Lamm, 1911), 3–5.
106. See Hillel J. Kieval, "Representation and Knowledge in Medieval and Modern Accounts of Jewish Ritual Murder," *Jewish Social Studies* 1, 1 (1994): 52–72. See also, Hermann L. Strack, *The Jew and Human Sacrifice: Human Blood and Jewish Ritual, an Historical and Sociological Inquiry* (London: Cope & Fenwick, 1909). For a contemporary antisemitic account see Carl Mommert, *Der Ritualmord: Bei den Talmud-Juden* (Leipzig: E. Haberland, 1905).
107. Biberfeld, *Halsschnitt, nicht Hirnzertrümmerung!* 38.
108. In England, it was widely believed that because of the nature of his crimes, and owing to the fact that they had been committed in London's heavily Jewish East End, Jack the Ripper was, by profession, a shochet. See Sander L. Gilman, *The Jews' Body* (New York: Routledge, 1995), esp. 119.
109. See the two articles "Die Blutlüge vor Gericht" and "Der Knabenmord in Xanten," *Allgemeine Zeitung des Judentums* 56 (1892): 338–343.
110. Stern, *Das Schächten*, 22.
111. Loewi's remarks are to be found in *Jüdische Stimmen gegen das Schächten*, 9–10.
112. See *Gutachten (II) betreffend das jüdisch-rituelle Schlachtverfahren* (n.p.: Freien Vereinigung für die Interessen des othodoxen Judentums, 1913).
113. Isak Unna, *Das Schächten vom Standpunkt der Religion und des Tierschutzes* (Berlin: Reichszentrale für Schächtangelegenheiten, 1931), 28.
114. See the comments by Max Freudenthal (1868–1937), a Reform rabbi in Nuremberg, who urged Reform Jews to battle on behalf of their Orthodox co-

religonists against the anti-shehitah campaign. W. Gunther Plaut, *The Growth of Reform Judaism* (New York: World Union for Progressive Judaism, 1965), 266–267.
115. The various testimonials were also reprinted in Swiss and Austrian reports.
116. Unna, *Das Schächten*, 17.
117. Leopold Zung, *Gutachten über die Beschneidung* (Frankfurt am Main, 1844); Jacob Katz, "The Struggle over Preserving the Rite of Circumcision in the First Part of the Nineteenth Century" in his *Divine Law in Human Hands: Case Studies in Halakhic Flexibility* (Jerusalem: Magnes Press, 1998), 320–356; and Lawrence A. Hoffman, *Covenant of Blood: Circumcision and Gender in Rabbinic Judaism* (Chicago: University of Chicago Press, 1996), 2–9.
118. Benedikt de Spinoza, *A Theologico-Political Treatise and Political Treatise* (New York: Dover, 1951), 56.
119. Katz, *Out of the Ghetto*, 77.
120. H. E. G. Paulus, *Die Jüdische National absonderung nach Ursprung, Folgen und Besserungsmitteln* (Heidelberg: C.F. Winter, 1831), 74–79.
121. Richard Andree, *Zur Volkskunde der Juden* (Bielefeld: Velhagen & Klasing, 1881), 153.
122. In fact, in 1878 a Jewish doctor named Rosenzweig proposed that a national law be passed purely out of sanitary considerations that would have required German Christians be circumcised. Andree, *Volkskunde der Juden*, 163.
123. Falk Wiesemann, "Die Präsentation der 'Hygiene der Juden' auf Hygiene-Ausstellungen in Deutschland," in *Hygiene und Judentum*, ed. Nora Goldenbogen, Susanne Hahn, Caris-Petra Heidel, and Albrecht Scholz (Dresden: Verein für regionale Politik und Geschichte Dresden, 1995), 16–22.
124. Bamberger, "Die Hygiene der Beschneidung," in *Hygiene der Juden*, ed. Max Grunwald (Dresden: Historischen Abteilung der Internationalen Hygiene-Ausstellung, 1911), 109–110.
125. *Rabbinischer Gutachten über die Beschneidung* (Frankfurt am Main: I. F. Bach, 1844). See also Ben Rabbi, *Die Lehre von der Beschneidung der Israeliten: in ihrer mosaischen Reinheit dargestellt und entwickelt* (Stuttgart: Hallberger, 1844).
126. Joseph Bergson, *Die Beschneidung vom historischen, kritischen und medicinischen Standpunkt mit Bezug auf die neuesten Debatten und Reformvorschläge* (Berlin: Scherk, 1844), 44–85. For a contemporary account that also deals with the medical aspects of brit milah, see M. G. Salomon, *Die Beschneidung: historisch und medizinisch beleuchtet* (Braunschweig: F. Vieweg, 1844). On circumcision as an act of bodily marking among warring peoples, see Johann Heinrich Ferdinand von Autenrieth, *Abhandlung über den Ursprung der Beschneidung bei wilden und halbwilden Völkern, mit Beziehung auf die Beschneidung der Israeliten* (Tübingen: H. Laupp, 1829).
127. Bergson, *Die Beschneidung*, 106–107.
128. Bergson, *Die Beschneidung*, 114–118, 123.

129. See D. Salomon, *Kurzgefasste Abhandlung von der Phimosis, Paraphimosis und einigen andern Krankheiten der Vorhaut des männlichen Gliedes, mit Beschreibung der verschiedenen Operationsmethoden und der Beschneidung der Israeliten* (Quedlinburg: Basse, 1833).
130. Bergson, *Die Beschneidung*, 119–122. Such was also the opinion of Bergson's contemporary, Gideon Brecher, a physician at the Jewish hospital in Prossnitz. See his *Die Beschneidung der Israeliten von der historischen, praktisch-operativen und ritualen Seite* (Vienna: F.E. von Schmid and J.J. Busch, 1845), 48. See also Abraham Glassberg, ed., *Die Beschneidung in ihrer geschichtlichen, ethnographischen, religiösen und medicinischen Bedeutung* (Berlin: C. Boas, 1896), 27.
131. Bergson, *Die Beschneidung*, 108–109.
132. Henri Baptiste Grégoire, *Essay on the Physical, Moral, and Political Reformation of the Jews* (London: C. Forster, Poultry, 1791), 43.
133. R. Pott, "Über die Gefahren der rituellen Beschneidung," *Münchener medicinischer Wochenschrift* 45, 4 (25 January 1898): 108–111.
134. Philipp Münz, "Ueber die Vortheile der rituellen Beschneidung. Eine Erwiderung," *Münchener medicinischer Wochenschrift* 45, 9 (March 1, 1898): 264–266. Münz was also adamant that circumcision for Jews be seen as the "holiest and most important religious commandment, a foundational pillar of the whole religion" (264). See also Gustav Löffler, *Die Beschneidung im Lichte der Medizin: Vier Vorträge* (Frankfurt am Main: L. Golde, 1912).
135. Joseph Hyrtl, *Lehrbuch der Anatomie des Menschen: Mit Rücksicht auf physiologische Begründung und praktische Anwendung* (Vienna: Braumüller, 1885), 801; Jean Baptiste Joly, *Histoire de la Circoncision: Étude Critique du Manuel Opératoire des Musulams et des Israélites*, 2. éd. (Paris: Sociéte d'éditions scientifiques, 1899), 34; and Nicolo Barrucco, *Die sexuelle Neurasthenie und ihre Beziehung zu den Krankheiten der Geschlechtsorgane*, trans. Ralf Wichmann (Berlin: Salle, 1899).
136. *Jewish Encyclopedia*, vol. 4, 101.
137. Felix Theilhaber, "Zur Lehre von dem Zusammenhang der sozialen Stellung und der Rasse mit der Entstehung der Uteruscarcinome" (Inaugural Dissertation, Munich: K.K. Ludwigs-Maximilians Universität, 1910); and Felix Theilhaber, *Die Beschneidung* (Berlin: Louis Lamm, 1927).
138. Carl Alexander, *Die hygienische Bedeutung der Beschneidung* (Breslau: Th. Schatzky, 1902), 6–8, 12.
139. For a discussion of these various issues see M. Rawitski, "Ueber die Nutzlichkeit des Vorhautschnittes bei Neugeborenen," in *Die Beschneidung*, ed. A. Glassberg (Berlin: C. Boas, 1896), xviii–xxviii; and Julius Jaffe, *Die rituelle Beschneidung im Lichte der Antiseptischen Chirurgie mit Berücksichtigung der Religiösen Vorschriften* (Leipzig: Gustav Fock, 1886), 2–8.
140. Samuel Weissenberg, "Hygiene in Brauch und Sitte der Juden," in *Hygiene der Juden*, ed. Max Grunwald (Dresden: Historischen Abteilung der Internationalen Hygiene-Ausstellung, 1911), 37.

141. Jaffe, *Die rituelle Beschneidung,* 8; Münz, "Vortheile der rituellen Beschneidung," 264; S. N. Kutna, "Studien über Beschneidung," *Monatschrift für Geschichte und Wissenschaft des Judentums* 45 (1901): 353–361, 433–453, esp. 434, 444–445, 448–453; Alexander, *Bedeutung der Beschneidung* 10; and Bamberger, "Die Hygiene der Beschneidung," 104.
142. George L. Mosse, *Nationalism and Sexuality: Respectability and Abnormal Sexuality in Modern Europe* (New York: Howard Fertig, 1985), 11; and George L. Mosse, *The Image of Man: The Creation of Modern Masculinity* (New York: Oxford University Press, 1996), 27, 60–62.
143. For the most comprehensive treatment see Jacob Katz, "The Controversy over the *Mezizah:* The Unrestricted Execution of the Rite of Circumcision," in his *Divine Law in Human Hands,* 357–402.
144. I. M. Arluck and I. J. Winocouroff, "Zur Frage über die Ansteckung an Tuberkulose jüdischer Kinder während der Beschneidung," *Beiträge zur Klinik der Tuberkulose* 22, 3 (1912), supplementary volume 342.
145. Bamberger, "Die Hygiene der Beschneidung," 108.
146. Emanuel Rosenbaum, *Meziza: Ist sie religiös geboten? Wirkt sie heilend oder schädlich?* (Frankfurt am Main: Sänger & Friedberg, 1913), 32.
147. Rosenbaum, *Meziza,* 34–39.
148. Rosenbaum, *Meziza,* 40–41.
149. See Joseph Grinvald, *Die rituelle Circumcission (Beschneidung) : operativ und rituell bearbeitet* (Frankfurt am Main: Kauffmann, 1892); and Otakar Klein, Sidon Efraim Karol and Eva Kosakova, "Brit Milah: Theologisch-Historische und Medizinische Ansichten," in *Medizinische Wissenschaften und Judentum,* ed. Nora Goldenbogen, Susanne Hahn, Caris-Petra Heidel, and Albrecht Scholz (Dresden: Verein für regionale Politik und Geschichte Dresden, 1996), 62–69.
150. Bamberger, "Die Hygiene der Beschneidung," 104.
151. Bamberger, "Die Hygiene der Beschneidung," 106.
152. One prominent German opponent of circumcision decried the act as fit for Africa, but not modern Germany. See Hermann Ploss, "Geschichtliches und ethnologisches über Knabenbeschneidung," *Deutsches Archiv für Geschichte der Medicin und medicinische Geographie* 8, 3 (1885): 100.
153. Paul Ascherson, "Über angeborenen Mangel der Vorhaut bei beschnitten Völkern," *Verhandlungen der berliner Gesellschaft für Anthropologie* (1888): 126–130.
154. Kutna, "Studien über Beschneidung," 446–447.
155. Pulzer, *Political Anti-Semitism,* 225.

## CHAPTER 7. BEFORE THE STORM

1. For a general overview of Jews in modern German medicine see Werner F. Kümmel, "Jüdische Ärzte in Deutschland zwischen Emanzipation und 'Ausschaltung,'" in *Richard Koch und die ärztliche Diagnose,* ed. Gert Preiser (Hildesheim: Olms Weidmann, 1988), 15–47.

2. Jacob Lestschinsky, *Das wirtschaftliche Schicksal des deutschen Judentums: Aufstieg, Wandlung, Krise, Ausblick* (Berlin: Energiadruck, 1932), 100.
3. Werner F. Kümmel, "Vom 'unnütz verlogen Volk' zum 'volksfremden Denken': Polemik gegen jüdische Ärzte im Wandel der Geschichte," in *Medizin und Antisemitismus: Historische Aspekte des Antisemitismus in der Ärzteschaft*, ed. Herbert Bareuther et al. (Münster: LIT, 1998), 37–38.
4. Jack L. Wertheimer, "The 'Ausländerfrage' at Institutions of Higher Learning: A Controversy over Russian Jewish Students in Imperial Germany," *Leo Baeck Institute Yearbook* 27 (1982), 187–215; and Jack L. Wertheimer, "Between Tsar and Kaiser — The Radicalisation of Russian Jewish University Students in Germany," *Leo Baeck Institute Yearbook* 28 (1983), 329–349.
5. David Preston, "Science, Society, and the German Jews: 1870–1933" (Ph.D. diss., University of Illinois at Urbana-Champaign, 1971), 106.
6. In fact, ever since the eighteenth century, Jews had chosen to attend a given university partly based on its proximity to Poland. Monika Richarz, "Soziale Voraussetzungen des Medizinstudiums von Juden im 18. und 19. Jahrhundert," in *Medizinische Bildung und Judentum,* ed. Albrecht Scholz and Caris-Petra Heidel (Dresden: DDP Goldenbogen, 1998), 7.
7. On German medicine in Baden see Arleen Marcia Tuchman, *Science, Medicine, and the State in Germany: The Case of Baden, 1815–1871* (New York: Oxford University Press, 1993).
8. Monika Richarz, "Demographic Developments," in *German-Jewish History in Modern Times,* vol. 3, ed. Michael A. Meyer (New York: Columbia University Press, 1997), 31.
9. Avraham Barkai, "Population Decline and Economic Stagnation," in *German-Jewish History in Modern Times,* vol. 4, ed. Michael A. Meyer, pp. 33, 37. For general background on Vienna see Erna Lesky, *The Vienna Medical School in the Nineteenth Century* (Baltimore: Johns Hopkins University Press, 1976). Similarly disproportionate figures are to be found in Eastern Europe where, after World War I, for example, 40 percent of Poland's physicians (2,965 out of 7,310) were Jews. Moreover, as in Germany and Austria, the figures are more marked when broken down according to city. In Cracow, Jews constituted 61 percent of physicians, while they were 66.3 percent in Warsaw, 70.5 percent in Lvov, 74 percent in Vilna, and 82.8 percent in Lodz, Poland's second largest city. Raphael Mahler, "Jews in Public Service and the Liberal Professions in Poland, 1918–1939," *Jewish Social Studies* 6 (1944): 324–326.
10. Norbert Kampe, *Studenten und 'Judenfrage' im Deutschen Kaiserreich. Die Entstehung einer akademischen Trägerschicht des Antisemitismus* (Göttingen: Vandenhoeck & Ruprecht, 1988), 83, 92.
11. On German women entering the field of medicine see Beate Ziegler, *Weibliche Ärzte und Krankenkassen. Anfänge ärztlicher Berufstätigkeit von Frauen in Berlin 1893–1935* (Weinheim: Deutsche Studien Verlag, 1993).

12. Atina Grossman, *Reforming Sex: The German Movement for Birth Control and Abortion Reform, 1920–1950* (New York: Oxford University Press, 1995), 49; Harriet Pass Friedenreich, "Jewish Women in Medicine in the Early 20th Century in Central Europe," in *Jews and Medicine: Religion, Culture, Science*, ed. Natalia Berger (Tel Aviv: Beth Hatefutsoth, 1995), 185–193.
13. Richarz, "Demographic Developments," 55; and Arthur Ruppin, *The Jews of Today* (London: Henry Holt, 1913), 126.
14. Preston, "Science, Society, and the German Jews," 105; and Richarz, "Demographic Developments," 56.
15. Richarz, "Soziale Voraussetzungen des Medizinstudiums von Juden," 12. Avraham Barkai makes the case that one of the primary reasons for the early migration of Jews from the countryside to the cities in Germany was to obtain excellent educational opportunities. See his "The German Jews at the Start of Industrialization: Structural Change and Mobility," in *Revolution and Evolution: 1848 in German-Jewish History*, ed. Werner E. Mosse et al. (Tübingen: J.C.B. Mohr, 1981), 123–149.
16. Pulzer, *Political Anti-Semitism*, 11.
17. Lestschinsky, *Das wirtschaftliche Schicksal des deutschen Judentums*, 85; and Barkai, "Population Decline and Economic Stagnation," 34–35.
18. Kümmel, "Polemik gegen jüdische Ärzte," 38.
19. Hermann Zondek, *Auf Festem Fusse: Erinnerungen eines jüdischen Klinikers* (Stuttgart: Deutsche Verlags-Anstalt, 1973), 48.
20. Shulamit Volkov, *Judisches Leben und Antisemitismus im 19. und 20. Jahrhundert* (München: C.H. Beck, 1990), 146–165.
21. *Standard Edition of the Complete Psychological Works of Sigmund Freud*, trans. and ed. James Strachey, vol. 4, *The Interpretation of Dreams* (London: Hogarth Press, 1995), 136–140. For the story of Freud's academic appointment and the strings he had to pull to make it happen see Peter Gay, *Freud: A Life for Our Time* (New York: Norton, 1988), 136–139.
22. "Vermischtes," *Mitteilungen aus dem Verein zur Abwehr des Antisemitismus* 14, 26 (1904): 204. Thomas Rainer Ehrke, "Antisemitismus in der Medizin im Spiegel der '*Mitteilungen aus dem Verein zur Abwehr des Antisemitismus*' (1891–1931)" (Ph.D. Diss., Mainz, 1978), 35–36.
23. "Vermischtes," *Mitteilungen aus dem Verein zur Abwehr des Antisemitismus* 15, 33 (1905): 262–263.
24. "Die Berufung von Juden zu ordentlichen Professoren an den medizinischen Fakultäten Deutschlands," *Mitteilungen aus dem Verein zur Abwehr des Antisemitismus* 18, 44 (1908): 339–340. The quotation appears on p. 339.
25. Fritz Stern, *Einstein's German World* (Princeton: Princeton University Press, 1999), 13–34.
26. "Vermischtes," *Mitteilungen aus dem Verein zur Abwehr des Antisemitismus* 18, 49 (1908): 383; Ehrke, "Antisemitismus in der Medizin," 39–40; Henry E.

Sigerist, *Civilization and Disease* (Chicago: University of Chicago Press, 1942), 176.
27. Quoted in Dennis B. Klein, *Jewish Origins of the Psychoanalytic Movement* (Chicago: University of Chicago Press, 1985), 49.
28. Theodor Billroth, *Über das Lehren und Lernen der medizinischen Wissenschaften an den Universitäten der deutschen Nation nebst allgemeinen Bemerkungen über Universitäten: Eine culturhistorische Studie* (Vienna: Carl Gerold's Sohn, 1876), 148–152. Klein, *Jewish Origins*, 50.
29. Billroth, *Universitäten der deutschen Nation*, 152–154fn; and quoted in Klein, *Jewish Origins*, 51.
30. Klein, *Jewish Origins*, 51–52.
31. George Sylvester Viereck, *Glimpses of the Great* (New York: Macaulay, 1930), 30.
32. Steven Beller, *Vienna and the Jews, 1867–1938: A Cultural History* (Cambridge: Cambridge University Press, 1993), 191–192.
33. Amos Elon, *Herzl* (New York: Holt, Rinehart and Winston, 1975), 60–61.
34. Quoted in Klein, *Jewish Origins*, 55–56.
35. Quoted in Klein, *Jewish Origins*, 56.
36. Anonymous, "Warum Salzburg eine katholische Universität haben muß," *Mitteilungen aus dem Verein zur Abwehr des Antisemitismus* 21, 17 (1911): 126.
37. Sol Liptzin, *Arthur Schnitzler* (Riverside, CA: Ariadne Press, 1995), 118–141.
38. Arthur Schnitzler, *Dr. Bernhardi* (New York: Simon and Schuster, 1928), 31.
39. Schnitzler, *Dr. Bernhardi*, 95.
40. Bruce Thompson, *Schnitzler's Vienna: Image of a Society* (London: Routledge, 1990), 160–176. According to Thompson, Schnitzler himself recognized the parallels with the Dreyfus Affair.
41. H. R. Klieneberger, "Arthur Schnitzler and the Jewish Question," *Forum for Modern Language Studies* 19 (1983): 261–273.
42. See Martin Swales' introduction to *Arthur Schnitzler: Professor Bernhardi* (Oxford: Pergamon Press, 1972), 5–7; and Mark Luprecht, *'What People Call Pessimism': Sigmund Freud, Arthur Schnitzler, and the Nineteenth-Century Controversy at the University of Vienna Medical School* (Riverside, CA: Ariadne Press, 1991).
43. Robert S. Wistrich, *The Jews of Vienna in the Age of Franz Joseph* (Oxford: Oxford University Press, 1990), 205.
44. "Ueber antisemitische Skandale im niederoesterreichischen Landtage," *Mitteilungen aus dem Verein zur Abwehr des Antisemitismus* 2, 40 (1892): 330–331; "The Emperor of Austria on Anti-Semitism," *Jewish Chronicle* (Oct. 7, 1892) 8; and Wistrich, *Jews of Vienna*, 178.
45. Ehrke, "Antisemitismus in der Medizin," 42–43.
46. Elon, *Herzl*, 162.
47. John W. Boyer, *Political Radicalism in Late Imperial Vienna: Origins of the Christian Social Movement, 1848–1897* (Chicago: University of Chicago Press, 1981);

Pulzer, *Political Anti-Semitism;* Ivar Oxaal, Michael Pollack, and Gerhard Botz, eds., *Jews, Antisemitism and Culture in Vienna* (London: Routledge and Kegan Paul, 1987); Werner Jochmann, *Gesellschaftskrise und Judenfeindschaft in Deutschland, 1870–1945* (Hamburg: Hans Christians, 1988), 30–98; and the comparative study by Albert Lichtbau, *Antisemitismus und soziale Spannung in Berlin und Wien 1867–1914* (Berlin: Metropol, 1994).

48. Gay, *Freud,* 16.
49. Theodor Herzl, *The Diaries of Theodor Herzl,* ed. and trans. Marvin Lowenthal (London: Victor Gollancz, 1958), 69.
50. Keith H. Pickus, *Constructing Modern Identities: Jewish University Students in Germany, 1815–1914* (Detroit: Wayne State University Press, 1999); Ehrke, "Antisemitismus in der Medizin," 43–46; and Pulzer, *Political Anti-Semitism,* 244–250.
51. George L. Mosse, *The Crisis of German Ideology: Intellectual Origins of the Third Reich* (New York: Grosset & Dunlap, 1964), 112; and Helmut Berding, *Moderner Antisemitismus in Deutschland* (Frankfurt: Suhrkamp, 1988), 103.
52. Jacob Katz, *From Prejudice to Destruction: Anti-Semitism, 1700–1933* (Cambridge, MA: Harvard University Press, 1980), 304.
53. Theodor Fritsch, *Handbuch der Judenfrage,* 28th ed. (Hamburg: Sleipner, 1919), 365.
54. Fritsch, *Handbuch der Judenfrage,* 365.
55. Kampe, *Studenten und 'Judenfrage' im Deutschen Kaiserreich,* 64, 66.
56. Ruppin, *Jews of Today,* 130–131; and Bernhard Breslauer, *Die Zurücksetzung der Juden an den Universitäten Deutschlands* (Berlin: Berthold Levy, 1911), 14–15.
57. Wilfried Teicher, "Der Anteil der jüdischen Ärzte an der Spezialisierung im ersten Drittel dieses Jahrhunderts in Preußen," in *Medizinische Wissenschaft und Judentum,* ed. Nora Goldenbogen et al. (Dresden: Verein für regionale Politik und Geschichte Dresden, 1996), 14–29.
58. "Die Zurücksetzung der Juden im Heere," *Mitteilungen aus dem Verein zur Abwehr des Antisemitismus* 18, 45 (1908): 349–350. The quotation appears on p. 350; and "Pastor Ritschke: Breslau und die jüdischen Militärärzte," *Mitteilungen aus dem Verein zur Abwehr des Antisemitismus* 19, 1 (1909): 6.
59. "Jüdische Militärärzte," *Mitteilungen aus dem Verein zur Abwehr des Antisemitismus* 4, 24 (1894): 187.
60. "Jüdische Militärärzte," *Mitteilungen aus dem Verein zur Abwehr des Antisemitismus* 8, 8 (1898): 63.
61. Ehrke, "Antisemitismus in der Medizin," 68.
62. "Sanitätsoffiziere und Antisemitismus," *Mitteilungen aus dem Verein zur Abwehr des Antisemitismus* 7, 3 (1897): 23.
63. Ehrke, "Antisemitismus in der Medizin," 79.
64. Lewy, "Antisemitismus und Medizin," *Im deutschen Reich* 5, 1 (1899): 8–9.

65. See the memoirs of Paul Rosenstein, *Narben bleiben Zurück: Die Lebenserinerungen des großen jüdischen Chirurgen* (Munich: Kindler and Schiermeyer, 1954), 66–67.
66. On Jews and aesthetic surgery see Sander L. Gilman, *Making the Body Beautiful: A Cultural History of Aesthetic Surgery* (Princeton, NJ: Princeton University Press, 1999).
67. Fritz Ringer, *The Decline of the German Mandarins: The German Academic Community, 1890–1933* (Cambridge, MA: Harvard University Press, 1969), 240.
68. Hans-Heinz Eulner, "Das Spezialistentum in der ärztlichen Praxis" in *Der Arzt und der Kranke in der Gesellschaft des 19. Jahrhunderts,* eds. Walter Artelt and Walter Rüegge (Stuttgart: Ferdinand Enke, 1967), 17–34.
69. Claudia Huerkamp, "The Making of the Modern Medical Profession, 1800–1914: Prussian Doctors in the 19th Century," in *German Professions, 1800–1950,* ed. Geoffery Cocks and Konrad H. Jarausch (New York: Oxford University Press, 1990), 66–84.
70. Teichner, "Spezialisierung," 22.
71. Claudia Huerkamp, *Der Aufsteig der Ärzte im 19. Jahrhundert: Vom gelehrten Stand zum professionellen Experten: Das Beispiel Preußens* (Göttingen: Vandenhoeck & Ruprecht, 1985), 12.
72. Huerkamp, "Modern Medical Profession," 72.
73. As these arguments applied to physics, see Alan D. Beyerchen, *Scientists under Hitler: Politics and the Physics Community in the Third Reich* (New Haven: Yale University Press, 1977).
74. Fritsch, *Handbuch der Judenfrage,* 365.
75. Fritsch, *Handbuch der Judenfrage,* 368.
76. Lewy, "Antisemitismus und Medizin," 12.
77. Philip Gillon, ed., *Recollections of a Medical Doctor in Jerusalem: From Professor Julius J. Kleeberg's Notebooks 1930–1938* (Basel: Karger, 1992), 3.
78. Lewy, "Antisemitismus und Medizin," 11.
79. For examples of Nazi era advertisements calling for "Aryan" physicians see Proctor, *Racial Hygiene,* 162.
80. Ehrke, "Antisemitismus in der Medizin," 52–62.
81. Evelyn R. Benson, "Nursing in Germany: A Historical Study of the Jewish Presence," *Nursing History Review* 3 (1995): 189–200; Dr. K., "Jüdische Krankenpflegerinnen," *Die Welt* 5, 4 (1901): 8–9.
82. Lewy, "Antisemitismus und Medizin," 7.
83. For what follows, I rely on Henry E. Sigerist, "From Bismark to Beveridge: Developments and Trends in Social Security Legislation," *Bulletin of the History of Medicine* 13, 4 (1943): 365–388; Huerkamp, *Der Aufsteig,* 194–240; Reinhard Spree, *Health and Social Class in Imperial Germany: A Social History of Mortality, Morbidity, and Inequality* (Oxford: Berg Press, 1988), 160–177; and Alfons

Labisch, "From Traditional Individualism to Collective Professionalism: State, Patient, Compulsory Health Insurance, and the Panel Doctor Question in Germany, 1883–1931," in Manfred Berg and Geoffrey Cocks, eds., *Medicine and Modernity: Public Health and Medical Care in Nineteenth- and Twentieth-Century Germany* (Cambridge: Cambridge University Press, 1997), 35–54.

84. Sigerist, "From Bismark to Beveridge," 387.
85. Huerkamp, "Modern Medical Profession," 76.
86. For what follows see Michael H. Kater, "Professionalization and Socialization of Physicians in Wilhelmine and Weimar Germany," *Journal of Contemporary History* 20 (1985): 677–701, esp. 678–682.
87. Kater, "Professionalization and Socialization of Physicians," 680.
88. Kater, "Professionalization and Socialization of Physicians," 681.
89. On the epidemic see Richard J. Evans, *Death in Hamburg: Society and Politics in the Cholera Years, 1830–1910* (New York: Oxford University Press, 1987), 390–395. For Jewish mortality rates from cholera epidemics in the late nineteenth century see Fishberg, *The Jews,* 279–281.
90. Ehrke, "Antisemitismus in der Medizin," 85; "Die Judenfrage und die . . . Cholera," *Die Welt* 12, 41 (1908): 13. For more antisemitic press accounts from Hamburg on the cholera epidemic see Daniela Kasischke-Wurm, *Antisemitismus im Spiegel der Hamburger Presse während des Kaiserreichs (1884–1914)* (Hamburg: LIT, 1997), 133–145.
91. "Die Cholera und die Juden," *Mitteilungen aus dem Verein zur Abwehr des Antisemitismus* 2, 37 (1892): 304.
92. See Claudia Huerkamp, "The History of Smallpox Vaccination in Germany: A First Step in the Medicalization of the General Public," *Journal of Contemporary History* 20 (1985): 617–635; "Ueber antisemitische Skandale im niederösterreichischen Landtage," *Mitteilungen aus dem Verein zur Abwehr des Antisemitismus* 2, 40 (1892): 330–331; "Die Vivisektionsdebatte im niederösterreichischen Landtage," *Mitteilungen aus dem Verein zur Abwehr des Antisemitismus* 18, 45 (1903): 357; and on animal experimentation see Lewy, "Antisemitismus und Medizin," 4–5.
93. "Das Impfgesetz — ein jüdisches Produkt," *Mitteilungen aus dem Verein zur Abwehr des Antisemitismus* 6, 25 (1896): 193–194. The citation appears on p. 194. See also "Impfung — Juden — Hunde," *Mitteilungen aus dem Verein zur Abwehr des Antisemitismus* 21 (1911): 180.
94. "Jüdische Aerzte," *Mitteilungen aus dem Verein zur Abwehr des Antisemitismus* 4, 43 (1894): 338.
95. Oskar Panizza, *The Operated Jew,* Jack Zipes, trans. (London: Routledge, 1991), 72–73.
96. "Die Pest in Wien," *Mitteilungen aus dem Verein zur Abwehr des Antisemitismus* 8, 44 (1898): 351–352.
97. Lewy, "Antisemitismus und Medizin," 4.

98. Lewy, "Antisemitismus und Medizin," 1–5.
99. For the general impact of the war on German medicine see Paul Weindling, *Health, Race and German Politics Between National Unification and Nazism, 1870–1945* (Cambridge: Cambridge University Press, 1989), 281–304.
100. Kater, "Professionalization," 684–686.
101. Egmont Zechlin, *Die deutsche Politik und die Juden im Ersten Weltkrieg* (Göttingen: Vandenhoeck und Ruprecht, 1969).
102. Werner Jochmann, "Die Ausbreitung des Antisemitismus," in *Deutsches Judentum in Krieg und Revolution 1916–1923*, ed. Werner E. Mosse (Tübingen: J.C.B. Mohr, 1971), 409–510.
103. Michael H. Kater, "Physicians in Crisis at the End of the Weimar Republic," in *Unemployment and the Great Depression in Weimar Germany*, ed. Peter D. Stachura (New York: St. Martin's Press, 1986), 49–77; Michael Kater, "Hitler's Early Doctors: Nazi Physicians in Predepression Germany," *Journal of Modern History* 59 (1987): 25–52. Weindling, *Health, Race and German Politics*, 305–488. For the way nazification worked within the heavily Jewish medical specialty of dermatology, see A. Hollander, "The Tribulations of Jewish Dermapathologists under the Nazi Regime," *American Journal of Dermapathology* 8 (1983): 1926; and Wolfgang Weyers, *Death of Medicine in Nazi Germany: Dermatology and Dermapathology under the Swastika* (Philadelphia: Ardor Scribendi, 1998), esp. 45–125.
104. On volkish thought see George L. Mosse, *The Crisis of German Ideology: Intellectual Origins of the Third Reich* (New York: Grosset and Dunlap, 1964); and George L. Mosse, *Nazi Culture* (New York: Schocken, 1988), 75–78.
105. In addition to the relevant works mentioned elsewhere in the endnotes see Robert Jay Lifton, *The Nazi Doctors: Medical Killing and the Psychology of Genocide* (New York: Basic Books, 1986); Johanna Bleker and Norbert Jachertz, eds., *Medizin im Dritten Reich* (Cologne: Deutscher Ärzte-Verlag, 1989); Gerhard Baader and Ulrich Schultz, eds., *Medizin und Nationalsozialismus: Tabuisierte Vergangenheit—Ungebrochene Tradition?* 4th ed. (Frankfurt: Mabuse Verlag, 1989); Achim Thom and Genadij I. Caregorodcev, eds., *Medizin unterm Hakenkreuz* (Berlin: Volk und Gesundheit, 1989); Barbara Bromberger, Hans Mausbach, and Klaus-Dieter Thomann, *Medizin, Faschismus und Widerstand* (Frankfurt: Mabuse Verlag, 1990); Hartmut M. Hanauske-Abel, "Not a Slippery Slope or a Sudden Subversion: German Medicine and National Socialism in 1933," *British Medical Journal* 313 (1996): 1453–1463; and Ernst Klee, *Auschwitz, die NS-Medizin und ihre Opfer* (Frankfurt: Fischer, 1997).
106. For what follows I have relied upon Werner F. Kümmel, "Die Ausschaltung rassisch und politisch mißliebige Ärzte," in *Ärzte im Nationalsozialismus*, ed. Fridolf Kudlien (Cologne: Kiepenheuer & Witsch, 1985), 56–82; Proctor, *Racial Hygiene*, 131–176; Michael H. Kater, *Doctors under Hitler* (Chapel Hill: University of North Carolina Press, 1989), 177–206; Michael H. Kater, "Un-

resolved Questions of German Medicine and Medical History in the Past and Present," *Central European History* 25, 4 (1992): 407–423; and Bareuther et al., *Medizin und Antisemitismus*.

107. "Die Vertreter der Ärzteschaft beim Reichskanzler," *Deutsches Ärzteblatt* 62, 15 (1933): 153–154. Also quoted in Hanauske-Abel, "Not a Slippery Slope," 1459.
108. Hanauske-Abel, "Not a Slippery Slope," 1460.
109. Dagmar Hartung von Doetinchem und Rolf Winau, eds., *Zerstörte Fortschritte Das Jüdische Krankenhaus in Berlin* (Berlin: Hentrich, 1989), 146–215; and Rivka Elkin, "The Survival of the Jewish Hospital in Berlin, 1938–1945," *Leo Baeck Institute Yearbook* 38 (1993): 157–192.

## CONCLUSION

1. Richard B. Goldschmidt, *In and Out of the Ivory Tower* (Seattle: University of Washington Press, 1960), 56.
2. Paul R. Mendes-Flohr and Jehuda Reinharz, eds., *Jew in the Modern World* (New York: Oxford University Press, 1995), 267–268.
3. Peter A. Bochnik, *Die mächtigen Diener. Die Medizin und die Entwicklung von Frauenfeindlichkeit und Antisemitismus in der europäischen Geschichte* (Hamburg: Rowohlt, 1985), 43.
4. Michael Kater, "Unresolved Questions of German Medicine and Medical History in the Past and Present," *Central European History* 25 (1992): 415–423.

# INDEX

alcoholism, 108–17: assimilation, 114–17; cultural issues, 112–13, 115–16, 303*nn37,38;* nutrition, 205; sobriety in Jewish community, 109–10; syphilis, 110, 176, 182; tuberculosis, 130

antisemitism: caricatures of Jews, 52–53, 257–59; converts, 54–58, 286*n85;* medicalization of, 146, 149, 245–46, 254–58; medical research and, 259–61; medical specialization and, 251–53; post–World War I, 261–62; racist literature, 48–50, 54–58, 257–59; Third Reich, 11–12, 262–64. *See also* body image; medical profession headings; stereotypes

assimilation: alcoholism, 114–17; *brit milah,* 223, 231–33; Jewish self-hatred, 180–82, 184; *kashrut,* 202, 323*n44;* language, 168, 317*n66;* mental illness, 152, 159, 163–66, 170–72, 175–78

Association of Socialist Physicians, 11–12

Becker, Rafael, 167–68, 175–83
Benedikt, Moritz, 164–68, 170
Bergson, Joseph, 225–27
Billroth, Theodor, 240–43
blood libel, 51, 57, 220–21
body image: feminization of, 9, 68, 146–50, 313*nn153,158;* Jewish nationhood and, 105; physical weakness, 9, 142–43, 267–68, 307*n77;* in psychiatry, 158, 184, 315*n32*, 317*n69;* tuberculosis, 126. *See also brit milah;* mental illness; sexual behavior; stereotypes

*brit milah:* assimilation, 223, 231–33; diabetes, 228; German state regulation of circumcision, 224–25; hygienic basis of, 225, 228–30, 328*n126; metsitsah,* 131–32, 225–27, 229–30; *mohelim,* 224, 230–31; Reform Judaism, 224–25; science, 225–27; separatism, 222–23, 231–33; sexual behavior, 149, 227–29; sexual identity, 145–49; state regulation of circumcision, 224–25; tuberculosis, 229

Charcot, Jean-Martin, 156–57, 315*n29*
Christian-Jewish relations: blood libel, 51, 57, 220–21; Christian physicians and, 37, 51; Church bans on Jewish physicians, 17, 21, 36, 280*n9;* Jews treating Christian patients, 17–26, 47–51, 57, 277*n51;* theological debates, 187–89, 321*n7*
circumcision. *See brit milah*
commercialization of medicine, 249–50
Committee for the Defense Against Antisemitic Attacks, 212

# INDEX

community health care, Jewish, 37–44, 89, 193–94, 281*n17*
converts, 54–58, 173–174, 286*n85*

death rituals: burial, 97–104, 298*n114*, 299*n125*; determining signs of death, 95–97, 297*n105*, 298*n111*; *Scheintod* (apparent death), 95–97, 298*n107*
Dembo, Isaac, 212–19
diabetes, 132–42: *brit milah,* 228; incidence in Jewish community, 132–34; *kashrut,* 204–5; marriage patterns and, 134–36; nutrition, 140–41, 204–5
Diaspora, 9, 159–60, 166–67, 175, 267–68
dietary laws. See *kashrut*

education, medical: in Austria, 240–46; in Germany, 44–45, 59–63, 234–36, 240; in Middle Ages, 16–17; Padua University (Italy), 28–30; restrictions on Jewish academics, 239–40; traditional Judaism and, 7–8, 29–30, 265–66; Vienna medical school, 240–43; women, 20–21. *See also* medical profession headings; physicians, Jewish
Engländer, Martin, 170–72
epidemics, 257–59

family, Jewish, 118–23, 129–30, 165, 172
feldshers, 86–88, 265
folk medicine, 86–88, 92, 250–51, 265
Freud, Sigmund, 156–57, 239–40, 243, 315*nn20,29*, 319*n95*
Fritsch, Theodor, 247–48, 252–53

Gintzburger, Benjamin Wolff, 191–92, 194

*Hasidim,* 91–92, 296*n87*
*Haskalah:* acculturation, 64–65, 90–94, 289*n6*, 297*n95*; burial controversy, 95–104, 298*n114*; folk medicine, opposition to, 86–89, 91–92, 296*n88*; health and hygiene, Jewish, 69–77, 161–62, 170, 317*n69*; medicine, professionalization of, 82–86, 89–90, 294*n60*; public health education, 80–82, 92; *Scheintod* (apparent death), 95–97, 297*n105*, 298*nn107,111*
health and hygiene, Jewish: *brit milah,* 228–30; environment, 12, 114–15, 127, 171–72; *Haskalah,* 69–77; health care, Jewish communal, 37–40, 89, 281*n17*; Jewish law, 194–96; *kashrut,* 198–201; *mikvaot,* 192–94; nutrition, 69–73; physical inactivity, 74–76, 137, 172; poverty and, 67–68, 171; public health policy, 194–96; *shehitah,* 216–17; stereotypes of "Jewish" illnesses, 149–50, 176, 271*n4*, 272*n5*; tuberculosis, 129–30. *See also* death rituals
health care, Jewish communal, 37–40, 89, 281*n17*
health insurance, 254–56
heredity, 155–57, 201, 315*n29*
Herz, Marcus, 92–104
Herzl, Theodor, 243, 246
Hirsch, Salomon Zvi *(Yudisher Teriyak),* 58, 287*n99*
Hoppe, Hugh, 110, 114, 130–31

International Hygiene Exhibition (Dresden), 223–24
Israel, state of, 268
Italy, medicine in, 28–30, 41, 43–44, 279*n63*, 284*n49*

Jews, Eastern European: education, traditional, 83, 167, 175; medical education in Germany, 234–36, 240, 331*n9*; mental illness, 159, 162, 165–70, 173, 175; Poland, 41–44, 282*n29*, 288*n111*, 331*n9*; poverty, 168,

171; religious observance, 84, 177; tensions with Western European Jews, 184; Theodor Billroth and, 241–43

Jews, French, 68, 157–58, 290*n16*

Jews, Western European: assimilation of, 168–69; mental illness, 153, 159, 162, 171–72, 175–76; religious observance, 178–81; tensions with Eastern European Jews, 184

Judaism, Orthodox: *kashrut*, 204; mental illness, 165–66, 317*n69*; psychoanalysis, 179; *shehitah*, 212, 221

Judaism, Reform: *brit milah*, 224–25; *kashrut*, 200–201, 324*n48*; *shehitah*, 209–10, 221, 327*n114*

Judaism, traditional: burial customs of, 98, 101; education, 74–75, 83, 167, 175; Haskalah, 65–66; medical education, 7–8, 29–30, 265–66; mental health, 165; science, 30–31, 199; secular knowledge and, 29–32, 41–43, 279*n70*

*Judenkrankheit*. *See* diabetes

Kant, Immanuel, 111, 187

*kashrut*: assimilation, 202, 323*n44;* diabetes, 204–5; German Jewish attitudes toward, 198–200, 219; moral aspects of, 202–3; nutrition, 203–5; Reform Judaism, 200–201, 324*n48;* scientific dimensions of, 201–4; tuberculosis, 130, 216

Krafft-Ebing, Richard von, 154–55, 171, 314*n17*

Kraus, Karl, 151, 171, 313*n1*

licensing, medical, 15–16, 38, 89

lifestyle, Jewish: disease, 4, 137–40, 271*n4*, 272*n5;* education, traditional, 74–75, 83, 167, 175; family, 118–23, 129–30, 165, 172; healthful nature of, 112–13, 175–77; marriage, 134–36, 155–56; mental illness, 167–68, 171–72, 181; nutrition, 291*nn25,26,* 69–74, 202, 290*n6;* occupations, 120–21, 138–39, 170–72, 236–37; physical inactivity, 74–76, 137, 172; sexual behavior, 155, 165, 174–75, 192, 227–28

Lueger, Karl, 246, 259

Luther, Martin, 48

magical healing, 22–24, 35–36, 49, 92, 277*nn47,51*

Marcuze, Moishe, 77–79, 83–88, 91–92, 293*n45*

marriage, Jewish, 134–36, 155–56

medical literature: in Hebrew, 14–16, 34–36, 273*n5,* 275*n16;* Jewish medical history, 191–92, 197; Jews as translators of, 15–16, 274*n14;* popular medical guides, 80–82, 92; in Yiddish, 78–79

medical profession, Austrian, 240–46

medical profession, German: antisemitism, 52–57, 246–47, 252–53; commercialization of, 254–56; general practitioner, 252; health insurance, 254–56; overcrowding and unemployment in, 51, 247–48, 262; restrictions on Jewish advancement, 220, 239, 253; Third Reich, 11–12, 262–64

medical specialization: antisemitism, 251–53; gendering of, 261; and the general practitioner, 251; Jewish physicians in, 249–50, 252, 261; patient attitudes toward, 251

Mendelssohn, Moses, 77, 97, 162–63

mental illness: assimilation, 152, 159, 163–66, 170–72, 175–78; asylums, Jewish, 179, 182; of converts, 173–74; Eastern European Jews, 159, 162, 165–70, 173; education, traditional, 83, 167, 172, 175; heredity, 155–57, 201, 315*n29;* incidence among Jews, 152–53, 176, 182;

# INDEX

mental illness (*continued*)
Jewish self-hatred, 107–8, 180–81, 184; lifestyle, 167–68, 171–72, 181; marriage patterns, Jewish, 134–36, 155–56; neuroses, 139–41, 149–50, 163–66, 171–72; racial basis of, 154–55, 182–83, 314*n17*, 315*n32*; religious observance, 162, 177–81, 184, 319*n95*; stereotypes of Jewish psychiatric patients, 163–64; syphilis, 166, 182

Middle Ages: Church bans on Jewish physicians, 17, 21, 36, 280*n9*; Italy, medicine in, 28–30; *Judensau*, 52–53, 285*n78*; magical healing, 22–24, 35–36, 49; medical education, 14–17, 274*n9*; mystique of Jewish physicians, 21, 27–28

midwifery, 85–86

*mikvaot*, 192–94

*mohelim*, 224

nationhood, Jewish: body image, 105, 300*n1*; Diaspora, 9, 159–60, 166–67, 267–68; homeland, 178, 180. *See also* Zionism

Nazi Physicians' League, 11

Nossig, Alfred, 194–96

nurses, Jewish, 253–54

nutrition: alcoholism, 205; diabetes, 140–41, 204–5; eating habits, 291*nn25,26*, 69–74, 202, 290*n6*; *kashrut*, 203–5; masculinization of, 205

Oppenheim, Herman, 169–70, 173, 317*n69*, 318*n72*

Pasmanik, Daniel, 181–82

patients, Jewish, 123–25, 129, 163

physicians, Jewish: Christians and, 17–26, 36–37, 47–51, 57, 277*n47*, 277*n51*; Church bans on treatment by, 17, 21, 36, 280*n9*; communal responsibilities of, 37–40, 43–44; *Haskalah*, 65–66, 79; Jewish patients and, 123–25, 129, 163; licensing, 15–16, 19, 38; magical healing, 22–24, 35–36; medical research, 159–61, 259–61; medical specialization, 251–53; in the Middle Ages, 13–17, 21, 27–30, 36, 280*n9*; in popular Jewish culture, 66–67; rabbis and, 30–31, 41–42; responses to antisemitism, 57–58, 155–57; salaries of, 39–40; as social elites, 42, 61, 237–38; stereotypes of, 27–28, 46–50, 52–53, 277*n47*; Third Reich persecution, 11–12, 262–64; women practioners, 20–21. *See also* psychiatry

Poland, 41–44, 182, 282*n29*, 288*n111*, 331*n9*

poverty, 67–68, 168, 171

Preuss, Julius, 196–97, 322*n37*

psychiatry, 158–61, 171, 174, 184, 315*n32*, 317*n69*

rabbis, 30–31, 41–42

racist literature, 48–49, 54, 257–59

Rank, Otto, 147, 174–75

Reichmann, Frieda, 179

ritual animal slaughter. *See shehitah*

Sabbath, 112–13, 205, 325*n70*

Schnitzler, Arthur (*Professor Bernhardi*), 244–45

science: *brit milah* and, 225–27; Judaism and, 30–31, 186, 199, 266, 279*n70*; *shehitah* and, 211–15, 218, 221–22, 326*n97*

sexual behavior, 155, 165, 174–75, 192, 227–28

*shehitah*: Christian animal slaughter compared with, 215–19; German opposition to, 208–12, 218–22, 327*n101*; humaneness of, 206–8, 213–15; hygiene, 216–17; Jewish

342

views on, 209–12, 221, 327*n114*; scientific support for, 211–15, 218, 221–22, 326*n97*; Swiss opposition to, 208–11
Spanish Inquisition, 27–29
stereotypes: caricatures of Jews, 52–53, 257–59, 285*n78*; feminization of, 9, 68, 313*nn153,158*; feminization of Jewish body, 146–48; of "Jewish" illnesses, 149–50, 176, 271*n4*, 272*n5*; of Jewish physicians, 27–28, 46–50, 52–54, 277*n47*; Jews in the military, 249, 261, 307*n77*; of mental illness, 163–65, 176; of the sickly Jew, 76, 105–8, 175, 300*n1*
Streicher, Julius, 269
suicide, 115
Switzerland, 208–11
syphilis: alcoholism, 110, 176, 182; assimilation and, 176–77; *brit milah*, 229; mental illness, 166, 182; sexual activity, 192, 227–28

Third Reich, 11–12, 262–64
Treumundt, Christian, 52–54
tuberculosis, 126–32: body image, 126; *brit milah*, 229; environment, 126–28, 130; hygiene, 129–30; *kashrut*, 130, 216; *metsitsah*, 131–32; mortality, 127, 130–31, 138; spas, 136–37

Vienna medical school, 240–43
Vital statistics, 117–26

Weininger, Otto, 147–48, 313*n151*
Wessely, Naphtali Herz, 64–65
Wittels, Fritz, 173–74, 175, 318*n86*
Wolf, Elcan Isaac, 69–77, 161–62, 170, 317*n69*
women: child-rearing, 120–24, 304*n50*; mental illness, 165; midwifery, 85–86; misogyny in medicine, 146, 311*n140*; nurses, 253–54; physicians, 20–21, 235–36, 278*n61*; pregnancy, 75–76, 120, 121, 192; work, 120, 121

Zionism: Jewish health, 8–9, 78, 107, 140, 180–84, 196; medicine, 8, 181–82, 253–54; mental illness and Jewish identity, 159–60, 167–68, 175–81